CRITICAL CARE
EXAMINATION
REVIEW

THIRD EDITION

Healing from The Heart
You: The Owner's
Manual

Mehmet C. Oz author

Janet Kirby referred above
talked re: mother + father's stroke
@ Sacramento train station

§ coleathome @ hotmail.
com

CRITICAL CARE

EXAMINATION

R E V I E W

Third Edition

Laura Gasparis Vonfrolio, RN, PhD, CEN, CCRN
Publisher, REVOLUTION - *The Journal of Nurse Empowerment*
President, Education Enterprises & Power Publications
Staten Island, New York
1-800-331-6534

Joanne Noone, RN, MSN, CS, CCRN
Assistant Professor of Nursing
Kauai Community College
Lihue, Hawaii

ISBN: 0-9627246-9-6

Cover Design: Adam Blyn, Pamela Carrasco
Copy Editor: Elizabeth Wallace

Published by
Power Publications
56 McArthur Avenue
Staten Island, New York 10312
1-800-331-6534

654321

Contents

Acknowledgements

To the memory of my beloved, Dad, James Gasparis.

First, I'd like to extend loving gratitude to my Mom, Fay Gasparis, whose constant nurturing, support, and secretarial expertise have made this book possible.

Second, a sincere and special thanks to my husband, Charles T. Vonfrolio, M.D., for his continuous encouragement and understanding throughout this endeavor.

L.G.V.

To Kevin

I wish to thank my nursing colleagues, who have taught me the art of nursing and passed on to me their love for critical care nursing. I'm grateful to my co-author, Laura Gasparis Vonfrolio, who believed in me enough to include me in this endeavor and who constantly spurs me on to further achievement. Special thanks to my husband, Kevin Noone, for his sustaining support, and to my family, especially my late father, Hugh Barr, for creating an environment for independence and achievement.

J.N.

INTRODUCTION

Critical Care Examination Review is designed primarily to help experienced critical care nurses pass the American Association of Critical Care Nurses' (AACN) certification examination (the CCRN examination). Information contained in this book reflects the content of the AACN's *Core Curriculum for Critical Care Nursing,* on which the CCRN examination is based. Nurses required to take hospital certification examinations in order to work in critical care areas and those enrolled in continuing education courses in critical care will also find this book useful. It can help them pass the required test and provide them with knowledge required to function as a critical care nurse.

This review book covers cardiovascular, respiratory, neurologic, renal, gastrointestinal, endocrine, hematologic and immunologic, and multi-system patient care problems. Answers provide the rationale for the correct choice and, where appropriate, explain why the other choices are incorrect.

You should begin with the first question of each chapter and progress in sequence. Do not skip from one question to another. As you progress, you will build on knowledge obtained from the previous answer's explanation.

About the CCRN Certification Examination

The CCRN Certification Examination was last revised in 1991; the new version was first administered in February, 1992 (consult AACN for any subsequent changes). The examination tests nursing judgment as applied to actual patient situations, although you should study basic anatomy, physiology, and pathophysiology as a basis for making evaluative decisions. The CCRN test is not organized by body systems as in this book; that is, a cardiovascular question may follow a neurology question. You may also see a patient situation followed by three related questions, each one referring to a different system or subject. We organized this book by systems to make it an easier study guide; the learner can review those areas in which he or she feels weakest and progress accordingly.

The CCRN Certification Examination lasts 4 hours and comprises 200 questions, weighted as follows:

Section	Percent of Questions on CCRN exam	Number of Questions on CCRN exam
Cardiovascular	39%	78
Respiratory	22%	44
Neurologic	8%	16
Renal	5%	10
Gastrointestinal	8%	16
Endocrine	4%	8
Hematologic and Immunologic	4%	8
Multisystem	10%	20
	100%	**200**

Psychosocial components of critical care are subsumed under each system in the certification examination.

The number of review questions for each subject area in this book was determined by two factors: (1) the weight given a specific area on the CCRN examination and (2) the amount of information test takers need in each area to pass the CCRN examination.

The number of review questions in this book is as follows:

Section	Number of Questions
Cardiovascular	187
Respiratory	135
Neurologic	120
Renal	98
Gastrointestinal	90
Endocrine	103
Hematologic and Immunologic	75
Multisystem Patient Care Problems	30
	838

Although the test begins at 9:00 a.m., you are expected to be at the test center by 8:00 a.m. Test takers are seated alphabetically in various rooms, with two proctors usually present in each room. Be sure to bring two forms of identification to the examination; for example, any photo I.D. and your test admission ticket. You'll also need at least two #2 pencils. Bring calipers with you if you need them to decipher a rhythm, although only a few rhythm strips usually appear on the CCRN examination. A nonprinting calculator is also allowed.

Immediately before the test, you'll have time to review the instructions for filling out the answer sheet. Your test results may be delayed if you don't follow these instructions precisely. The test comes in a sealed booklet. Do not break the seal before you are told to do so. After the test begins, the proctors periodically will write the time remaining on a blackboard.

Test-Taking Tips

*Get a good night's sleep the night before the test. Being rested will give you an advantage that you won't have if you're exhausted.

*When you see the test for the first time, scan the first page for a question you can easily answer. This will give you the confidence you need to approach the test without panic.

*Check the answer sheet frequently during the test to make sure you aren't making small but serious errors, such as answering Question #2 in Question #3's box. Such an error will affect your overall test score.

*Keep the first answer you choose. It is probably right. The more you fret over which answer to select, the more indecisive you can become. If you don't know an answer, come back to that question later. Try to narrow your choices to the point where your choice has fair odds of being correct. For example, if you can narrow your choices to two answers and then guess, you have a 50% chance of being correct.

*Eat a salty breakfast. Salt increases mental alertness.

Try to relax. Overwhelming anxiety will hamper you. Don't let this test intimidate you, even though it's important for you to pass. Also remember, you've prepared well for this test if you have studied this book. And if you've taken the test before, you've already had a valuable test-taking experience.

We hope our efforts increase your knowledge and help you pass the test, and we look forward to your comments on our book.

Laura Gasparis Vonfrolio
Joanne Noone

CHAPTER 1

CARDIOVASCULAR SYSTEM

1. The most important functional structure within the cardiac muscle is:

    A. Sarcotubular system
    B. Intercalated discs
    C. Syncytium
    D. Sarcoplasmic reticulum

2. Which coronary vessel supplies blood to the atrioventricular (AV) node?

    A. Right coronary artery
    B. Coronary sinus artery
    C. Left anterior descending artery
    D. Nodal artery

3. Which coronary artery supplies the anterior-septal wall of the left ventricle?

    A. Right coronary artery
    B. Left circumflex artery
    C. Nodal artery
    D. Left anterior descending artery

4. The resting membrane potential (RMP) is primarily the result of:

    A. An electrical charge of +80 to +90 mV for myocardial muscle fibers
    B. A higher intracellular sodium ion concentration
    C. A negative extracellular charge and positive intracellular charge
    D. The sodium pump mechanism

5. Coronary perfusion takes place:

A. During systole
B. During diastole
C. Equally during diastole and systole
D. Continuously

6. The most important determinant of coronary artery blood flow is:

A. Systolic blood pressure
B. Heart rate
C. Preload
D. Afterload

7. Diastole is _____ of the cardiac cycle.

A. 2/3
B. 1/3
C. 1/2
D. 3/4

8. Where is the base of the heart located?

A. Left 5th intercostal space medial to the midclavicular line
B. Left 5th intercostal space close to the sternum
C. Same location as the point of maximal impulse (PMI)
D. 2nd intercostal space close to the sternum

9. The beginning of systole is accompanied by which heart sound?

A. S_1
B. S_2
C. S_3
D. S_4

10. In reference to the second heart sound (S₂), which statement is *false?*

   A. Produced when the aortic and the pulmonic valves close
   B. Occurs at the end of ventricular systole
   C. May be heard best with the diaphragm of the stethoscope
   D. Produced when the mitral and the tricuspid valves close

11. Which of the following is an abnormal heart sound?

   A. Fixed split of S_2
   B. Physiologic split of S_2
   C. S_3 in a child
   D. S_2 split on inspiration

12. The nurse may auscultate a ventricular gallop (S_3) in patients with:

   A. Congestive heart failure
   B. Pericarditis
   C. Mitral stenosis
   D. Aortic stenosis

13. All of the following are true statements about a ventricular gallop (S_3) *except:*

   A. Sound is low-pitched and heard best with the diaphragm of the stethoscope
   B. Sound occurs during the early phase of ventricular filling
   C. Sound occurs because of resistance to ventricular filling resulting from decreased compliance of the ventricle
   D. Sound is best heard at the apex with the patient in the left lateral position

14. The fourth heart sound (S_4):

   A. Occurs after ventricular contraction
   B. Is best heard with the diaphragm of the stethoscope
   C. Is a normal finding in children
   D. Occurs during atrial contraction

15. An S_4 may occur in patients with:

A. Myocardial infarction
B. Mitral stenosis
C. Aortic insufficiency
D. Tricuspid stenosis

16. The sound of a heart murmur is produced by:

A. The closing of heart valves
B. The turbulence of abnormal blood flow
C. The vibration of valve structures of chamber walls
D. The opening of diseased valves

17. The nurse would auscultate the valve areas by listening:

A. Directly over each valve
B. Along the bony ridge of the sternal angle
C. At the base and apex for a total of 1 minute
D. In the direction of blood flow, at the intercostal spaces

18. A murmur heard best at the apex may be related to a:

A. Mitral valve defect
B. Tricuspid valve defect
C. Stenotic aortic valve
D. Regurgitant pulmonic valve

19. Regurgitant blood flow across which valves will cause a systolic murmur?

A. Mitral and aortic
B. Tricuspid and pulmonic
C. Mitral and tricuspid
D. Pulmonic and aortic

20. All of the following are systolic murmurs *except:*

A. Mitral stenosis
B. Tricuspid insufficiency
C. Aortic stenosis
D. Mitral insufficiency

21. In a patient with a recent myocardial infarction, a pansystolic murmur loudest at the apex and associated with a thrill may indicate:

A. Aortic stenosis
B. Aortic insufficiency
C. Tricuspid insufficiency
D. Mitral insufficiency

22. Regurgitant blood flow across which valves will cause a diastolic murmur:

A. Mitral and aortic
B. Tricuspid and pulmonic
C. Mitral and tricuspid
D. Pulmonic and aortic

23. Forward blood flow across which stenotic valves will cause a diastolic murmur?

A. Mitral and aortic
B. Tricuspid and pulmonic
C. Mitral and tricuspid
D. Pulmonic and aortic

24. The two imaginary lines that intersect on the chest to determine the phlebostatic axis are:

A. Midsternal line and the 4th intercostal space (ICS)
B. Midaxillary line and the 2nd ICS
C. Midaxillary line and the 4th ICS
D. Midclavicular chest line and the 4th ICS to the side of chest

25. If the transducer level is lower than the phlebostatic axis during pulmonary arterial pressure monitoring:

    A.   The readings will be falsely high
    B.   An "overwedge" waveform will appear
    C.   The curve will be dampened
    D.   Catheter "fling" will occur on the waveform

Case Study

Questions 26-32 refer to the following case study:

Mr.S., who has a history of congestive heart failure, is admitted to your unit with a medical diagnosis of sepsis and dehydration. Initial assessment reveals intravascular depletion. A pulmonary artery catheter is inserted.

26. The proximal lumen of a pulmonary artery catheter inserted in Mr. S. is correctly positioned when it is in the:

    A.   Right atrium
    B.   Right ventricle
    C.   Pulmonary artery
    D.   Pulmonary capillary

27. In which area of the heart would the pulmonary artery catheter be most likely to cause dysrhythmias?

    A.   Right atrium
    B.   Right ventricle
    C.   Pulmonary artery
    D.   Pulmonary capillary

28. Which of the following interventions would be used *first* to correct dysrhythmias associated with catheter insertion?

    A.   Administration of lidocaine
    B.   Defibrillation
    C.   Withdrawal of catheter tip
    D.   Cardioversion

29. Which of the following hemodynamic measurements is taken with the balloon inflated?

    A. Pulmonary capillary wedge pressure (PCWP)
    B. Cardiac output
    C. Pulmonary artery pressure (PAP)
    D. Mixed venous O_2 saturation

30. Flotation of a pulmonary catheter into a wedge (PCWP) position increases the risk of :

    A. Dysrhythmias
    B. Pulmonary infarction
    C. Pneumothorax
    D. Infection

31. Prolonged inflation of the catheter balloon increases the risk of:

    A. Dysrhythmias
    B. Air embolism
    C. Pneumothorax
    D. Pulmonary hemorrhage

32. If the pulmonary artery catheter in Mr. S. was reading 30/14 and then you noticed the continuous reading of 30/4, you would suspect:

    A. Decreased diastolic pressure due to beneficial effect of medications
    B. Decreased pulmonary artery pressure due to increased anoxia
    C. Catheter moved into the right ventricle
    D. Catheter advanced distally

33. Which of the following pressures are within normal limits?

   A. PAP=34/24, W=12
   B. PAP=30/20, W=10
   C. PAP=28/28, W=20
   D. PAP=24/14, W=12

34. Which of the following most accurately indicates changes in left ventricular pressure?

   A. Central venous pressure
   B. Pulmonary capillary wedge pressure
   C. Systemic arterial blood pressure
   D. Pulmonary artery pressure

35. A normal wedge pressure, increased pulmonary artery pressures, and evidence of right ventricular failure would most likely indicate:

   A. Cardiac tamponade
   B. Left ventricular failure
   C. Myocardial infarction
   D. Pulmonary embolism

36. Which of the following results in an elevated pulmonary artery pressure and a normal wedge pressure?

   A. Pulmonary hypertension
   B. Pulmonary edema
   C. Left ventricular failure
   D. Constrictive pericarditis

37. Mr.C., age 48, was admitted with increasing dyspnea and swollen feet. Upon Swan-Ganz catheterization, his pressures were as follows: right atrial=20, right ventricular=70/22, pulmonary artery=70/36, and pulmonary capillary wedge=12. His condition would be diagnosed as:

A. Congestive heart failure
B. Cardiac tamponade
C. Pulmonary hypertension
D. Hypovolemia

38. Cardiac index is calculated by dividing the cardiac output by the:

A. Mean arterial pressure
B. Patient's body surface area
C. Patient's weight
D. Pulmonary capillary wedge pressure

39. Preload may be described as follows:

A. The stretch produced within the myocardium at the end of diastole
B. The volume in ventricles during systole
C. The back-up of pressure in the systemic circulation
D. The amount of blood returning to the heart

40. Afterload may be described as follows:

A. The measurement of the left ventricular end-diastolic pressure
B. The amount of force of ventricular contraction
C. The impedance of ejection of blood from the left ventricle
D. The amount of blood remaining in the left ventricle after systole

41. Afterload is indicated best by the measurement of:

 A. Pulmonary capillary wedge pressure
 B. Stroke volume
 C. Systemic vascular resistance
 D. Ejection fraction

Case Study

Questions 42-46 refer to the following case study:

Mr.A. is admitted to the critical care unit with an acute anterior wall myocardial infarction (MI). A Swan-Ganz catheter is inserted.

42. The following blood gas samplings for Mr. A were obtained during Swan-Ganz insertion: right atrial O_2 saturation, 75%; right ventricular, 94%; and pulmonary artery, 94%. This is diagnostic of:

 A. Atrial septal defect
 B. Cardiac tamponade
 C. Ventricular septal defect
 D. Pulmonary embolus

43. Occlusion of the left anterior descending coronary artery may produce all of the following *except*:

 A. Massive left ventricular infarction
 B. Anterior infarction
 C. Septal infarction
 D. Right bundle branch block

44. The nurse would anticipate Mr.A.'s 12-lead ECG to show:

 A. ST elevations in V_5 and V_6
 B. Q waves in II and a VL
 C. ST elevations in II, III and aVF
 D. ST elevations in V_1 and V_2

45. Which complication would be *least* likely to occur in the patient with an acute anterior wall myocardial infarction?

A. Mobitz II heart block
B. Mitral insufficiency
C. Right bundle branch block
D. Ventricular aneurysm

46. Which dysrhythmia is the most significant in an acute myocardial infarction?

A. Atrial fibrillation
B. Premature ventricular contractions
C. First degree atrioventricular block
D. Premature junctional contraction

Case Study

Questions 47-51 continue the previous case study.

The patient, Mr. A, suddenly develops complete heart block. A temporary pacemaker is inserted, and Mr. A. is scheduled for a permanent pacemaker.

47. Which of the following definitions of temporary pacemaker components is *incorrect?*

A. Proximal electrode: paces the myocardium
B. Pacemaker catheter: contains two electrodes
C. Output control: regulates energy output
D. Rate control: regulates frequency of pacing

48. Which is *least* likely to contribute to the inability of a permanent pacemaker to sense the patient's rhythm?

A. Battery failure
B. Improper position of catheter
C. Faulty sensing mechanism
D. Electromagnetic interference

49.   What is the first action the nurse should take if Mr.A.'s temporary pacemaker is not sensing?

    A.   Position the patient on his left side
    B.   Check the sensitivity control
    C.   Turn up the energy output
    D.   Turn off the pacemaker

50.   Which of the following conditions necessitates a higher energy output (milliamps) for a temporary pacemaker?

    A.   Digitalis toxicity
    B.   Hypokalemia
    C.   Atrioventricular block
    D.   Ventricular dysrhythmias

51.   Mr. A. has a VVI pacemaker. What does the first initial of this pacemaker indicate?

    A.   The location of the catheter
    B.   Which chamber is sensed
    C.   The mode of the pacemaker
    D.   Which chamber is paced

Case Study
Questions 52-61 refer to the following case study:

Mr.I. is admitted with an inferior wall infarction. His blood pressure is 110/70 and his pulse is 62. He is presently pain-free.

52.   Which of the following is least helpful in diagnosing an acute myocardial infarction (MI)?

    A.   Patient's history
    B.   Physical examination
    C.   Enzyme studies
    D.   Serial ECGs

53. The isoenzymes most specific for cardiac muscle damage are:

    A. CPK-MB and LDH_1
    B. CPK-MM and LDH_3
    C. CPK-MM and LDH_1
    D. CPK-MB and LDH_3

54. In evaluating LDH isoenzymes, which report would indicate myocardial damage?

    A. LDH_5 greater than LDH_4
    B. LDH_2 greater than LDH_1
    C. LDH_1 greater than LDH_2
    D. LDH_4 greater than LDH_5

55. The enzyme that returns to normal level 7 to 10 days after myocardial damage is:

    A. SGPT
    B. CPK
    C. LDH
    D. SGOT

56. The inferior wall MI in Mr.I. will show indicative changes in leads:

    A. V_1 to V_4
    B. $V_{1,}$ aVL
    C. $V_{5,}$ V_6
    D. II, III, aVF

57. An inferior wall MI most likely results from occlusion of which artery?

    A. Anterior descending
    B. Right coronary
    C. Circumflex
    D. Left main coronary

58. The dysrhythmia shown below is:

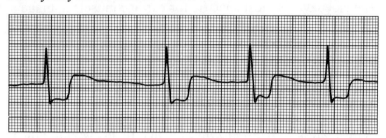

    A. Atrial flutter with variable conduction to the ventricles
    B. Atrial fibrillation
    C. Supraventricular tachycardia
    D. Junctional tachycardia

59. When Mr.I. develops the above dysrhythmia, the nurse would expect which of the following to occur?

    A. Ventricular irritability
    B. Syncope
    C. Widening pulse pressure
    D. Decreased cardiac output

60. The most common complication of an MI is:

    A. Dysrhythmia
    B. Congestive heart failure
    C. Cardiogenic shock
    D. Pulmonary embolism

61. The nurse could expect Mr.I. to develop all of the following complications *except*:

    A. Mobitz II heart block
    B. Sinus bradycardia
    C. Sick sinus syndrome
    D. Idioventricular rhythm

62. Which of the following would be typical of right ventricular failure?

    A.   Pulmonary capillary wedge pressure greater than 25mm Hg
    B.   Jugular venous distention 2 cm above the clavicle
    C.   Bilateral moist rales
    D.   Hepatosplenomegaly

63. Which of the following statements about jugular venous pressure is *false?*

    A.   Examination of the jugular veins provides important information about cardiac compensation
    B.   Internal jugular pulsations give a more accurate pressure than do external jugular pulsations
    C.   When examining for jugular venous pressure, the nurse must elevate the head of the bed 30 degrees
    D.   Pulsations should be absent while the patient is lying flat

64. Hepatojugular reflux suggests:

    A.   Chronic liver condition
    B.   Obstructive lung disease
    C.   Congestive heart failure
    D.   Acute liver dysfunction

Case Study

Questions 65-68 refer to the following case study:

Mr.L. is admitted to the critical care unit with dyspnea and short ness of breath on exertion. He has a history of chronic obstructive pulmonary disease (COPD). Chest X-ray confirms a diagnosis of congestive heart failure. A pulmonary artery catheter is inserted.

65. Which factor would *not* place Mr.L. at risk for left ventricular failure?

    A.   Pulmonary hypertension
    B.   Cardiomyopathy
    C.   Aortic stenosis
    D.   Acute myocardial infarction

66. Which is *not* an early sign of CHF?

    A.   Increase in central venous pressure (CVP) reading
    B.   Fine, moist crackles at lung bases
    C. S_3 heart sound
    D.   Tachycardia

67. The clinical presentation of Mr.L. with *left* ventricular failure includes:

    A.   Nocturnal dyspnea
    B.   Bounding pulses
    C.   Hepatosplenomegaly
    D.   Pitting edema

68. Which of the following hemodynamic parameters would indicate left ventricular failure in a patient with COPD?

    A.   PAP-54/22, PCWP-14
    B.   PAP-48/26, PCWP-16
    C.   PAP-22/12, PCWP-16
    D.   PAP-48/26, PCWP-20

69. Which patient is *least* at risk for developing cardiogenic shock?

    A.   A 24-year-old with cardiac tamponade from a stab wound to the heart
    B.   A 72-year-old with a history of heart disease who has developed a dysrhythmia
    C.   A 55-year-old with acute pericarditis who underwent cardiac surgery 3 weeks ago
    D.   A 44-year-old with an anterolateral wall myocardial infarction

16

70. In cardiogenic shock, which physiologic compensatory mechanisms occur to increase blood pressure and cardiac output?

    A. Increasing heart rate and increasing force of contraction
    B. Increasing heart rate and decreasing preload
    C. Decreasing preload and decreasing afterload
    D. Decreasing heart rate and decreasing preload

Case Study
Questions 71-82 refer to the following case study:

Mrs.C. is admitted to the critical care unit with crushing chest pain. An ECG reveals a massive infarction. She is hypotensive, diaphoretic, and oliguric. A diagnosis of cardiogenic shock is made.

71. Clinical manifestations of Mr.C.'s cardiogenic shock would include all of the following *except:*

    A. Distended neck veins
    B. Pulmonary congestion
    C. S_3 heart sound
    D. Low central venous pressure

72. In a patient with an acute myocardial infarction, an early assessment finding that may indicate cardiogenic shock is:

    A. S_3 heart sound
    B. Bilateral crackles heard throughout inspiration
    C. Warm, diaphoretic skin
    D. Urine output of 30 ml in 1 hour

73. One of the earliest clinical signs of cardiogenic shock is:

    A. Tachycardia
    B. Cyanosis
    C. Fluffy-white chest X-ray
    D. Hypotension

74. Vasodilator therapy is instituted for Mrs.C. Vasodilator therapy exerts a therapeutic effect in cardiogenic shock by:

   A.   Decreasing venous return
   B.   Reducing peripheral vascular resistance
   C.   Enhancing cardiac output
   D.   All of the above

75. Another beneficial effect of vasodilator therapy that Mrs.C. should be assessed for is:

   A.   Decreased pulmonary capillary wedge pressure
   B.   Increased pulmonary artery pressure
   C.   Increased systemic vascular resistance
   D.   Decreased cardiac output

76. While Mrs.C. is in cardiogenic shock, another beneficial effect of vasodilator therapy is:

   A.   Increased systemic vascular resistance
   B.   Decreased preload and afterload
   C.   Increased pulmonary artery pressure
   D.   Increased pulmonary vascular resistance

77. The effectiveness of vasodilator therapy may be most immediately indicated by:

   A. PaO_2
   B.   Vital signs
   C. $PaCO_2$
   D.   Urine output

78. Dopamine is added to Mrs.C.'s therapeutic regimen. The therapeutic outcome of inotropic agents used to manage the patient in cardiogenic shock is:

   A.   Vasodilation
   B.   Improved tissue perfusion
   C.   Increased heart rate
   D.   Decreased force of myocardial contractility

79. Which of the following medications would be most effective if prescribed for Mrs.C. to decrease preload and afterload?

A. Dopamine
B. Nitroprusside
C. Dobutamine
D. Digoxin

80. Which is the first parameter to respond to intravenous Lasix?

A. Urine output
B. PCWP
C. Breath sounds
D. Chest X-rays

81. Positive inotropic agents are used to:

A. Improve tissue perfusion
B. Decrease water loss through the kidney
C. Increase heart rate
D. Vasodilate vessels

82. The treatment *least* effective in protecting the myocardium from further damage is:

A. Decreasing peripheral vascular resistance
B. Decreasing ventricular preload
C. Increasing left ventricular afterload
D. Increasing cardiac output

Case Study
Questions 83-87 continue the previous case study.

Twelve hours after Mrs.C. is admitted, an intra-aortic balloon pump (IABP) is inserted. Her status has improved as a result of this measure.

83. Which of the following is *true* concerning the IABP?

    A. Increases left ventricular pressure
    B. Increases PCWP
    C. Increased coronary artery perfusion
    D. Increases afterload

84. The therapeutic effects of the IABP include all of the following *except:*

    A. Increased cardiac output
    B. Increased cardiac afterload
    C. Decreased myocardial O_2 consumption
    D. Increased aortic pressure

85. A nursing measure that would be *inappropriate* while the IABP is inserted would be to:

    A. Perform passive range-of-motion exercises four times a day
    B. Monitor pulses frequently
    C. Keep the head of the bed elevated 45 to 60 degrees
    D. Administer antipyretics for temperature above 101°F.

86. The intra-aortic balloon pump is:

    A. Deflated during systole
    B. Inflated during systole
    C. Deflated during diastole
    D. None of the above

87. IABP therapy is contraindicated for which of the following?

    A. Papillary muscle rupture
    B. Incompetent aortic valve
    C. Left ventricular failure after bypass
    D. Unstable angina refractory to the medical regimen

Questions 88-93 refer to the following case study:

Mr. A., age 54, has a history of angina pectoris. He has been having frequent chest pain, necessitating increased sublingual doses of nitroglycerin. ST depressions are noted on his ECG.

88. A patient with typical anginal pain such as Mr. A.'s may describe it as:

A. A vague ache over the left side of the chest
B. A tight, oppressive substernal pain radiating to the left arm
C. A severe, sharp pain around the sternum radiating up both sides of the neck
D. An intense, shooting pain from the left side of the chest radiating to the left arm

89. All of the following are true regarding angina pectoris *except:*

A. Pain may radiate to shoulders, arms, or jaw
B. Relief from nitroglycerin may take as long as 1 hour
C. Pain gradually subsides with rest
D. ST depressions may be seen during an attack

90. Which of the following would *not* precipitate an anginal episode?

A. Hypokalemia
B. Physical activity
C. Smoking
D. Heavy meals

91. ST depression indicates:

A. Ischemia
B. Injury
C. Necrosis
D. Pericarditis

92. The pathologic changes found on an ECG to indicate myocardial ischemia are:

    A.   ST elevation
    B.   ST segment depression and T wave elevation
    C.   Q wave formation
    D.   ST segment depression and T wave inversion

93. The nurse auscultates an S_4 gallop during her assessment of Mr.A. The appearance of an S_4 gallop during an anginal episode signifies:

    A.   Congestive heart failure
    B.   Decreased compliance of ischemic zone
    C.   Aortic stenosis
    D.   Increased left ventricular filling volume

94. The nurse may expect a patient with Prinzmetal's angina to experience:

    A.   Chest pain at rest
    B.   Chest pain always relieved by nitrates
    C.   No ECG changes during the episode
    D.   Cyanotic episodes

95. Which of the following statements is *false* regarding Prinzmetal's angina?

    A.   It is the result of coronary artery spasm
    B.   Calcium blockers are the pharmacological treatment
    C.   It occurs in 5% to 10% of angina cases
    D.   Surgical intervention is warranted

Case Study

Questions 96-101 refer to the following case study:

Mr.K., age 39, is admitted to the intensive care unit (ICU) after a motor vehicle accident. He suffered a rib fracture when his chest hit the steering wheel. His diagnosis is pericardial tamponade.

96. In assessing Mr.K, the nurse would observe:

    A. Narrowing pulse pressure
    B. Decreased wedge pressure
    C. Decreased central venous pressure
    D. Decreased pulse

97. Which is *not* characteristic of pericardial tamponade?

    A. Rise in central venous pressure
    B. Pulsus paradoxus
    C. Distant heart sounds
    D. Widening pulse pressure

98. Pulsus paradoxus can be defined as:

    A. An absence of pulse during expiration
    B. A decrease of 20 mm Hg in arterial systolic pressure on expiration during auscultation of blood pressure
    C. A drop of more than 10 mm Hg in arterial systolic pressure on inspiration
    D. A drop of 20 mm Hg in arterial systolic pressure on deep inspiratory effort

99. The nurse may observe pulsus paradoxus in patients with all of the following *except:*

    A. Patent ductus arteriosus
    B. Severe pulmonary emphysema
    C. Cardiac tamponade
    D. Hypovolemic shock

100. An emergency pericardiocentesis is performed on Mr.K. All of the following are common complications of pericardiocentesis *except:*

A. Ventricular perforation
B. Pneumothorax
C. Complete heart block
D. Ventricular fibrillation

101. A nursing responsibility during pericardiocentesis for cardiac tamponade is to:

A. Prepare an infusion of isoproterenol (Isuprel)
B. Monitor the patient's ECG tracings in a V lead
C. Place the patient flat, if possible
D. Encourage the patient to perform Valsalva's maneuver, if possible

Case Study

Mr.S., a 54-year-old man with a known history of coronary artery disease, is admitted with progressively worsening angina pectoris. Tests were done to delineate the extent of his disease and to deter mine if he is a candidate for coronary artery bypass grafting (CABG).

102. Which of the following is *not* an invasive diagnostic technique for cardiac assessment?

A. His bundle ECG
B. Ventriculography
C. Vectorcardiography
D. Aortography

103. Technetium phosphate imaging is performed on Mr.S. This test:

    A.   Uses cold spot imaging
    B.   Determines coronary artery blockage
    C.   Calculates left ventricular ejection fraction
    D.   Specifies the area of myocardial damage

104. Which patient is the *least* appropriate candidate for angioplasty? The patient with:

    A.   New-onset angina
    B.   Single vessel disease
    C.   Multiple areas of obstruction in a single vessel
    D.   An ejection fraction of 50%

105. Indications for CABG for Mr.S. would include all of the following *except:*

    A.   New transmural myocardial infarction
    B.   Chronic disabling angina pectoris
    C.   Unstable angina unresponsive to medical therapy
    D.   Occlusion of the left main coronary artery

106. Which of the following findings would *not* be a contraindication for CABG when selecting a candidate?

    A.   Poor left ventricular function
    B.   Recent myocardial infarction
    C.   Distal coronary artery disease
    D.   History of an old MI

107. Which condition contraindicates CABG?

    A.   Recent angioplasty
    B.   Subendocardial myocardial infarction
    C.   Preoperative ejection fraction of 10% without angina
    D.   Malignant dysrhythmias

108. Mr.S. undergoes CABG. Postoperatively, the nurse would assess him for complications. Which would be *least* likely to occur?

   A. Graft occlusion
   B. Perioperative infarction
   C. Numbness of donor leg
   D. Progression of atherosclerotic process

109. Physiologic effects of cardiopulmonary bypass include all of the following *except:*

   A. Fever spikes
   B. Hemodilution
   C. Clotting abnormalities
   D. Third-space fluid shifting

110. Because of rapid metabolic and temperature changes during the postoperative period, the nurse should check Mr.S. for:

   A. Dysrhythmias
   B. Heparin rebound
   C. Hyperkalemia
   D. Hyperthermia

111. The rationale for inserting a temporary pacemaker during CABG is to:

   A. Treat trifascicular block, which commonly occurs
   B. Optimize cardiac output
   C. Override tachydysrhythmias
   D. Test stress by rapid atrial pacing

112. All postoperative cardiac patients develop:

   A. Confusion
   B. Pericarditis
   C. Hypokalemia
   D. Atelectasis

113. A nursing intervention for a patient experiencing pain from pericarditis would be to:

    A. Instruct the patient on the importance of bed rest
    B. Take the patient's blood pressure before giving nitro-glycerin for pericardial pain
    C. Encourage the patient to sit up and lean forward
    D. Encourage the patient to breathe deeply

114. Pericarditis may be suspected if the patient's ECG shows:

    A. First-degree AV block
    B. Prominent U wave
    C. Prominent R wave
    D. ST elevations

115. Which of the following statements is *true* about cardiopulmonary resuscitation in the immediate postoperative cardiac surgery patient?

    A. Abdominal instead of sternal thrusts must be used
    B. Defibrillator may not be set higher than 200 joules
    C. The chest may be compressed only 1/2 inch
    D. Open-chest cardiac massage must be performed

Case Study

Questions 116-119 refer to the following study:

Mr.M. a 26-year-old man, sustained severe abdominal injuries in an automobile accident. When he is admitted to the intensive care unit (ICU), his blood pressure is 80/50 mm Hg, his heart rate is 130 beats/minute, and his respiratory rate is 30 breaths/minute.

116. Which of the following phrases best describes shock?

    A. The inability of the body to excrete metabolic waste products
    B. The collapse of the respiratory system
    C. The collapse of the sympathetic nervous system
    D. A state of inadequate tissue perfusion

117. Which of the following nursing actions is *inappropriate* during the initial stabilization of Mr.M.?

    A. Administering oxygen therapy
    B. Applying medical antishock trousers (MAST)
    C. Placing the patient in the Trendelenburg position
    D. Infusing lactated Ringer's solution via a large-bore I.V. line

118. At the time of Mr. M.'s admission, assessment findings most indicative of hypovolemic shock include:

    A. Pulsus paradoxus
    B. A hemoglobin value of 10/dl, hematocrit value of 38%
    C. A widening pulse pressure
    D. A central venous pressure (CVP) above 4 mm Hg

119. Patient assessment data that suggest hypovolemia as a cause of shock include:

    A. Decreased central venous pressure and distended neck veins only while the patient is supine
    B. Increased urine sodium level and a urine specific gravity of 1.010
    C. Decreased pulse pressure
    D. Tachycardia with ventricular gallop (S_3)

120. An indication of shock is a drop in systolic blood pressure below:

A. 100 mm Hg
B. 96 mm Hg
C. 90 mm Hg
D. 80 mm Hg

121. The most common result of shock is:

A. Metabolic acidosis
B. Respiratory acidosis
C. Metabolic alkalosis
D. Hypovolemia

122. Fluid replacement in the hypovolemic patient is *best* gauged by which parameter?

A. Blood pressure
B. Pulmonary capillary wedge pressure
C. Systemic vascular resistance
D. Pulmonary artery pressure

123. Which of the following is a consequence of multiple transfusions?

A. Brudzinski's sign
B. Chvostek's sign
C. Cullen's sign
D. Babinski's sign

Case Study

Questions 124-127 refer to the following case study:

Mr.B. presents with chest pain that lasts more than 30 minutes and that is unresponsive to sublingual nitroglycerin. In addition, ST elevation is present in leads II, III and aVF. Thrombolytic therapy is instituted.

124. Which is *not* an indication for thrombolytic therapy?

  A. An occluded arteriovenous fistula
  B. Subendocardial myocardial infarction (MI)
  C. Pulmonary embolus
  D. Peripheral arterial occlusion

125. A thrombolytic agent used in the first few hours of an MI is:

  A. Heparin
  B. Streptokinase (Streptase)
  C. Thrombokinase
  D. Warfarin (Coumadin)

126. Thrombolytic therapy is contraindicated in a recent:

  A. Deep vein thrombosis
  B. Pulmonary emboli
  C. Cerebrovascular accident (CVA)
  D. Coronary occlusion

127. Mr.B.'s thrombolytic therapy should be discontinued if which of the following occurs?

  A. Low-grade fever
  B. Vomiting
  C. Dyspnea
  D. Relief of chest pain

Case Study

Questions 128-131 continue the previous case study.

Another thrombolytic therapy that may be instituted for Mr.B. involves tissue plasminogen activator (t-PA).

128. The nurse administering t-PA must monitor Mr.B. for all of the following *except:*

A. Peripheral thrombosis
B. Myocardial reperfusion
C. Bleeding complications
D. Coronary reocclusion

129. Before initiating t-PA therapy, the nurse must establish a mini-mum of how many intravenous infusions?

A. One
B. Two
C. Three
D. Four

130. The total dose of t-PA, as approved by the Food and Drug Administration (FDA), is:

A. 50 mg
B. 100 mg
C. 200 mg
D. 500 mg

131. Which finding in Mr.B. would *not* indicate reperfusion during t-PA infusion?

A. Drop in arterial blood pressure
B. Resolution of ST segment elevation
C. Ventricular tachycardia
D. Dramatic reduction in chest pain

Case Study

Questions 132-133 refer to the following case study:

Mr.F. has been admitted with an acute anterior wall MI. He continues to have intermittent chest pain relieved with morphine sulfate 5 mg. I.V. push. His blood pressure is 130/70 and his pulse is 110 beats per minute.

31

132. Which of the following is not a complication of an acute myocar
dial infarction (MI)?

A. Myocarditis
B. Dressler's syndrome
C. Ventricular aneurysm
D. Papillary muscle rupture

133. Suddenly, Mr.F. develops ventricular tachycardia. He is pulseless.
Your immediate response would be to:

A. Defibrillate with 200 joules
B. Defibrillate with 300 joules
C. Administer lidocaine 100- mg bolus
D. Perform a precordial thump

Case Study

Questions 134-135 refer to the following case study:

Mr.Q. is admitted to the critical care unit with an acute inferior-posterior wall MI. He is having frequent premature ventricular contractions. You are about to administer lidocaine.

134. During prophylactic administration of lidocaine, after what time
interval should the second bolus be given to Mr.Q.?

A. 2 minutes
B. 5 minutes
C. 10 minutes
D. 15 minutes

135. The recommended dosages of lidocaine should be decreased by
50% in all of the following conditions *except:*

A. Confusion
B. Congestive heart failure
C. Shock
D. Hepatic disease

Questions 136-138 refer to the following case study:

Mr.Q. is on a 2 mg/minute drip of lidocaine. His cardiac monitor alarm goes off. The monitor shows ventricular tachycardia. He has a pulse but is hemodynamically unstable.

136. The nurse's first response would be to:

    A. Administer lidocaine 100 mg I.V. bolus
    B. Defibrillate with 200 joules
    C. Administer a precordial thump
    D. Perform immediate synchronized cardioversion with 100 to 200 joules

137. Mr.Q.'s rhythm progresses to ventricular fibrillation. After three defibrillation attempts, which medication should be administered first?

    A. Sodium bicarbonate
    B. Epinephrine 1 mg I.V.
    C. Lidocaine 100 mg I.V. bolus
    D. Atropine 0.5 mg I.V.

138. During the code, Mr.Q.'s monitor shows sinus bradycardia, but no pulse is present. Pulseless electrical activity (PEA) is diagnosed. Initial treatment should be to administer:

    A. Calcium chloride
    B. Epinephrine
    C. Atropine
    D. Sodium bicarbonate

139. The PR interval can be defined as:

A. The interval for conduction from the sinus node to the AV (atrioventricular) node
B. The amount of time necessary for atrial depolarization
C. The interval measuring AV conduction time
D. The measurement from the beginning of the P wave to the end of the QRS complex

140. The dysrhythmia shown below can be interpreted as:

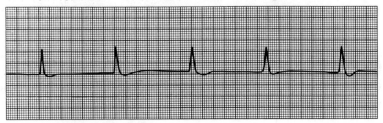

A. Atrial fibrillation
B. Controlled atrial fibrillation
C. Sinus bradycardia
D. Junctional rhythm

141. Sick sinus syndrome includes:

A. Cardiac standstill
B. Bradycardia-tachycardia syndrome
C. Complete heart block
D. Stokes-Adams syndrome

142. Second-degree AV block (Mobitz Type II) is *not* caused by:

A. Digitalis toxicity
B. Acute myocardial infarction
C. Hypokalemia
D. Coronary artery disease

143. Which dysrhythmia does *not* respond to carotid sinus massage?

    A. Ventricular tachycardia
    B. Paroxysmal atrial tachycardia
    C. Atrial flutter
    D. Atrial fibrillation

144. Your patient's cardiac monitor displays the strip below. Recent history includes an inferior wall MI. Blood pressure is stable and asymptomatic. Which of the following would be the *least* likely choice for therapy:

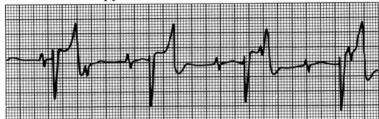

    A. Temporary pacemaker
    B. Permanent pacemaker
    C. Atropine
    D. Isuprel drip

145. The rhythm strip shown below indicates:

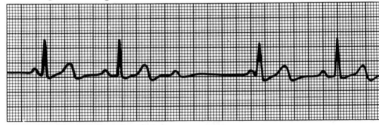

    A. Sinus dysrhythmia
    B. First-degree AV block
    C. Second-degree AV block (Mobitz Type I or Wenckebach)
    D. Second-degree AV block (Mobitz Type II)

146. The dysrhythmia shown below indicates:

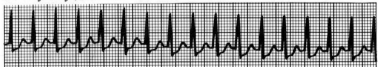

    A.   Sinus tachycardia
    B.   Ventricular tachycardia
    C.   Atrial flutter 2:1
    D.   Supraventricular tachycardia

147. Progressive prolongation of the PR interval followed by a blocked P wave describes:

    A.   Sinus arrest
    B.   First-degree AV block
    C.   Second-degree AV block (Mobitz Type I or Wenckebach)
    D.   Second-degree AV block (Mobitz Type II)

148. An early P wave not followed by a QRS complex is known as:

    A.   Sinus arrest
    B.   Blocked premature atrial contraction
    C.   Ventricular escape
    D.   Second-degree AV block (Mobitz Type II)

149. Hyperkalemia may be identified electrocardiographically by all of the following *except:*

    A.   Prominent U wave
    B.   Peaked T wave
    C.   Widened QRS complex
    D.   Diminished P wave amplitude

150. A common complication of Wolff-Parkinson-White syndrome may include all the following *except*:

    A.   Third-degree AV block
    B.   Atrial fibrillation
    C.   Ventricular fibrillation
    D.   Paroxysmal atrial tachycardia

151. The drug of choice for idiopathic hypertrophic subaortic stenosis (IHSS) is:

A. Digoxin
B. Inderal
C. Lidocaine
D. Dobutamine

152. Which drug may prolong the QT interval?

A. Isoproterenol (Isuprel)
B. Atropine
C. Disopyramide (Norpace)
D. Epinephrine

153. The most potent vasoconstrictor known is:

A. Angiotensin II
B. Bradykinin
C. Renin
D. Dopamine

154. Which condition would stimulate renin secretion?

A. Increased blood supply to the renal tubules
B. Decreased blood pressure
C. Decreased sympathetic output
D. Increased sodium concentration

155. The nurse may detect pulsus magnus in a patient with:

A. Thyrotoxicosis
B. Cardiac tamponade
C. Aortic stenosis
D. Congestive heart failure

156. Which valve is most commonly involved in infective endocarditis?

    A.   Tricuspid
    B.   Pulmonic
    C.   Mitral
    D.   Aortic

157. Hypertension causes a reflex bradycardia from stimulation of:

    A.   Adrenergic receptors
    B.   Baroreceptors
    C.   Alpha receptors
    D.   Beta receptors

158. Malignant hypertension is characterized by a diastolic blood pressure over:

    A.   90 mm Hg
    B.   100 mm Hg
    C.   110 mm Hg
    D.   140 mm Hg

159. The earliest clue in assessing for a dissecting aortic aneurysm would most likely be:

    A.   Diaphoresis
    B.   Back pain
    C.   Dependent edema
    D.   Crackles

Case Study:

Mr. V., 57, is admitted to the ICU with a diagnosis of acute lateral wall myocardial infarction. Upon admission to the ICU, the nurse assesses him to be quite anxious.

Questions 160 -166 refer to the above case study.

160. Which of the following symptoms would support the assessment of anxiety?

    A.   Increased urinary frequency
    B.   Bradycardia
    C.   Muscle weakness
    D.   Flushed Skin

161. Although initially stable upon admission, Mr. V.'s blood pressure and urine output have decreased over the last two hours. The physician decides to place a pulmonary artery catheter to aid in hemodynamic assessment, obtains consent and leaves the room to set up. Mr. V. begins to ask questions, which leads the nurse to conclude that he does not understand the information just given by the physician. The nurse should:

    A.   Answer Mr. V.'s questions
    B.   Notify the supervisor
    C.   Notify the physician
    D.   Do nothing because the consent is already signed

162. During pulmonary artery catheter placement, the correct lead to monitor Mr. V. is:

    A.   Lead II
    B.   Lead III
    C.   Lead V_1
    D.   Lead V_6

163. The reason to monitor in this lead is to observe for which complication?

    A.   Ventricular dysrhythmias
    B.   RBBB
    C.   LBBB
    D.   Septal perforation

164. As the catheter is floated from the pulmonary artery to the pulmonary capillary wedge position, the mean PCWP is 24mm HG with the following waveform.

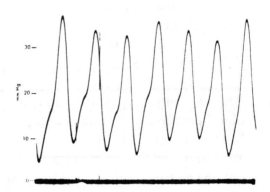

The correct interpretation of this data is:
A.   An elevated PCWP from pump failure
B.   Curling of the catheter is the pulmonary artery
C.   Curling of the catheter back into the right ventricle
D.   A large V wave

165. The above situation is a result of:

A.   Papillary muscle rupture
B.   Ventricular septal defect
C.   Cardiogenic shock
D.   Right ventricular failure

166. After the procedure, Mr. V.'s rhythm changes into a wide QRS tachycardia. The physician is unable to determine whether the rhythm is of venticular or atrial origin. In situations like this, it is best to administer:

A.   Lidocaine
B.   Procainamide
C.   Verapamil
D.   Adenosine

Case Study:

Mr. L., 66 years old, is admitted with an acute inferior wall MI.

Questions 167-173 refer to the above situation.

167. During the admission history, Mr. L. tells the nurse that he has been told that he is a "Type A" personality. Which comparative statement about Type A and B behaviors during hospitalization foran acute myocardial infarction is true?

    A. Type B behavior uses denial as a defense mechanism more often

    B. Type A behavior is associated with shorter hospitalization

    C. Type B personalities are more concerned with death

    D. Type B personalities tend to exhibit more Type A behaviors during hospitalization

168. His blood pressure drops two hours after admission, although his lungs remain clear to auscultation. He has positive JVD, which increases on inspiration. It would be most appropriate at this time to:

    A. Obtain a right precordial lead tracing

    B. Continuously monitor in lead III

    C. Continuously monitor in lead V_1

    D. Obtain a direct posterior lead tracing

169. The physician places a pulmonary artery catheter to guide therapy. Anticipated readings would be:

    A. RA pressure = 4 mm Hg; PCWP = 4 mm Hg

    B. RA pressure = 20 mm Hg; PCWP = 4 mm Hg

    C. RA pressure = 4 mm Hg; PCWP = 20 mm Hg

    D. RA pressure = 20 mm Hg; PCWP = 20 mm Hg

170. Correct therapy at this time would include:

    A.   Intraaortic balloon pump
    B.   Volume expansion
    C.   Vasodilator therapy
    D.   All of the above

171. They physician orders an intravenous bolus of furosemide (Lasix) for Mr. L. The nurse feels that furosemide would be unsafe in this situation and that dopamine (Intropin) is indicated. If, after questioning the order, the nurse is told to give furosemide, she should:

    A.   Refuse to give the furosemide
    B.   Give the dopamine instead
    C.   Give the furosemide
    D.   Ask another physician

172. During his first few days of hopitalization, Mr. L. exhibits signs of denial. At this time, patients with a myocardial infarction may experience a positive correlation between denial and;

    A.   More complications
    B.   A better survival rate
    C.   An increase in mortality
    D.   More psychological problems

173. In creating a teaching plan for Mr. L., the nurse realizes he is more likely to comply with a medical regimen if:

    A.   His family expects him to comply
    B.   He values the regimen
    C.   He intends to comply
    D.   He is informed about the regimen

Ms. N., 68, is admitted to the ICU with chest pain. She has a history of angina and ventricular dysrhythmia. Two weeks ago she was started on quinidine gluconate.

Questions 174 - 177 refer to the above situation.

174. Ms. N.'s EKG shows deep T wave inversion in leads V_2 and V_3 but is otherwise normal. This finding is consistent with:

   A. Posterior wall MI
   B. Pericarditis
   C. Anterioseptal MI
   D. Wellen's syndrome

175. Which electrocardiographic parameter should be monitored with quinidine therapy?

   A. PR interval
   B. Electrical axis
   C. QT interval
   D. Heart rate

176. Ms. N.'s rhythm deteriorates into the following dysrhythmia, which is correctly interpreted as:

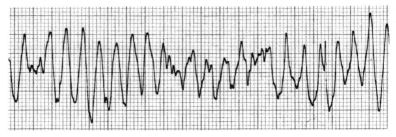

   A. Atrial fibrillation with an accessory pathway
   B. Torsade de pointes
   C. Ventricular tachycardia
   D. Ventricular fibrillation

177. The treatment of choice for this dysrhythmia is:

    A.   Adenosine
    B.   Cardioversion
    C.   Defibrillation
    D.   Magnesium

Case Study
Questions 178-181 refer to the following case study:

Mr. F., age 43, is admitted to the ICU. He has had chest pain for the last 2 hours and ST elevation in V_1 - V_4. Acute anterior-wall myocardial infarction is diag nosed. The physician plans to administer t-PA (tissue plasminogen activator)

178. Which statement about t-PA and streptokinase is *true?*

    A.   They are equally effective
    B.   They both activate circulating and fibrin-bound plasminogen
    C.   Only t-PA depletes clotting factors
    D.   The half-life of t-PA is considerably shorter than that of streptokinase

179. Which of the following patients is most likely to be excluded from t-PA therapy?

    A.   The patient was given streptokinase after a previous myocardial infarction with successful reperfusion
    B.   The patient is 77 years old and on coumadin therapy at home
    C.   The patient has had a recent streptococcal upper respiratory infection
    D.   The patient has had chest pain for no more than 5 hours

180. Which laboratory value change may occur after t-PA therapy?

    A.   Elevated fibrin split products
    B.   Decreased fibrinogen
    C.   Increased partial thromboplastin time
    D.   Increased prothrombin time

181. Which of the following indicates successful reperfusion after t-PA therapy?

    A.   Negative creatine phosphoskinase (CPK) isoenzymes
    B.   Q wave formation
    C.   Atrial fibrillation
    D.   Accelerated idioventricular rhythm

Case Study
Questions 182-187 refer to the following case study:

Mrs. R., age 52, is admitted to the ICU, awaiting a cardiac transplantation. She has a history of idiopathic cardiomyopathy.

182. An absolute contraindication to heart transplantation found during preoperative evaluation would be:

    A.   Irreversible pulmonary hypertension
    B.   Chronic obstructive pulmonary disease
    C.   Recurrent ventricular dysrhythmias
    D.   Diabetes mellitus

183. Signs of acute rejection Mrs. R. should be assessed for post-operatively include:

    A.   Ischemia documented on ECG
    B.   Lung crackles, gallop heart rhythm
    C.   Hypertension, bradycardia
    D.   Swelling at incision site

184. Acute rejection in cardiac transplantation is diagnosed by:

A. ECG
B. Chest X-ray
C. Echocardiography
D. Endomyocardial biopsy

185. Mrs. R. is started on cyclosporine (Sandimmune) postoperatively. In assessing for complications related to this drug therapy, the nurse should monitor Mrs. R.'s

A. Blood glucose
B. Serum creatinine
C. Serum amylase
D. Serum magnesium

186. A frequent postoperative cardiac transplant nursing diagnosis Mrs. R. should be assessed for is:

A. Powerlessness
B. Body image disturbance
C. Ineffective denial
D. Hopelessness

187. Which statement by Mrs. R. demonstrates correct under standing regarding her heart rate/rhythm post-transplant?

A. "There should be no change in my heart rate or rhythm because of the transplant"
B. "I have a pacemaker now to help my heart beat effectively"
C. "My heart beats more rapidly because of irritability from scar tissue"
D. "My heart rate rises more slowly now when I begin activity or exercise"

1.   **Correct answer - C**

Cardiac muscle differs from skeletal muscle because it has more mitochondria; thus, more adenosine triphosphate (ATP) is generated incardiac muscle. The cardiac muscle fibers are connected to one another by intercalated discs, forming a lattice arrangement called a functional syncytium. This syncytium is important in allowing rapid simultaneous depolarization throughout the heartmuscle.

2.   **Correct answer - A**

In 80% of the population, the right coronary artery supplies the atrioventricular (AV) node. In the remaining 20%, the left circumflex artery supplies blood to the AV node. The right coronary artery also supplies the sinus node in 55% of the population, and the left circumflex, the other 45%

3.   **Correct answer - D**

The left anterior descending artery (LAD) supplies the anterior part of the intraventricular septum, the anterior wall of the left ventricle, the right bundle branch, and the anterior superior divi-sion of the left bundle branch. The LAD is a branch of the left coronary artery. The right   coronary artery supplies the sinus node in 55% of the popula-tion, the atrio ventricular node in 90% of the population, and the inferior-posterior wall of the left ventricle.

4.   **Correct answer - D**

The resting membrane potential (RMP), -80 to -90 mV for myocardial muscle fibers, is primarily the result of the sodium pump mechanism. Sodium ion concentration is higher outside the cell and potassium ion concentration is higher inside the cell. The positively charged sodium keeps the outside of the cell more positively charged than the intracellular space.Concentrations of sodium and potassium are controlled by the sodium pump, which regulates concentrations of these cations in the resting membrane.

5. **Correct answer - B**

Most blood flow in the coronary arteries of the left ventricular myocardium occurs during ventricular diastole. During ventricular systole, the pressure exerted on the intramuscularportions of the coronary vessels by contracting myocardial fibers helps impede coronary blood flow.

6. **Correct answer - B**

Because coronary blood flow occurs during diastole, the amount of time in diastole affects coronary perfusion. Therefore, heart rate is the most important determinant of coronary artery blood flow.

7. **Correct answer - A**
$$S + 2 \times D = \frac{X}{3} = MAP$$

Diastole is two-thirds of the cardiac cycle. For this reason, the average of the systolic and diastolic pressures is not used to calculate mean arterial pressure. Instead, mean arterial pressure is determined by adding the systolic pressure to twice the diastolic pressure and dividing that total by three. The mean arterial pressure, therefore, is closer to the diastolic pressure than to the systolic pressure.

8. **Correct answer - D**

The base of the heart comprises two areas: the aortic area, or the right 2nd intercostal space close to the sternum, and the pulmonic area, the left 2nd intercostal space close to the sternum. The left 5th intercostal space medial to the midclavicular line is called the mitral area. The left 5th intercostal space close to the sternum is called the tricuspid area. The point of maximal impulse (PMI) is usually found in the left 5th intercostal space and is 2-3/4" to 3-1/2" (7 to 9 cm) lateral to the midsternal line.

9. **Correct answer - A**

S_1 marks the onset of ventricular systole. The first heart sound, S_1 is produced when the mitral and tricuspid valves close. When ventricu

S₁ = M + T closing

S₂ = A + Pulmonic close

lar systole ends, the aortic and pulmonic valves close, producing an S_2 heart sound. S_3 and S_4 are considered abnormal heart sounds in an adult.

10. **Correct answer - D**

Closure of the mitral and tricuspid valves produces an S_1. An S_2 heart sound is heard when the aortic and the pulmonic valves close, marking the end of ventricular systole and the beginning of ventricular diastole. An S_2 may be heard best with the diaphragm of the stethoscope at the base of the heart. *A + P closure* *2nd i. space*

11. **Correct answer - A**

CHF

A fixed split of S_2 is an abnormal heart sound. Asynchronous closure of the aortic and pulmonic valves causes persistent splitting of A_2 and P_2 during inspiration and expiration. When ventricular systole ends, the aortic valve normally closes before the pulmonic valve. During expiration, the interval between the two sounds is small. Because the ear cannot distinguish between them, the two sounds are heard as one. During inspiration, however, intrathoracic pressure decreases and venous return to the right ventricle increases - prolonging right ventricular systole and delaying pulmonic valve closure - so that a physiologic split of S_2 is normal. A third heartsound (S_3) in children is normal and usually disappears when they sit or stand. An S_3 in adults usually indicates a disease, such as congestive heart failure

12. **Correct answer - A**   *S₃ - Vent. gallop*

A third heart sound (S_3) heard in an adult is called a ventricular gallop. Pathologic, it is often the first clinical sign of congestive heart failure. *LEFT* An S_3 occurs during the early, rapid phase of ventricular filling because of an increase in left ventricular diastolic pressure and a noncompliant, stiff ventricle. Pericarditis often causes an extracardiac sound called a pericardial rub. Mitral stenosis produces a diastolic heart murmur, and aortic stenosis, a systolic heart murmur, neither is a heart sound

13. **Correct answer - A**

An S_3 is a low-pitched sound best heard with the bell of the stethoscope placed at the apex of the heart and the patient in the left lateral position. This position brings the ventricle up against the chest wall. Again, an S_3 occurs during the early, rapid phase of ventricular filling, resulting from an increase in volume load or a decrease in left ventricular compliance.

14. **Correct answer - D**

The fourth heart sound (S_4), called an atrial gallop, is caused by vibrations produced in late ventricular diastole, during atrial contraction of blood into a ventricle that resists filling. Like an S_3, it is best heard with the bell of the stethoscope at the apex of the heart with the patient in the left lateral position.

15. **Correct answer - A**

An S_4 is commonly heard in patients with hypertension, aortic stenosis, heart failure, or myocardial infarction. An S_4 may also be heard in a patient during an attack of angina pectoris. Mitral stenosis, aortic insufficiency, and tricuspid stenosis are diastolic murmurs and have no connection with an S_4 heart sound.

16. **Correct answer - B**

The turbulence of abnormal blood flow within the heart produces the sounds of a heart murmur - vibratory sounds of increased duration. Sounds of turbulence are termed murmurs when they emanate from passage of blood across heart valves.

17. **Correct answer - D**

The nurse auscultates the valve areas by listening in the direction of blood flow. The principal areas of cardiac auscultation to determine murmur locations include the mitral valve at the apex (5th left intercostal space), tricuspid valve at the left lower sternal border, pulmonic valve at the base of the heart (2nd left intercostal space), and aortic valve at the base of the heart (2nd right intercostal space).

Insufficiency = backflow = REGURGE

18. **Correct answer - A**

A murmur heard best at the apex may be related to a mitral valve defect. Murmurs of the mitral valve, such as the systolic murmur of mitral insufficiency or the diastolic murmur of mitral stenosis, are loudest at the apex.

19. **Correct answer - C**

Regurgitant blood flow across the mitral and tricuspid valves will cause a systolic murmur. During ventricular systole, the mitral and tricuspid valves should be closed to prevent backflow of blood into the atria. When the mitral and tricuspid valves are closed incompetently during systole, the backflow of blood produces a systolic murmur known as mitral or tricuspid regurgitation or insufficiency.

20. **Correct answer - A**

Heart murmurs result from turbulent blood flow. Clinically, two main factors produce murmurs: stenosis, or high rates of blood flow through a constricted valve, and insufficiency, or backflow of blood through an incompetent valve. Murmurs are described according to position in the cardiac cycle-systolic or diastolic. Mitral insufficiency, tricuspid insufficiency, aortic stenosis, and p u l m o n i c *Syst* stenosis are systolic murmurs produced when the ventricles contract. Mitral stenosis, tricuspid stenosis, pulmonic insufficiency, and aortic *Diast* insufficiency are diastolic murmurs produced when the ventricles are filling.

21. **Correct answer - D**

Mitral insufficiency is a pansystolic (throughout systole) murmur heard loudest at the apex of the heart and often associated with a thrill. It usually occurs as a complication of myocardial ischemia or infarction. When the papillary muscles and chordae tendineae - the structures that support the mitral valve leaflets - are injured, incomplete valvular closure occurs. An incompetent valve allows blood to reflux into the left atrium during ventricular systole, generating turbulence and, thus, the murmur of mitral insufficiency.

22.   **Correct answer - D**

Regurgitant blood flow across the pulmonic and aortic valves will cause a diastolic murmur. During ventricular diastole, the pulmonic and aortic valves close. If they are diseased and cannot close completely, backflow of blood through these valves produces diastolic murmurs of pulmonic and aortic regurgitation or insufficiency.

23.   **Correct answer - C**

The forward flow of blood through stenotic mitral and tricuspid valves during ventricular diastole produces the murmurs of mitral and tricuspid stenosis. These murmurs occur as blood is squeezed from the atria into the ventricles and must pass through a narrow lumen caused by stenotic valves.

24.   **Correct answer - C**

With the patient in the supine position, the phlebostatic axis intersects a line drawn along the 4th intercostal space and a line drawn along the midaxillary line. This reference point was first described to identify the area of the right atrium for measurement of central venous pressure. It is now also used for placement of transducers when measuring pulmonary capillary wedge pressure.

25.   **Correct answer - A**

Readings will be falsely high if the transducer level is lower than the phlebostatic axis during pulmonary artery pressure monitoring. This is caused by the additional pressure, or weight, of the fluid within the catheter and tubing, also known as hydrostatic pressure. When the phlebostatic axis and transducer level are at the same height, effects of hydrostatic pressure are negated. Catheter fling will occur on the waveform when the tip of the balloon flotation catheter is close to the pulmonic valve. The turbulence caused by the valve opening and closing results in a chaotic, spiking waveform known as a catheter fling.

26.   Correct answer - A

The (proximal lumen) of a pulmonary artery catheter is correctly positioned when it is in the right atrium. This lumen is used for fluid administration, blood sampling, and monitoring of right atrial pressure, which is needed to calculate systemic vascular resistance.

See 29. 2nd answer: there is a proximal + a distal lumen!!

27.   Correct answer - B

The pulmonary artery catheter would most likely cause dysrhythmias in the right ventricle The physician should be notified when a right ventricular waveform is identified so that the catheter can be repositioned promptly.

28.   Correct answer - C

Withdrawing the catheter tip from the right ventricle would be the first and simplest intervention to correct a dysrhythmia caused by catheter insertion. If unsuccessful, then defibrillation, cardioversion, or lidocaine administration could be used to terminate the dysrhythmia.

29.   Correct answer - A

Measurement of pulmonary capillary wedge pressure (PCWP) is taken with the balloon inflated. This occludes right ventricular pressures, allowing the catheter to read pulmonary venous pressures, which indirectly measure left ventricular pressures. The balloon is deflated when measuring pulmonary artery pressures or cardiac output and when withdrawing blood to evaluate mixed venous O_2 saturation.

PA pressures must be Read in the PA not the atrium see 26.

30. **Correct answer - B**

Flotation of a pulmonary catheter into the wedge position increases the risk of pulmonary infarction. Although deflated, the catheter still occludes blood flow through the capillary, causing small areas of infarction.

31. **Correct answer - D**

Prolonged inflation of the catheter balloon increases ᵗʰᴱ risk of pulmonary hemorrhage. An inflated balloon presses against fragile capillary vessels and may rupture them if inflated too long. Suspect this if hemoptysis appears in the patient.

32. **Correct answer - C**

A sudden drop in the diastolic pressure during hemodynamic monitoring indicates the catheter has moved back to the right ventricle. Normally, right ventricular and pulmonary artery systolic pressures are equal. However, during diastole, the pulmonic valve closes, separating the right ventricle from the pulmonary artery. Right ventricular diastolic pressure, then, is lower (normally 0 to 5 mm Hg) because it reflects right atrial pressure, a low pressure chamber. Pulmonary artery diastolic pressure is higher (normally 8 to 12 mm Hg) because it reflects left ventricular pressure, a higher pressure chamber.

33. **Correct answer - D**

Normal pulmonary artery systolic pressure is between 20 and 30 mm Hg; normal pulmonary artery diastolic pressure is between 8 and 14 mm Hg; and normal pulmonary capillary wedge pressure is between 8 and 14 mm Hg. Pulmonary artery diastolic and capillary wedge pressures should be similar in the absence of disease.

34. **Correct answer - B**

Pulmonary capillary wedge pressure is the most accurate indicator of changes in left ventricular pressure. In the wedge position, right ventricular pressures are occluded and forward pressures in the

54

pulmonary vasculature are measured. These reflect the heart's left ventricular end-diastolic pressure because an open system exists from the tip of the catheter to the left ventricle as the mitral valve is opened during diastole.

35.   Correct answer - D

A normal wedge pressure, increased pulmonary artery pressures, and signs of right ventricular failure may indicate a pulmonary embolus. Because the pulmonary vasculature is situated between the right and left sides of the heart, respiratory disease would raise right ventricular pressures. Wedge pressure, a reflection of left ventricular pressures, would not be elevated.

36.   Correct answer - A

Pulmonary hypertension would result in an elevated pulmonary artery pressure and a normal wedge pressure. In pulmonary edema and left ventricular failure, both pressures would be elevated. In constrictive pericarditis, the entire heart is compressed, elevating all pressures.

37.   Correct answer - C

An elevated right ventricular pressure and a normal wedge pressure indicate pulmonary hypertension. Increasing dyspnea and swollen feet also suggest right ventricular failure. In congestive heart failure, *Left* the wedge pressure would be high, although right ventricular pressure may not be high initially. In cardiac tamponade, pericardial fluid would elevate all pressures within the heart. Pressures would be low in hypovolemia.

(R) Vent fail : symptoms dyspnea + edema
Pulmhtn : ↑ RV pressure - ↑ PA press.
("Embolic) + normal wedge (PCW)

38.   Correct answer - B

$$CI = \frac{CO}{BSA}$$

Cardiac index is calculated by dividing the cardiac output by the patient's body surface area, measured in meters squared (m^2). Because the index relates cardiac output to body size, it reflects body requirements more accurately than cardiac output does. Normal cardiac index is 2.5 to 3.5 liters/minute/m^2. Body surface area charts

[handwritten at top: PCWP | X PRE LOAD = LV Volume – VENOUS RETURN | AFTER LOAD = PRESSURE + PC wedge P. pressure]

can be found in most cardiac textbooks.

39.   Correct answer - A   *[handwritten: PRELOAD - STRETCH End. V. diastole]*

Preload may be described best as the stretch produced within the myocardium at the end of ventricular diastole. According to Starling's law, the more a myocardial fiber stretches in diastole, the more it contracts in systole. The volume in ventricles after diastole, called the end-diastolic volume, reflects the heart's contractile ability. The back-up of pressure in the systemic circulation, called systemic vascular resistance, refers to afterload. The amount of blood return-ing to the heart, called venous return, is a prime factor affecting preload.

[handwritten: mitral valve (PV + ↓ VENA CAVA) Tri-cuspid]

40.   Correct answer - C

[handwritten: MAP & SVR]

Afterload may be described best as the impedance to ejection of blood from the left ventricle. This is clinically represented by the mean arterial pressure and systemic vascular resistance. The measurement of the left ventricular end-diastolic pressure is the clinical represen-tation of preload and is indirectly determined *[handwritten: monitored]* by the pulmonary capillary wedge pressure. The amount of force of ventricular contraction is called contractility. The amount of blood remaining in the left ventricle after systole is called the left ventricular end-systolic volume, or residual volume.

41.   Correct answer - C

Measurement of systemic vascular resistance best indicates after-load. The higher the pressure in the systemic circulation, the greater the impedance of ejection (afterload). The pulmonary capillary wedge pressure indirectly reflects left ventricular end-diastolic pres-sure, referring to preload. Stroke volume is the amount of blood ejected by the ventricle with each cardiac contraction, referring to contractility. Ejection fraction is the percentage of the left ventricular end-diastolic volume ejected during each cardiac cycle.

56

42. Correct answer -C

Oxygen saturations in the right of the heart reflect deoxygenated blood returning from the body and are usually about 75% saturated. An abnormally high reading, such as that in the example, reflects a left-to-right shunt, with oxygenated blood returning to the right side of the heart. Because this abnormal reading starts in the right ventricle, a ventricular septal defect would be suspected.

43. Correct answer - A

[handwritten: LCA × LAD, ANT WALL, SEPTAL, RBBB → infarction]

The left coronary artery branches into the left anterior descending artery, which supplies the anterior part of the interventricular septum, the anterior wall of the left ventricle, the right bundle branch, and the anterior superior division of the left bundle branch. Thus, occlusion of the left anterior descending artery may result in an anterior wall infarction, a septal infarction, and a right bundle branch block.

44. Correct answer - D

The nurse would anticipate a 12-lead ECG of a patient with an anterior wall MI to show ST elevations in leads V_1 and V_2 with reciprocal ST depressions in leads II, III and a VF.

45. Correct answer - B

[handwritten: ANT WALL infarct = Mobitz II h.b., RBBB b.b.b., Vent aneurysm]

A complication least likely to occur in a patient with an anterior wall MI would be mitral insufficiency - a systolic murmur most likely seen in an inferior wall MI patient. A Mobitz II heart block, right bundle branch block (RBBB), and ventricular aneurysm would most likely develop in the patient with an anterior wall MI.

46. Correct answer - B

Premature ventricular contractions are the most significant dysrhythmias in an acute myocardial infarction. Irritability of the ischemic tissue is caused by intracellular potassium depletion (causing an elevated extracellular potassium level), inability of the ischemic area to repolarize (causing electrical current flows from the ischemic

57

tissue), and sympathetic discharge in response to myocardial damage. Irritability may cause ectopic firing from the ventricular cells, resulting in ventricular tachycardia or ventricular fibrillation, both lethal dysrhythmias.

47. **Correct answer - A** *Prox - senses*
Dist - paces

The pacemaker catheter contains two electrodes: the proximal (which senses the patient's inherent rhythm) and the distal (which paces the myocardium). The output control regulates energy output delivered to the distal electrode, measured in milliamperes. The rate control regulates pacing frequency, measured in beats per minute.

48. **Correct answer - D**

Electromagnetic interference rarely causes hazards with newer permanent pacemakers. (However, in temporary pacemakers, electrocautery may override the sensing mechanisms.) Battery failure, improper catheter position, a faulty sensing mechanism, and a lead wire fracture can result in sensing failure.

49. **Correct answer - B**

If the patient's temporary pacemaker is not sensing, the nurse should first check the sensitivity control, a simple yet often over looked intervention. The dial may have inadvertently been turned to a fixed rate. If this is not the case and the patient's rhythm is adequate, the nurse should turn off the pacemaker temporarily (to prevent ventricular fibrillation from R-on-T phenomenon) and notify the physician. If the patient's rhythm is inadequate, turning up the energy output or positioning the patient on the left side may help. The electrode may have moved, and increasing the voltage may cause capture. If this is unsuccessful, positioning the patient on his left side may help move the catheter back into position. Either intervention is a temporary measure; the nurse must notify the physician to reposition the catheter.

50.   **Correct answer - B**   ↓ K⁺ depresses heart

Hypokalemia necessitates a higher energy output for a temporary pacemaker, presumably because of its depressant effects on the myocardium. Myocardial ischemia or necrosis may cause the same problem. Necrotic tissue does not carry impulses, whereas ischemic tissue's capacity to respond to electrical stimulation is impaired.

51.   **Correct answer - D**

Pacemaker types are written as a three-letter code. The first initial refers to the chamber paced, the second to the sensing chamber, and the third to the mode of response. Thus, a VVI pacemaker is one that has ventricular pacing and sensing and inhibited mode (demand). The following initials are used: V = ventricular, A = atrium, D = double chamber, I = inhibited, T = triggered, and O = not applicable.

52.   **Correct answer - B**

The physical examination is least helpful in diagnosing an acute myocardial infarction (MI). Physical findings - such as gallops, murmurs, crackles, or hypotension - rarely occur during the early stages of an MI and can indicate various diseases. Any two of three factors - history of MI, positive enzyme studies, or positive ECG - confirm the diagnosis.

53.   **Correct answer - A**

The isoenzymes most specific for cardiac muscle damage are CPK-MB and LDH1. The heart is the only organ that contains more than a trace amount of CPK-MB. CPK-MB is undetectable in the absence of myocardial damage (so isoenzyme assays will read 100% CPK-MB), but levels can reach 15% if myocardial necrosis occurs. LDH1 is released during myocardial damage but also is found in other organs - such as the kidneys and stomach - and in erythrocytes. Although not as organ-specific as CPK-MB, LDH1 has a delayed peak, so its measurement is useful in patients presenting to the emergency room more than 48 hours after onset of symptoms.

54. **Correct answer - C**

A report of LDH_1 greater than LDH_2 indicates myocardial damage. Normally, LDH_2 is greater than LDH_1. If an LDH_1 rich organ other than the heart is damaged, LDH_2 usually rises. Damage to the heart or erythrocytes would not cause a rise in LDH_2. Therefore, to prevent erythrocyte damage, one should not hemolyze an LDH isoenzyme specimen.

[handwritten: ONSET PEAK LDH - 12-24 hrs 72 hrs 3 DAYS]

55. **Correct answer - C** *[handwritten: CPK - 4-6 hrs 12-20 — 1 → 1 day]*

LDH returns to normal 7 to 10 days after an infarction. The onset of LDH elevation occurs 12 to 24 hours after tissue damage and peaks at 72 hours. CPK begins to rise 4 to 6 hours after infarction, with a peak by 12 to 20 hours, and usually returns to normal by the 2nd or 3rd day. SGOT starts to increase in about 6 to 8 hours, peaks in 18 to 36 hours, and tapers off about the 4th to 6th day. SGPT is more specific for liver disease but may rise if the myocar-dial damage is accompanied by shock or severe congestive heart failure that results in liver congestion or damage.

56. **Correct answer - D**

An inferior wall MI will show indicative changes in leads II, III and aVF because these leads look at the inferior wall. Changes in leads V_1 to V_4 indicate an anterior-septal infarction because these leads look at the front of the heart, most specifically the septum. Changes in V_1, a VL, V_5 and V_6 indicate a lateral wall infarction because these leads look at the heart from the lateral side of the left ventricle.

[handwritten: 80% RCA → inferior + SA node dominant Posterior AV node R vent.]

57. **Correct answer - B**

[handwritten left margin: L CIRC. LV lateral in all]

Occlusion of the right coronary artery will most likely result in an inferior wall MI. About 80% of the population has right dominant circulation (the right coronary artery supplies the inferior and posterior walls of the heart, the sinoatrial and atrioventricular nodes, and the right ventricle). The remaining 20% has left dominant circulation (the left circumflex supplies the inferior and posterior walls). The circumflex artery supplies the lateral wall of the left ventricle in all persons. The circumflex is one branch of the left main coronary

[handwritten: 20% LCA Circumflex dominant]

LCA ⟨ L cir.
         ⟨ LAD

artery; the other branch is the left anterior descending artery, which
supplies the anterior wall of the left ventricle and the septum.

58.   Correct answer - B

The interpretation of this strip is atrial fibrillation. The criteria for
this dysrhythmia are absence of P waves and irregular QRS complexes. The strip does not reflect junctional or supraventricular
tachycardia because these dysrhythmias have regular QRS complexes. This dysrhythmia is not atrial flutter because no flutter waves
appear on the strip.

59.   Correct answer - D

The hemodynamic consequences of atrial fibrillation may be severe.
Cardiac output is significantly compromised by the rapid ventricular
response and by the loss of a synchronized atrial beat, or atrial kick.
Cardiac output can decrease by as much as 30% when atrial fibrillation occurs in a patient with significant heart disease.

① Dysrhythmias   ③ Shock
60.   Correct answer - A ② CHF   ④

Dysrhythmias are the most common complication of an acute MI.
Nearly all patients with acute MI experience transient rhythm alterations. Congestive heart failure is the next most common complication, usually occurring if the heart's pumping performance is impaired. Cardiogenic shock, the most serious complication, occurs in
about 15% of patients hospitalized with an acute infarction. Pulmonary embolism results from formation of mural thrombi on a
hypokinetic myocardium or as a result of bed rest (from peripheral
thrombus). It may be a more frequent complication than previously
thought because it can go clinically undetected, and its signs and
symptoms mimic those of the MI.

61.   Correct answer - A

The nurse could expect the patient with an inferior wall MI to develop
sinus bradycardia, sick sinus syndrome, or idioventricular rhythm.
These result from ischemia to the sinus and atrioventricular nodes, as
the right coronary artery supplies these structures and the inferior wall

61

of the left ventricle. Mobitz II heart block would most likely result as a complication in the patient with an anterior wall MI.

62.   **Correct answer - D**

Hepatosplenomegaly would reflect right ventricular failure. Other clinical signs include dependent pitting edema, jugular venous distention greater than 3 cm above the sternal angle, and elevated central venous pressure readings. A pulmonary capillary wedge pressure (PCWP) above 25 mm Hg and bilateral moist crackles reflect left ventricular failure.

63.   **Correct answer - D**

Examination of the jugular veins and their pulsations allows an accurate estimation of central venous pressure and therefore gives important information about cardiac compensation. The internal jugular pulsations provide a more accurate reading than external jugular pulsations. When examining for jugular venous pressure, the nurse should elevate the head of the bed 30 degrees. When the patient is in a horizontal position, jugular venous pulsations should be present; if they are absent, blood volume depletion may be suspected.

64.   **Correct answer - C**

A hepatojugular reflux is elicited by exerting firm and sustained pressure with your hand over the patient's right upper quadrant for 30 to 60 seconds. Watch for increased jugular venous pressure during this maneuver. A rise of more than 1 cm is abnormal (a positive hepatojugular reflux) and suggests congestive heart failure.

65.   **Correct answer - A**

Pulmonary hypertension results in an enlarged right ventricle, which may progress to right ventricular failure. Cardiomyopathy, aortic stenosis, and acute myocardial infarction would predispose a patient to left ventricular failure.

66.   Correct answer - A

A diseased left ventricle cannot pump blood returning from the lungs into systemic circulation; this decreases cardiac output, and the patient's heart rate increases to compensate. An S_3 may appear, indicating heart failure. Lung pressure increases because of blood accumulation, and crackles may be auscultated. Increased central venous pressure (CVP) is a late sign of left ventricular failure. As lung pressure continues to increase, producing pulmonary edema, increases in right ventricular pressure produce an elevated CVP.

67.   Correct answer - A

Clinical presentation of a patient with left ventricular failure would include nocturnal dyspnea, along with other signs and symptoms, such as tachycardia, diaphoresis, crackles, pallor, gallop rhythm, and elevated pulmonary artery diastolic and pulmonary capillary wedge pressure (PCWP). Bounding pulses, hepatosplenomegaly, and pitting edema would be present in the patient with right ventricular failure.

68.   Correct answer - D

A pulmonary artery pressure (PAP) of 48/26, a PCWP of 20 would reflect an increase in left ventricular end-diastolic pressure (LVEDP), such as in left ventricular failure.

69.   Correct answer C

The postoperative cardiac patient with acute pericarditis is least likely to develop cardiogenic shock. Cardiogenic shock is a vicious cycle that involves loss of myocardial contractility; resultant hemodynamic and metabolic reflex mechanisms cause further ischemia and the deterioration of contractility. Acute pericarditis, an inflammation of the pericardium, has a self-limiting, short-term clinical course when related to an acute myocardial infarction or cardiac surgery. The cause is not irritation but an autoimmune response lasting 2 to 6 weeks. Pericardial effusion usually does not develop. Pain, the most characteristic symptom of acute pericarditis, usually can be alleviated by leaning forward. A pericardial friction rub is the most important physical finding. Most commonly, cardiogenic shock occurs as a complication of a myocardial infarction, especially when at least 40% of the left ventricle is necrotic and ischemic. When the heart's ability to pump blood declines, the risk of cardiogenic shock increases. This occurs in conditions that produce deficient cardiac filling, such as cardiac tamponade and dysrhythmias in a compromised patient.

70.   Correct answer - A

In cardiogenic shock, the sympathetic nervous system is activated physiologically to compensate for the failing heart. Catecholamines, such as epinephrine, increase heart rate and force of contraction in an attempt to maintain cardiac output and blood pressure. These mechanisms are doomed to fail because they increase the workload of the heart, which cannot take the added stress.

71.   Correct answer - D

The clinical manifestations of cardiogenic shock result from the heart's impaired contractility, which decreases cardiac output and elevates left ventricular end-diastolic pressure (LVEDP). The reduced cardiac output impairs perfusion to the vital organs and peripheral tissues. Thus, the patient exhibits changes in sensorium, such as restlessness, anxiety, or confusion. The skin is cold and clammy from peripheral vasoconstriction. As the cardiac output declines, the pulse pressure narrows; peripheral pulses are rapid and thready. Systemic arterial pressure drops, and hypotension ensues. Urine output decreases as kidney perfusion declines. A rise in the LVEDP increases left atrial and pulmonary pressures, resulting in pulmonary congestion. Tachypnea, dyspnea, and pulmonary edema develop; an S_3 can be heard as the left ventricle fails and becomes overdistended during diastole. Increased pressures on the left side of the heart progress back through the pulmonary venous system into the right side of the heart. This increase in pulmonary pressure decreases the right ventricular performance and may result in right ventricular failure, which in turn produces an elevated CVP and jugular vein distention with hepatomegaly.

72.   Correct answer - A

An early assessment finding that may indicate cardiogenic shock in the patient with an acute MI is an S_3 heart sound. The patient with an acute MI is at high risk of developing cardiogenic shock because of a decrease in the contractile function of the left ventricle. Thus, early recognition of signs and symptoms of left ventricular failure is vital. Initially, the failing ventricle causes decreased cardiac output. The body compensates by increasing sympathetic stimulation to increase the heart rate and to shunt blood to vital organs via peripheral vasoconstriction. The skin is cool and clammy. Tachycardia and an increased afterload from vasoconstriction increase the cardiac work load and oxygen consumption. Decreased ventricular emptying during systole occurs, preload increases, and an S_3 may be heard. Pulmonary congestion then follows from the backward transmission of left ventricular pressure, resulting in dyspnea, orthopnea, and bilateral crackles. As left ventricular failure progresses, pulmonary congestion increases and cardiogenic shock ensues.

73.   Correct answer - A

One of the earliest signs of cardiogenic shock is tachycardia, as the sympathetic nervous system discharges to compensate for the cardiac insult. Cyanosis is a relatively late sign of shock and rather undependable. A fluffy-white chest X-ray and hypotension occur as the compensatory mechanisms fail to maintain cardiac output.

74.   Correct answer - D

Vasodilator therapy relaxes the systemic vessels, producing venous pooling of blood and decreasing venous return. Less blood enters the right side of the heart, resulting in decreased right atrial, ventricular, and pulmonary artery pressures. At the same time, lower pressure in the systemic circulation further reduces cardiac work load by decreasing the peripheral vascular resistance against which the left ventricle must eject its blood. Afterload - as measured by aortic systolic pressure - declines, and cardiac output increases.

Afterload is - pressure

65

75. Correct answer - A

Decreased pulmonary capillary wedge pressure (PCWP) indicates that the vasodilator is having a positive effect. Reduced left ventricular end diastolic pressure, as evidenced by decreased PCWP, results from increased cardiac output and decreased venous return to the heart. ① volume out ↑   ② volume in ↓

76. Correct answer - B

The beneficial effect of vasodilator therapy in managing cardiogenic shock is decreased preload and afterload. Vasodilator therapy reduces venous tone and increases venous capacitance. This decreases blood return to the heart, thereby lowering the LVEDP. Vasodilator therapy also reduces arterial vascular tone, which results in decreased impedance to left ventricular ejection (afterload); cardiac work load decreases, and cardiac output increases.

77. Correct answer - D

Effective vasodilator therapy improves cardiac output. Increased urine output reflects a generalized improvement in blood flow to the tissues, including the kidneys, and a reversal of the shock syndrome.

78. Correct answer - B

Inotropic agents improve tissue perfusion in the patient with cardiogenic shock. They increase the force of myocardial contraction; cardiac output increases because of enhanced contractility. Dopamine (Inotropin) is a sympathomimetic drug that has inotropic properties. Its vasopressor effects increase coronary blood flow, thereby improving tissue perfusion. The chronotropic effects of dopamine increase heart rate. This potential adverse effect limits its use because tachycardia increases myocardial oxygen consumption.

79. Correct answer - B

Nitroprusside has a balanced vasodilating effect on both arteries and veins, so it effectively decreases afterload and preload. Dopamine, dobutamine, and digoxin are primarily positive inotropic agents; that is, their main effect is to increase the heart's contractility.

80.   **Correct answer - B** n + L – vAsodilAToRs

Lasix has an initial immediate vasodilatory effect, causing venous pooling, decreasing pulmonary venous congestion, and decreasing pulmonary capillary wedge pressure. Lasix also has a later diuretic effect, reflected in an increase in urine output. Breath sounds and chest X-rays may take hours to improve.

81.   **Correct answer - A**

Inotropic agents increase the force of myocardial contraction, thereby improving tissue perfusion. A chronotropic agent increases heart rate.

82.   **Correct answer - C**

The goals of therapy for the patient in cardiogenic shock are to improve myocardial contractility, increase cardiac output, and reduce the myocardial demand for oxygen. Improvement of cardiovascular function is primarily managed by pharmacologic therapies. Nitroprusside (Nipride) and nitroglycerin (Tridil) are commonly used to decrease both preload (ventricular end-diastolic pressure) and afterload (vascular resistance). These vasodilators reduce blood return to the heart and decrease systemic peripheral vascular resistance. Cardiac output is further enhanced by a decrease in cardiac work load and oxygen demand and by complete emptying of the ventricles during systole. Vasodilator therapy is used with sympatho-mimetic drugs, such as dopamine (Inotropin) and dobutamine (Dobutrex). These vasopressors have an inotropic effect that enhances myocardial contractility and cardiac output.

83.   **Correct answer - C**

The intra-aortic balloon pump (IABP) increases coronary artery perfusion. When the balloon is inflated, it occludes about 80% of the thoracic aorta, thereby displacing the blood up toward the coronary arteries. Because the heart muscle derives its blood supply during diastole, balloon inflation provides more blood to the myocardium during diastole, thus increasing coronary artery perfusion.

84.   Correct answer - B

The therapeutic effect of the IABP is to increase cardiac output, decrease myocardial O_2 consumption, increase aortic pressure, and decrease cardiac afterload. The IABP, when deflated during systole, displaces blood volume in the aorta, which lowers aortic end-diastolic pressure and resistance to left ventricular ejection, decreasing after-load. Displacement of the blood volume allows more efficient pumping of the left ventricle, increases cardiac output, and decreases myocardial O_2 consumption. This preserves the already compromised myocardium.

85.   Correct answer - C

It would be inappropriate to elevate the head of the bed 45 to 60 degrees, as this may increase flexion of the hip - thereby occluding or kinking the IABP catheter at the insertion into the femoral artery. The head of the bed must be elevated no higher than 45 degrees. Performing passive range-of-motion (ROM) exercises, monitoring pulses, and administering antipyretics for a temperature above $101°$F. are appropriate actions. Remember to use salicylates with caution because the patient is anticoagulated while on the IABP.

86.   Correct answer - A

The intra-aortic balloon pump is deflated during systole and creates a potentially empty space to accommodate, without resistance, the stroke volume. This decreases impedance to left ventricular ejection (afterload) and decreases left ventricular work load.

87.   Correct answer - B

IAPB therapy is contraindicated in a patient with an incompetent aortic valve because balloon inflation would increase aortic regurgitation. Papillary muscle rupture causes mitral valve incompetence. Decreasing afterload through the use of IABP may save the patient's life until surgical repair of the mitral valve occurs. In left ventricular failure after bypass, IABP therapy provides circulatory assistance until recovery occurs. This method has significantly reduced postoperative mortality. IAPB therapy is also indicated for unstable angina refractory to the medical regimen. Increased coronary artery perfusion stops the angina promptly, increasing the ejection fraction and thereby stabilizing the patient.

88. Correct answer - B

Clinical presentation in the patient experiencing angina pectoris is precordial, middle, or lower sternal pain that may radiate to the shoulders, arms, neck, and jaw. The pain is usually described as burning, squeezing or heavy, not sharp or shooting. Characteristically, the pain begins on exertion, usually lasts 1 to 4 minutes, and subsides when precipitating factors are removed.

89. Correct answer - B

Nitroglycerin usually relieves the pain of angina pectoris within 45 to 90 seconds. If not, angina may have progressed to the unstable state or an infarction may be occurring.

Mental Humor Break

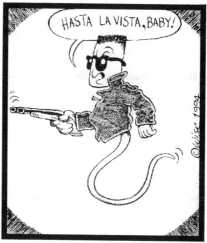

THE SPERMINATOR

90. **Correct answer - A**

The precipitating factors for angina pectoris are physical activity (not necessarily strenuous), emotional excitement, smoking, or heavy meals. Nocturnal angina (pain when the patient is in a recumbent position) may also be a precipitating factor.

91. **Correct answer - A**

ST depression indicates myocardial ischemia. Injury to the myocardium is evidenced electrocardiographically by an ST elevation. Myocardial necrosis is evidenced by a Q wave greater in width than 0.04 mm in two or more leads. Pericarditis presents with elevated ST segments throughout the chest leads.

92. **Correct answer - D**

The pathologic changes found on an ECG that indicate myocardial ischemia are ST segment depression and T wave inversion. ST elevation indicates injury, except in pericarditis. ST segment depression and T wave elevation in V_1 and V_2 may indicate posterior wall injury because of the mirror image one obtains when looking for posterior wall damage. Q wave formation is diagnostic of myocardial damage.

93. **Correct answer - B**

Although an S_4 results from an increase in left ventricular filling volume and is often heard in patients with congestive heart failure and aortic stenosis, an S_4 during an anginal episode signifies decreased compliance of the ischemic zone.

94. **Correct answer - A**

Prinzmetal's angina, also called atypical angina, is characterized electrocardiographically by ST elevation during the episode. Pain is unrelated to exertion and usually occurs at rest.

95. Correct answer - D

About 5% to 10% of angina pectoris cases result from coronary artery spasm. This syndrome, termed Prinzmetal's (variant) angina, is characterized by anginal pain at rest with associated ST segment elevation. Treatment consists of calcium channel-blocking agents. Surgical intervention for coronary artery spasm is not indicated, especially since the decrease in blood supply is due to spasms rather than atherosclerosis.

96. Correct answer - A

In assessing a patient with cardiac tamponade, the nurse would observe a narrowed pulse pressure. When fluid accumulates in the pericardium, the heart cannot fill completely during diastole. As a result, diastolic pressure rises, and the patient has elevated left (PCWP) and right (CVP) ventricular pressures. The pulse increases to maintain cardiac output.

97. Correct answer - D

Pulse pressure narrows because of the rise in diastolic filling pressure. An elevated CVP and pulsus paradoxus are common symptoms of tamponade. Heart sounds may be distant because they can be muffled by pericardial fluid.

inspiration ↓ venous return
↓ ↓ SV

98. Correct answer - C

Pulsus paradoxus can be defined as the absence of a pulse or no auscultation of Korotkoff sounds for more than 10 mm Hg in arterial systolic pressure during inspiration. A drop in pressure of less than 10 mm Hg is a normal response to inspiration. Inspiratory effort causes a rise in intrathoracic pressure, which compresses the great vessels to the heart and diminishes venous return to the heart. Also, inspiration causes pulmonary venous pooling, which further decreases blood return to the left side of the heart and, as a result, decreases stroke volume during inspiration.

99.   Correct answer - A

Pulsus paradoxus is not seen in patent ductus arteriosus but may be seen in severe pulmonary emphysema, cardiac tamponade, pericardial effusions, and hypovolemic shock.

100.   Correct answer - C

Heart block is not a complication of pericardiocentesis. Ventricular perforation can occur if the needle is advanced too far and ventricular fibrillation can result if the needle contacts the myocardium. Pneumothorax can occur if the needle is accidentally introduced into the pleural space.

101.   Correct answer - B

A precordial (V lead) ECG lead should be attached to the hub of the intracardiac needle. During pericardiocentesis, the ECG should be recording in the V lead. If the needle contacts the myocardium, an ST elevation will be recorded. During the procedure, a high Fowler's position will provide maximum comfort for the awake patient. Isoproterenol and Valsalva's maneuver are not indicated in the treatment of pericardial tamponade.

102.   Correct answer - C

Vectorcardiography is a form of electrocardiography that measures the direction and magnitude of electrical forces. It is more diagnostic than a normal ECG, especially for bundle branch blocks, fascicular blocks, and myocardial infarction. A His bundle ECG involves passing an electrode catheter into the right side of the heart and positioning it near the tricuspid valve. The catheter specifies the site of a conduction delay, such as the atrioventricular node, His bundle, or bundle branch. Ventriculography is a radiographic test that uses a contrast medium to evaluate ventricular function. Aortography is an arteriogram of the aorta used to diagnose aortic aneurysms, coarctation of the aorta, or aortic valve incompetency.

103. **Correct answer - D**

Technetium phosphate imaging specifies the area of myocardial damage; technetium phosphate accumulates in the area of damage, showing a hot spot. Thallium scintiography uses cold spot imaging to reveal perfusion defects. Coronary arteriography determines coronary artery blockage. A gated pool study, which uses a radionuclide dye, helps evaluate ventricular ejection fraction.

104. **Correct answer - C**

The patient with multiple areas of obstruction in a single vessel is the least appropriate candidate for angioplasty; less than 10% of patients with coronary artery disease are candidates for the procedure. To maximize success, patients with diffuse cardiac disease are not recommended for angioplasty. An ejection fraction of 50% shows good cardiac function and makes the patient a good candidate for bypass grafting, a possible complication of angioplasty.

105. **Correct answer - A**

Coronary artery bypass grafting (CABG) is most commonly recommended for patients with unstable, preinfarction, or chronic disabling angina pectoris unresponsive to medical therapy; a hemodynamically significant lesion of the left main coronary artery; three-vessel coronary artery disease; and continuing angina pectoris after myocardial infarction. Controversy persists about operating on a patient with a new transmural myocardial infarction. Experience has shown that, for a large transmural infarction, surgery is safer after the infarction heals.

106. **Correct answer - D**

Poor left ventricular function, a recent myocardial infarction, and distal coronary artery disease are contraindications for CABG. A history of an old MI is not a contraindication for this surgery.

107. Correct answer - C

An ejection fraction of 10% in the absence of angina is a contraindication to CABG because the patient has diminished myocardial function preoperatively and would have a poor prognosis. If angina is present, the ejection fraction may be low because of hypoperfusion to the myocardium. The ejection fraction may improve when the pain is relieved.

108. Correct answer - C

Numbness of the donor leg would be least likely to occur postoperatively in the patient who has undergone CABG. Complications would include graft occlusion, perioperative infarction (which occurs in 2% to 4% of patients postoperatively), and progression of the atherosclerotic process, because saphenous vein grafts are prone to atheromatous changes.

109. Correct answer - A

Physiologic effects of cardiopulmonary bypass include hemodilution, clotting abnormalities, and fluid shifts. Proteinuria may occur as a result of cardiopulmonary bypass. Decreased serum protein levels foster third-space fluid shifting into the interstitial spaces. Clotting abnormalities occur because the bypass machine is traumatic to the blood cells, especially the platelets. During the operation, platelet numbers drop to 40% to 50% of the preoperative level.

110. Correct answer - B

Postoperatively, the nurse should be alert for heparin rebound. The blood must be fully heparinized during extracorporeal circulation. Hypothermia, which develops during surgery, alters heparin metabolism. When the patient has been weaned off cardiopulmonary bypass, the heparin is reversed by the slow intravenous administration of protamine sulfate. Heparin reversal can cause patient complications, including heparin rebound. It is thought that heparin can return to the circulation postoperatively because the heparin and protamine are metabolized at different rates.

111. Correct answer - B

A temporary pacemaker is inserted during CABG to optimize cardiac output through manipulation of the heart rate. Since heart rate x stroke volume equals cardiac output, increasing the heart rate will optimize cardiac output of the hypodynamic post-operative left ventricle.

112. Correct answer - B

All postoperative cardiac patients develop pericarditis because of the pericardiotomy, which causes inflammation. Confusion, hypokalemia, and atelectasis may also result from surgery, but these can be prevented with careful treatment.

113. Correct answer - C

Pericardial pain is typically relieved by encouraging the patient to sit up and lean forward. The pain is usually aggravated by deep inspiration and relieved by anti-inflammatory agents rather than nitroglycerin. These three hallmarks differentiate pericardial pain from the pain of acute myocardial infarction (MI).

114. Correct answer - D

ST elevations in two or three of the standard leads and some or all of the precordial leads are characteristic changes in the ECG of a patient with pericarditis. This occurs early in the course, followed by ST segments returning to baseline and T wave flattening, then inversion, in all leads except aVR. The absence of Q waves, the loss of R wave voltage in V leads, and a general distribution of ST segment changes help to differentiate pericarditis from an acute MI.

115. Correct answer - D

Open-chest cardiac massage must be carried out in CPR for the post-operative cardiac surgery patient. Effective massage consists of compressing the heart between the sternum and spinal cord, increasing intrathoracic pressure. During cardiac surgery, the sternum is

75

broken to gain access to the mediastinum. Therefore, postoperatively, the sternum is not intact and would not provide effective chest compressions.

116. Correct answer - D

Shock is a syndrome characterized by impaired cellular metabolism from decreased blood flow - a state of inadequate tissue perfusion. The major pathophysiologic problem occurs in the microcirculation at the capillary level. Inadequate tissue perfusion and decreased oxygen delivery result in a constellation of physiologic responses. As shock develops, a fall in cardiac output triggers compensatory mechanisms as pressoreceptors are stimulated to cause vasoconstriction. The net effect is an increase in mean arterial pressure and a restriction of peripheral blood flow. The available circulating volume is shunted to perfuse vital organs. As peripheral vasoconstriction progresses, a marked reduction in oxygen delivery to the cells forces a switch from aerobic to anaerobic metabolism. Increased lactic acid is produced resulting in respiratory compensation; body-acid load is reduced by blowing off carbon dioxide. As a shock state continues, respiratory compensation fails and the progressive decline in pH from excessive lactate levels ensues. Metabolic acidosis causes impaired cellular function and impaired capillary permeability. Intravascular volume is further decreased as blood flows into capillary beds. The patient is now in the progressive state of shock as compensatory mechanisms fail to maintain an adequate cardiac output.

117. Correct answer - C

Initial management of a patient in shock involves provisions for airway and ventilation; maintenance of blood volume, pressure, and circulation; and maintenance of cellular oxygen consumption. Specific measures include oxygen therapy and administration of intravenous fluid, preferably lactated Ringer's solution via a large-bore I.V. line. Medical antishock trousers (MAST) can also be used in patients with leg or abdominal injuries who have signs and symptoms of hypovolemic shock. This will autotransfuse about 1,000 ml of blood, reduce blood loss by application of direct pressure, and immobilize leg injuries. The patient in shock should be flat, with only the legs elevated. The Trendelenburg position, once favored in managing shock, has been abandoned because it allows the diaphragm to migrate upward, thus compromising ventilation. Also, this position may cause a reflex inhibition of the pressoreceptor activity, thereby decreasing sympathetic stimulation and further compromising arterial blood pressure.

hypovolemia + Hgb loss of Bld

118. Correct answer - A

T Hgb "plasma

Pulsus paradoxus may be present in patients with hypovolemic shock. Its cardinal sign is an abnormal fall (greater than 10 mm Hg) in systolic blood pressure during inspiration. The systolic sound disappears during inspiration because of pulmonary vascular pooling caused by increased lung expansion and increased intrathoracic negative pressure. When intravascular depletion is present, as in hypovolemic shock, the fall of systolic block pressure during inspiration is exaggerated when venous return to the heart is compromised. The patient may also present with a narrowing pulse pressure, which indicates a fall in cardiac output, and a cardiovascular pressure (CVP) reading below 4, which indicates intravascular depletion. Any single hematocrit or hemoglobin value is an unreliable indicator of the patient's condition. Either an increase or decrease in hemoglobin values may signal hypovolemia; dropping values suggest whole blood loss, whereas rising values suggest loss of plasma. Acute blood loss may cause a significant drop in hemoglobin over 1 to 2 hours; however, in older patients, acute blood loss may not cause a significant drop for at least 12 hours.

119. Correct answer - C

Tilt Test - BP + HR Δ's
Pulse Pressure con = Striki Vol.

Patient assessment data suggesting hypovolemia as the cause of shock include an abnormal tilt test. This assessment tool indicates circulating blood volume loss by measuring blood pressure and pulse rate changes during patient position changes. Abnormal tilt test findings include improved blood pressure when the patient's legs are raised above heart level, or a 10 mm Hg or greater drop in systolic blood pressure between supine and sitting positions. Pulse pressure is a far better indicator of early shock than is blood pressure. Pulse pressure is related to cardiac stroke volume; thus, changes provide a good indication of blood flow. During the early stages of shock, the systolic pressure usually drops faster than the diastolic pressure, thereby narrowing or decreasing the pulse pressure. The hypovolemic patient will have flat neck veins when supine, a low CVP, decreased urine sodium level, and a high urine specific gravity. An S_3 is heard when left ventricular end-diastolic pressure (LVEDP) increases - as found in congestive heart failure (CHF) or cardiogenic shock. Tachycardia occurs in all forms of shock, as the heart attempts to increase cardiac output.

120.   **Correct answer - D**

An indication of shock is a drop in systolic blood pressure below 80 mm Hg. When the compensatory mechanism of vasoconstriction fails to maintain blood pressure, the decompensatory stage sets in and reflects a systolic pressure below 80 mm Hg.

121.   **Correct answer - A**

Metabolic acidosis, or lactic acidosis, is the most common result of shock. The fall in cardiac output causes poor delivery of oxygen to the tissues. Because oxygen is necessary for cellular metabolism, the cells attempt to get energy by the anaerobic process of glycolysis, which produces tremendous amounts of lactic acid. Removal of carbon dioxide from the tissues also is impaired; tissue carbon dioxide levels then rise and react with water in the cells to produce carbonic acid.

122.   **Correct answer - B**

Hemodynamic measurements obtained by pulmonary arterial catheters provide valuable information. Fluid replacement is monitored best by the pulmonary capillary wedge pressure (PCWP). If PCWP is low, the patient needs fluids. The systemic vascular resistance provides information for vasodilator or vasoconstrictor therapy. Pulmonary artery pressure approximates venous pressure within the lungs and may increase in pulmonary hypertension or hypoxia, regardless of the patient's fluid status.

123. Correct answer - B

Hypocalcemia is a potential problem during massive transfusions because citrate preservatives may bind ionized calcium. In fact, alkalosis may also develop after multiple transfusions, as sodium citrate is converted to sodium bicarbonate. Patients who have these electrolyte and acid-base imbalances may demonstrate Chvostek's sign, a facial twitching that occurs when the side of the face is tapped. Brudzinski's sign indicates meningeal irritation; both the upper legs at the hips and the lower legs at the knees are flexed in response to the path of flexion of the head and the neck on the chest. Babinski's sign, which is the dorsiflexion of the big toe upon scratching the bottom of the foot, indicates upper motor neuron dysfunction. Cullen's sign, ecchymosis around the umbilicus, usually is seen in hemorrhagic pancreatitis.

124. Correct answer - B

A subendocardial myocardial infarction (MI), typically a result of decreased perfusion from coronary artery spasm or hypotension, is not an indication for thrombolytic therapy. Subendocardial MIs usually do not occur with thrombotic occlusions. Indications for thrombolytic therapy include a transmural MI, an occluded arterio-venous fistula, pulmonary embolus, and peripheral arterial and venous occlusions.

125. Correct answer - B

Streptokinase is a nonenzymatic protein thrombolytic agent excreted by group C beta-hemolytic streptococci. Thrombolytic therapy is effective in treating massive pulmonary emboli, extensive deep vein thrombosis, and lysis of a thrombus-occluded arteriovenous cannula. Substantial evidence supports the use of streptokinase in treating acute MI in its early stages. Heparin and warfarin are anticoagulant agents. Thrombokinase does not exist.

126. Correct answer - C

Streptokinase is contraindicated in the patient with a recent cardiovascular accident (CVA), active GI bleeding, coagulation disorder, cardiac trauma or massage, intracranial neoplasm, severe hypertension, mitral valve disease with atrial fibrillation, subacute bacterial endocarditis, or acute or chronic renal or hepatic failure: streptokinase is also contraindicated in the patient who has undergone surgery within the past 10 days (including paracentesis, thoracentesis, and invasive biopsy). To avoid complications, a thorough assessment - including a detailed history, a physical examination, and laboratory studies - should be obtained before starting therapy. Anticoagulant or antiplatelet agents should not be given concurrently. Prothrombin time, partial thromboplastin time, thrombin time, and total platelet count should be measured before and during streptokinase.

127. Correct answer - C

Thrombolytic therapy should be discontinued immediately if the patient develops dyspnea, which may indicate a severe allergic reaction. Adverse reactions to streptokinase therapy include hemorrhagic complications with bleeding at I.V. sites, incision sites, and wounds. These can be treated with pressure and discontinuation of therapy. In severe hemorrhage, fresh frozen plasma can be administered and aminocaproic acid (Amicar) may be needed. Allergic reactions include urticaria, pruritus, headache, musculoskeletal pain, bronchospasm, edema, hypertension, and fever. Febrile reactions and mild allergic symptoms can be treated with acetaminophen, antihistamines, and steroids. Severe allergic reactions warrant discontinuation of the infusion. Rare adverse effects include delirium and tachycardia.

128. Correct answer - A

The nurse administering tissue plasminogen activator (t-PA) therapy must monitor the patient for myocardial reperfusion because t-PA opens closed coronary arteries about 70% of the time. Bleeding complications may occur because t-PA causes fibrin clot dissolution and coronary reocclusion. Peripheral thrombosis is not associated with t-PA therapy.

129. Correct answer - B

Before initiating t-PA therapy, the nurse must establish a minimum of two intravenous infusions: the t-PA infusion, and a continuous heparin infusion initiated during the first hour of t-PA therapy.

130. Correct answer - B

The total dose of t-PA, as approved by the Food and Drug Administration (FDA), is 100 mg. This dose is infused over 3 hours as follows: 60 mg over the first hour, with 6 to 10 mg given as an I.V. bolus over 1 to 2 minutes; 20 mg over the second hour; and 20 mg over the third hour.

131. Correct answer - A

Findings that indicate reperfusion during t-PA infusion include dramatic reduction in chest pain, resolution of ST segment elevation, and reperfusion dysrhythmias. These dysrhythmias include sinus bradycardia, accelerated idioventricular rhythm, ventricular tachycardia, heart block, and ventricular fibrillation.

132. Correct answer - A

Myocarditis is not a complication of an acute myocardial infarction. Myocarditis is an inflammatory disease of the myocardium and may be viral, protozoal (Chagas disease), or immunologic. Dressler's syndrome, a postinfarction pericarditis occurring in 2% to 5% of patients 1 to 4 weeks post-MI, is characterized by fever and pericardial effusion. Ventricular aneurysm and papillary muscle rupture are consequences of extensive left ventricular damage.

133. Correct answer - A

Ventricular tachycardia without a pulse should be treated similarly to ventricular fibrillation - by immediate unsynchronized defibrillation at 200 joules for the first attempt, 300 joules for the second, and 360 joules for the third. A precordial thump should be given for pulseless ventricular tachycardia only when a defibrillator is unavailable: although this maneuver may occasionally convert ventricular tachycardia to sinus rhythm, it is equally likely to convert the tachycardia to ventricular fibrillation.

134. Correct answer - C

Because the half-life of lidocaine's distribution phase is 8 minutes, the recommendation is to provide a second bolus after 10 minutes. This prevents a rapid decline of the plasma level and avoids toxic effects from rapid administration. However, for terminating dysrhythmias - rather than for prophylactic use - it may be necessary to give a second bolus 1 to 2 minutes after the first.

135. Correct answer - A

√ Lidocaine 50% when Liver junction impaired

Lidocaine is metabolized through the liver. Congestive heart failure, shock, and hepatic disease impair liver function. Thus, lidocaine dosages should be decreased by 50% in these disorders. Confusion is a toxic effect of lidocaine; its appearance should cause termination of the drug.

136. Correct answer - D

If the patient has a pulse but is hemodynamically unstable, immediate cardioversion with 100 to 200 joules must take precedence over antidysrhythmic therapy.

137. Correct answer - B

When a patient is in ventricular fibrillation and three defibrillation attempts have been made at 200, 300 and 360 joules, epinephrine 1 mg should be administered intravenously or via endotracheal tube.

138. Correct answer - B

If sinus bradycardia is evident on the monitor but no pulse is present, the patient is in pulseless electrical activity (PEA). The first priority is to resume CPR. Epinephrine 1 mg should be the first medication given, either intravenously or by endotracheal tube. This amount should be repeated at least every 5 minutes.

139. **Correct answer - C**

The PR interval measures atrioventricular conduction time. Representing passage of the electrical impulse from the atrium to the ventricular myocardium, the PR interval is measured from the beginning of the P wave to the beginning of the QRS complex (normally between 0.12 and 0.20 seconds).

140. **Correct answer - D**

The interpretation of this strip is junctional rhythm. The criterion for this dysrhythmia is the absence of upright P waves before each QRS complex or the presence of inverted P waves before the QRS complex. In junctional rhythm, the QRS complexes are regular, at the rate of 40 to 60 beats/minute.

141. **Correct answer - B**

Sick sinus syndrome is a general diagnostic category of sinus dysfunction that includes such rhythm disorders as sinus bradycardia or sinus arrest, sometimes interrupted by periods of rapid supraventricular dysrhythmias. These supraventricular dysrhythmias can include rapid atrial fibrillation or supraventricular tachycardia. Symptomatic bradycardia, termed Stokes-Adams syndrome because syncope may develop, is a neurologic syndrome rather than a rhythm disorder. Etiology appears related to cellular degeneration in the sinoatrial node, which results in alternating periods of bradycardia and tachycardia.

142. **Correct answer - C**

Second-degree atrioventricular (AV) block is characterized by an intermittent interruption or failure of AV conduction. In many cases, second-degree AV block is associated with administration of digitalis, coronary artery disease, or acute myocardial infarction (MI). On an ECG, hypokalemia presents with a prolonged QT interval and the appearance of a U wave.

hypok → prolonged QT + u

ATRIAL Tach?

143.   Correct answer - A

Each dysrhythmia responds differently to carotid sinus massage, depending on its nature and origin. Sinus tachycardia is slowed only transiently. In atrial tachycardia, either the ventricular rate slows because of an increased AV block, or sinus rhythm is restored. In atrial fibrillation or flutter, the ventricular rate invariably slows because of the increased AV block. In contrast, ventricular tachycardia does not respond to carotid sinus massage.

144.   Correct answer - B

When a third-degree AV block results from an inferior wall MI, the block usually occurs in the region of the AV node; inflammation or edema results from ischemia or infarction of the neighboring myocardium. The block isusually transient and treated with atropine, an isuprel drip, and a temporary transvenous pacemaker.

145.   Correct answer - C

The interpretation of this strip is a second-degree AV block (Wenckebach, or Mobitz Type I). The criterion for this dysrhythmia is a progressively prolonged PR interval that lasts until a QRS complex is dropped. The cycle then repeats itself. The criteria for sinus dysrhythmia are a constant PR interval; upright P waves, one for each QRS complex; and a gradually irregular RR interval. The criteria for a first-degree AV block are a PR interval greater than 0.2 second, a constant PR interval, and one P wave for each QRS complex. Lastly, the criteria for a second-degree AV block (Mobitz Type II) are a constant PR interval, random episodes of a P wave, and no QRS complex.

146.   Correct answer - D

The interpretation of this strip is supraventricular tachycardia. The criteria are a heart rate greater than 150 beats/minute, normal QRS complex (between 0.04 and 0.10 second), and, because of the rapid rate, P waves that run into the preceding T waves and appear as one wave. The strip does not indicate ventricular tachycardia because the QRS complex is normal; ventricular tachycardia presents with a wid-

84

ened QRS complex greater than 0.12 second. Atrial flutter with a 2:1 conduction presents with a heart rate of 150 beats/minute (the flutter waves during atrial flutter occur at a rate of 300/minute, and every second one is conducted).

147.   **Correct answer - C**

Progressive prolongation of the PR interval followed by a blocked P wave indicates second-degree AV block (Mobitz Type I). This is usually a transient rhythm, signaling a progression of the block from first-degree to third-degree. It occurs in acute myocardial infarction, digitalis toxicity, and degenerative disease of the AV node.

148.   **Correct answer - B**

An early P wave not followed by a QRS complex is called a blocked premature atrial contraction. This usually occurs because the P wave is so early that the ventricle is still refractory from the previous impulse and cannot accept the new stimulus.

149.   **Correct answer - A**

A prominent U wave following a T wave occurs in patients who are hypokalemic. Peaked T waves, widened QRS complexes, and diminished or lost P waves signal hyperkalemia.

150.   **Correct answer - A**

Wolff-Parkinson-White (WPW) syndrome results from an abnormal AV pathway between the atria and the ventricles. This syndrome leads to an accelerated conduction of the atrial impulses to the ventricles, giving rise to recurrent bouts of paroxysmal atrial tachycardia. WPW syndrome presents with a normal P wave, a shortened PR interval, and a widened QRS complex and often mimics ventricular tachycardia. Atrial fibrillation is also common with a rapid ventricular response because the delay at the AV mode is bypassed. This rapid dysrhythmia may deteriorate to ventricular fibrillation if not treated promptly.

151. Correct answer - B

A heart with idiopathic hypertrophic subaortic stenosis (IHSS) has an enlarged left ventricular septal wall, a reduced left ventricular outflow cavity, and a thickened and displaced mitral valve. Symptoms include breathlessness, weakness, and fatigue because of reduced compliance of the left ventricle. The patient may have frequent ischemic anginal attacks. The pharmacologic keystone of IHSS management is the beta-adrenergic blocking agent propranolol (Inderal). By specifically blocking the sympathetic receptors that stimulate heart rate, cardiac contractile force, and blood pressure, this drug automatically relieves ventricular obstruction. That is, by slowing the heart, it allows more time for diastolic filling and improves the ventricular volume vital to patients with obstructive cardiomyopathy.

152. Correct answer - C

Disopyramide (Norpace) is a Type I antiarrhythmic similar to procainamide and quinidine. Norpace, as with other Type I antiarrhythmics, may prolong the QT interval. Isuprel, atropine, and epinephrine may shorten the QT interval by increasing the heart rate.

153. Correct answer - A

Angiotensin II is the most potent vasoconstrictor known. It produces arterial constriction and raises systolic and diastolic pressures. Renin is a protease secreted by the kidney; this secretion causes the kidney to release angiotensin I. Angiotensin I converts to angiotensin II by the alveolar cells of the lungs. Bradykinin is a polypeptide that induces vasodilation. Dopamine is the immediate precursor of norepinephrine. Classified as a vasopressor, dopamine in low doses may exert vasodilator effects on renal and mesenteric vessels.

154. Correct answer - B

Decreased blood pressure stimulates renin secretion. Other causes of renin secretion are increased sympathetic output and decreased serum sodium concentration. However, increases in blood supply

RENIN ?

to the renal tubules and in sodium concentration would inhibit renin secretion

155.   Correct answer - A

Pulsus magnus is a strong, bounding pulse that results from an increased metabolic rate caused by thyrotoxicosis. Pulsus paradoxus, in which the pulse is absent during inspiration, occurs in cardiac tamponade. Pulsus parvus, a small, weak pulse, may be seen in aortic stenosis. Pulsus alternans, in which every other beat is weak, is characteristic of congestive heart failure.

156.   Correct answer - C

The mitral valve is the most common site for infective endocarditis, followed by the aortic valve. Infection of the tricuspid valve is rare but occurs among I.V. drug abusers. Pulmonic valve endocarditis is the rarest form of endocarditis.

157.   Correct answer - B

Hypertension causes a reflex bradycardia from stimulation of the baroreceptors. Increases in arterial pressure stimulate the vasopressor area of the vasomotor center, which then increases vagal tone and slows heart rate. Adrenergic receptors refer to postganglionic sympathetic fibers, which secrete norepinephrine. Alpha-and beta-adrenergic receptors, when stimulated, cause the heart rate to accelerate. Alpha receptors also cause vasoconstriction, whereas beta receptor stimulation results in vasodilation and a stronger cardiac contraction.

158.   Correct answer - D

Malignant hypertension is characterized by a diastolic blood pressure greater than 140 mm Hg. Other clinical presentations include retinopathy with hemorrhage and papilledema, impaired renal function, and hypertensive encephalopathy.

159.   Correct answer - B

Back pain may be an early clue when assessing for a dissecting aortic aneurysm. The pain may signal the onset of a dissection. Caused by blood leakage into the intima, the pain usually is described as excruciating and tearing and may migrate as the dissection progresses.

160.   Correct answer - A

Increased urinary frequency is associated with anxiety, which occurs when a perceived physical or psychological threat produces symptoms similar to fear. The autonomic nervous system is stimulated to protect oneself from the threat. Visceral reflexes, such as bladder micturition, are stimulated, and blood is shunted away from the brain, GI tract, skin and kidneys to allow the heart and muscles to work more effectively to protect the self. Associated signs and symptoms of unreality, faintness, anorexia, cool and clammy skin, and an overall decrease in urine output occur with artery catheter placement.anxiety as do tach- yocardia and increased muscle tension. Although the overall urine output is decreased, a smaller bladder volume is needed to stimulate micturition.

161.   Correct answer - C

If, after the physician has left, a patient does not understand the information just given by the physician during an informed consent, the nurse should notify the physician, who should return and answer the patient's questions. If the physician does not return, the nurse's supervisor should be called and the procedure delayed until further explanations are rendered. The nurse should not answer the patient's questions because she is then assuming the physician's role and expertise. If the patient has questions that the nurse is not a liberty to answer, an informed consent was probably not obtained.

162.   Correct answer - C

During pulmonary artery catheter placement, the patient should be monitored in lead V_1 to observe for the complication of right bundle branch block.

163.   Correct answer - B

Since the right bundle branch lies close to the endocardial surface of the right ventricle, it may easily be traumatized during pulmonary artery catheter placement.

164. **Correct answer - D**

The waveform represents a large V wave during pulmonary capillary wedge pressure monitoring. This waveform may be misinterpreted as a right ventricular or pulmonary artery tracing because of the abnormal elevations produced by the V wave.

165. **Correct answer - A**

A large V wave in the setting of an acute lateral wall MI results from mitral regurgitation as a result of papillary muscle ischemia or rupture.

166. **Correct answer - B**

Since procainamide has both atrial and ventricular antiarrhythmic properties, it should be used in the setting of a wide QRS tachycardia in which the origin of the arrhythmia is unknown. Treating ventricular tachycardia with verapamil may result in severe hypotension and ventricular fibrillation. Since lidocaine enhances AV conduction, using it in the setting of supraventricular tachycardia may increase the ventricular rate.

167. **Correct answer - B**

Type A behavior, associated with shorter hospital stays than Type B behavior, is characterized by time urgency, impatience, and aggressiveness; Type B personalities are more relaxed and introverted. Type A personalities are twice as likely to develop heart disease. During acute myocardial infarction, Type A personalities tend to deny illness and don't want to waste time in the hospital, especially if they don't feel sick. Therefore, while they tend to have shorter hospital stays, they run a greater risk of fatal complications resulting from their denial.

168. **Correct answer - A**

Mr. L is demostrating signs of isolated right ventricular failure, most likely as a result of right ventricular myocardial infarction, which occurs in about 1/3 of all inferior wall MIs. Obtaining a right precordial lead electrocardiogram would help to support the diagnosis, since right precordial lead changes disappear early, within about 10 hrs after the onset of chest pain. Typical changes of ST elevation usually appear in leads V_4R-V_6R. ventricular tachycardia with verapamil may result in severe hypotension and ventricular fibrillation. Since lidocaine enhances AV conduction, using it in the setting of supraventricular tachycardia may increase the ventricular rate.

169.   Correct answer - B
Since isolated right ventricle failure may occur, right atrial pressures are elevated. Since forward flow to the left side is decreased, pulmonary cpillary wedge pressures, as well as cardiac output, will be decreased.

170.   Correct answer - B

Volume expansion is indicated in the setting of right ventricular MI to increase forward flow to the left side of the heart, and to increase wedge pressure, cardiac output and blood pressure.

171.   Correct answer - A

If the nurse feels a medication to be unsafe, she should refuse to administer the medication, informing the physician and the nursing supervisor of this. The physician may administer the medication himself. If the setting of a right ventricular myocardial infarction, diuretics may worsen cardiac output and are containdicated. Inotropic agents, such as dopamine (Intropin) and dobutamine (Dobutrex) may aid in improving cardiac output and are, in fact, indicated in the setting of a right ventricular myocardial infarction. Of course, the nurse should carefully document all interactions with the physician.

172.   Correct answer - B

During the first days of hospitalization for acute myocardial infarction, a patient may experience a positive correlation between denial and a better survival rate. A defense mechanism that inhibits anxiety, denial may protect against heart stimulation that anxiety can produce. However, denial in the recovery phase - when the patient may be noncompliant and does not recognize signs of further cardiac events - may decrease survival probabilty.

173.   Correct answer - A

Patients whose families expect them to comply with a medical regimen are most likely to do so. One study of cardiac patients to determine compliance with diet, stress reduction, activity, and medication found that patients believed their family's expectations were higher than their own. Although patient values, intention, and knowledge are important, including the family in discharge teaching and rehabilitation can promote compliance and increase self-care.

174.   Correct answer - D

Deep T wave inversion in leads V_2-V_3 is consistent with Wellen's syndrome, which indicates a critical stenosis of the left anterior descending coronary artery. Associated signs inlcude little or no enzyme elevation, no Q wave formation, and little or no ST elevation. Wellen's syndrome is a warning sign for an impending acute anterior wall myocardial infarction.

175.   Correct answer - C

Patients on quinidine, a class IA antiarrhythmic, should have their QT interval monitored for prolongation, which may precipitate torsade de pointes. Other class IA antiarrhythmics are procainamide (Procan, Pronestyl) and disopyramide (Norpace).

176.   Correct answer - B

Torsade de pointes, or polymorphous ventricular tachycardia, has a twisting characteristic to the QRS complexes. This rhythm usually results from a prolonged QT interval. It is important to differentiate this dysrthmia from ventricular tachycardia or fibrillation because conventional therapy is usually ineffective.

177.   Correct answer - D

Magnesium sulfate is the treatment of choice for torsade de pointes. 1-2 gm is administerd over 1 to 2 minutes, followed by a continuous infusion of 0.5-1 gm/hr. Other treatment which may be effective include overdrive pacing and isoproterenol (Isuprel).

178.   Correct answer - D

The half life of t-PA is considerably shorter than that of streptokinase (5 minutes vs. 18 minutes). This is a benefit if bleeding occurs - the effects of thrombolysis can be quickly reversed. Clinical studies indicate that t-PA is 25% to 50% more effective in thrombolysis than streptokinase. Clot-specific, t-PA only activates fibrin-bound plasminogen. Streptokinase activates circulating plasminogen and can deplete clotting factors, producing a systemic lytic effect.

179.   Correct answer - B

A 77-year-old patient on Coumadin therapy is not usually a candidate for thrombolytic therapy because of increased risk of bleeding from previous anticoagulant use - specifically intracranial bleeding in patients over age 70. Previous use of streptokinase and recent exposure to streptococcus bacteria are contraindications for streptokinase (not t-PA) therapy, because of risk of allergic reaction. Currently, thrombolytic therapy may be administered from up to 6-12 hours after the onset of chest pain to preserve myocardial tissue.

180.   Correct answer - A

Because t-PA activates fibrin-bound plasminogen, the only laboratory value change should be elevated fibrin split products. Increased prothrombin and partial thromboplastin times and decreased fibrinogen may occur with streptokinase therapy.

181.   Correct answer - D

Noninvasive markers of successful reperfusion include relief of chest pain, normalization of ST segments, reperfusion dysrhythmias, and rapid rise of creatine phosphokinase (CPK) isoenzymes. Reperfusion dysrhythmias include accelerated idioventricular rhythm, sinus brady-cardia, premature ventricular ectopy, and ventricular tachycardia. A rapid rise of CPK isoenzymes occurs because the reperfused artery washes out the CPK enzymes, which are then released into the systemic circulation, after the onset of chest pain in order to preserve myocardium.

182.   Correct answer - A

Irreversible pulmonary hypertension is an absolute contraindication of heart transplantation since failure of the donor heart would occur immediately after transplantation. A heart-lung transplantation would then be necessary if irreversible pulmonary hypertension is docu-mented preoperatively Diabetes mellitus and chronic obstructive lung disease are relative contraindications, depending on the degree of impairment and disability. Recurrent ventricular dysrhythmias are actually an indication of heart transplantation.

183.   Correct answer - B

Signs of congestive heart failure may indicate the development of acute rejection postoperatively. Assess for tachycardia, lung crack-les, gallop heart rhythm, and hypotension. A fever may also develop.

184.   Correct answer - D

Endomyocardial biopsy, performed transvenously, remains the only definitive method for documenting acute rejection.

185.   Correct answer - B

Nephrotoxicity and hepatotoxicity are the two major side effects of cyclosporine therapy. Monitor for a rise in serum creatinine and liver enzymes.

186.   Correct answer - B

After a cardiac transplant, the problem of body image disturbance may appear. Not only due to the presence of an external scar, this problem may also result from the removal of such a vital organ as a heart along with receiving someone else's heart. Body image disturbance may cause the patient to withdraw and hamper normal coping mechanisms. Allowing the patient to discuss her feelings, while accepting her nonjudgementally, may foster her acceptance of the change.

187.   **Correct answer - D**

Because there is no direct connection between Mrs. R.'s native sinus pacemaker and her heart, her heart rate does not rise quickly in response to increased metabolic demands, such as exercise, activity or fever. Instead, a slow rise in heart rate will be seen due to an increase in circulating catecholeamines. Mrs. R. should be instructed to begin activity or exercise slowly to compensate for this change in physiology.

CHAPTER 2

RESPIRATORY SYSTEM

1. At sea level, the partial pressure of oxygen in the air is:

    A.   760 mm Hg
    B.   160 mm Hg
    C.   105 mm Hg
    D.   40 mm Hg

2. A patient in the intensive care unit has the following arterial blood gas results: pH = 7.31, PCO_2 = 35 mm Hg, and HCO_3 = 18 mEq/liter. What is the correct interpretation of these results?

    A.   Uncompensated respiratory acidosis
    B.   Compensated respiratory acidosis
    C.   Uncompensated metabolic acidosis
    D.   Compensated metabolic acidosis

3. An assessment of the patient would most likely reveal him to be:

    A.   Hyperventilating
    B.   Apneic
    C.   Wheezing
    D.   Cyanotic

4. The most probable cause for the above arterial blood gas results is:

    A.   Nasogastric suction
    B.   Neuromuscular disease
    C.   Diabetic ketoacidosis
    D.   Anxiety

Case Study
Questions 5-26 refer to the following case study:

Mr. S. is admitted with a medical diagnosis of emphysema with impending respiratory failure. He has the following arterial blood *gas results: pH = 7.35, PO2 = 60 mm Hg, PCO$_2$ = 47 mm Hg, and HCO$_3$ = 35 mEq/liter.*

5. The correct interpretation of the above arterial blood gas results is:

    A. Compensated metabolic alkalosis
    B. Compensated respiratory acidosis
    C. Compensated respiratory alkalosis
    D. Compensated metabolic acidosis

6. This acid-base imbalance is a chronic condition because:

    A. The patient has had the same arterial blood gases since admission
    B. The PCO$_2$ is elevated
    C. The HCO$_3$ is elevated
    D. The pH is normal

7. The physician orders administration of 50% oxygen by face mask to Mr. S. The nurse knows that this would most likely result in:

    A. Resolution of the problem
    B. A decrease in the PCO$_2$
    C. Oxygen toxicity
    D. Hypoventilation

8. Mr. S.'s respiratory control is most likely affected by a change in:

    A. pH
    B. O$_2$ saturation
    C. PO$_2$
    D. PCO$_2$

9. All of the following are involuntary regulators of respiration *except* the:

    A. Hydrogen ion concentration
    B. Cortex
    C. Carbon dioxide level
    D. Oxygen level

10. The nurse performs a respiratory assessment on Mr. S. She observes his chest to be barrel-shaped. All of the following are true about barrel chest *except:*

    A. It can be a congenital deformity
    B. It is an increase in the anteroposterior diameter of the chest
    C. It is a response to air trapping in the lungs
    D. It can be a normal response to aging

11. Chest percussion of a patient with emphysema will reveal which type of sound?

    A. Resonant
    B. Hyperresonant
    C. Dull
    D. Flat

12. Which of the following parameters increases in the patient with emphysema?

    A. Functional residual capacity
    B. Tidal volume
    C. Inspiratory reserve volume
    D. Vital capacity

13. The volume of gas remaining in the lungs after normal expiration is the:

   A. Functional residual capacity
   B. Residual volume
   C. Expiratory reserve volume
   D. Forced vital capacity

14. On physical assessment, the nurse would observe Mr. S. for all of the following systemic responses to chronic obstructive pulmonary disease (COPD) *except:*

   A. Splenomegaly
   B. Polycythemia
   C. Clubbing of the fingers
   D. Distended neck veins

15. Some of the physiologic changes in patients with COPD occur because chronic hypoxia causes:

   A. Decreased cardiac output
   B. Peripheral cyanosis
   C. Anemia
   D. Increased erythropoiesis

16. Due to increased fatigue with loss of appetite, Mr. S. is started on an enteral tube feeding. Which type of diet is recommended for Mr. S?

   A. High fat, low carbohydrate
   B. High protein, high carbohydrate
   C. Low fat, high carbohydrate
   D. Low fat, high protein

17. A pulmonary artery catheter is inserted into Mr. S. to document whether he has pulmonary hypertension. Hemodynamic changes resulting from pulmonary hypertension do not include an increase in:

    A. Right ventricular pressure
    B. Pulmonary artery pressure
    C. Pulmonary capillary wedge pressure
    D. Pulmonary vascular resistance

18. Mr. S. is still breathing spontaneously without the aid of a mechanical ventilator. Which expected effect does spontaneous breathing have on hemodynamic waveforms?

    A. There is a increase in waveform pressures during inspiration
    B. There is a decrease in waveform pressures during inspiration
    C. There is a increase in waveform pressures during expiration
    D. There is a decrease in waveform pressures during expiration

19. A mixed venous blood gas sample is drawn from the pulmonary artery catheter. A mixed venous PO_2 of 35 mm Hg indicates:

    A. Adequate tissue perfusion
    B. Low cardiac output
    C. Hypoxemia
    D. Chronic acidosis

20. A mixed venous blood sample:

    A. Is drawn from the right atrial port of a pulmonary artery catheter
    B. Is a sample of oxygenated blood
    C. Reflects ventilation and circulation
    D. Replaces the need for arterial blood gas samples

21. A typical change that you might expect to see on Mr. S.' ECG is:

    A.   Complete right bundle branch block
    B.   Left ventricular hypertrophy strain
    C.   Peaked P waves
    D.   Generalized ST elevation

22. If Mr. S. was found to have familial emphysema, this would be evidenced by a deficiency in:

    A.   Surfactant
    B.   Serum alpha antitrypsin
    C.   Mucus production
    D.   Lactic acid dehydrogenase

23. An electrolyte imbalance that Mr. S. would most likely develop as a result of chronic hypoxia is low:

    A.   Sodium
    B.   Chloride
    C.   Bicarbonate
    D.   Calcium

24. The most common cause of chronic obstructive pulmonary disease (COPD) is:

    A.   Occupation
    B.   Pollution
    C.   Smoking
    D.   Aging

25. Mr. S. is taught pursed-lip breathing because it:

    A.   Prevents air trapping
    B.   Causes airway collapse
    C.   Increases surface tension
    D.   Allows air to be quickly exhaled

26. As part of discharge teaching, the nurse cautions Mr. S. to avoid high altitudes. Which change in arterial blood gases would be expected if he travelled to such an area?

A. PO_2 would be higher
B. pH would be lower
C. PCO_2 would be higher
D. O_2 saturation would be lower

Case Study

Questions 27-42 refer to the following case study:

Mr. D. is admitted to the intensive care unit (ICU) with status asthmaticus, including episodes of supraventricular tachycardia and hypertension. On admission his arterial blood gas results on O_2 therapy of 35% by Venturi mask are pH, 7.50; PO_2, 104 mm Hg; PCO_2, 25 mm Hg; and HCO_3, 23 mEq/liter. At home, Mr. D. was taking theophylline and prednisone.

27. Room air PO_2 drops to 104 mm Hg in the alveolus because of the:

A. Diffusion gradient
B. Addition of water vapor and carbon dioxide
C. Partial pressure of nitrogen
D. Venous admixture from normal physiologic shunting

28. The correct arterial blood gas interpretation is:

A. Uncompensated respiratory alkalosis
B. Compensated respiratory alkalosis
C. Uncompensated metabolic alkalosis
D. Compensated metabolic alkalosis

29. The most probable cause for Mr. D.'s acid-base imbalance is:

A. Hypoventilation
B. Hyperventilation
C. Side effect of prednisone
D. Theophyline toxicity

30. Associated symptoms Mr. D. would probably experience are:

  A. Headache and somnolence
  B. Nausea and vomiting
  C. Decreased ventilation and constricted pupils
  D. Numbness and tingling of extremities

31. Which of the following best describes Venturi oxygen therapy?

  A. Accurate oxygen concentration occurs by mixing oxygen with entrained air
  B. Oxygen is conserved by rebreathing one-third of expired air from a reservoir bag
  C. Oxygen is delivered through tubing with two soft plastic tubes inserted into the nostrils
  D. 100% oxygen can be delivered

32. The nurse auscultates Mr. D.'s lungs and hears vesicular breath sounds. Vesicular breath sounds:

  A. Have a short expiration phase
  B. Are heard over the trachea
  C. Are a combination of bronchial and bronchovesicular sounds
  D. Suggest consolidation of lung tissue

33. The physician orders propranolol (Inderal) to treat Mr. D.'s tachycardia and hypertension. The nurse questions the order; she knows propranolol is contraindicated in asthma because it may cause:

  A. Bronchospasm
  B. Atelectasis
  C. Pneumonia
  D. Apnea

34. Mr. D. has a history of extrinsic asthma. His status asthmaticus was most likely precipitated by:

A. Hay fever
B. Smoke
C. Exercise
D. Respiratory infection

35. A repeat blood gas analysis reveals hypercapnia. Hypercapnia associated with asthma occurs:

A. During improvement of bronchospasm
B. During hyperventilation
C. During severe airway obstruction
D. As an early sign of an asthma attack

36. Mr. D. is intubated and placed on a volume ventilator, which delivers a preset volume when the ventilator is triggered. An important disadvantage of this type of ventilator is that:

A. It lacks adequate alarms
B. Hypoventilation ensues if set pressures are reached early in the respiratory cycle
C. Positive end-expiratory pressure cannot be initiated
D. The set tidal volume is delivered even if high inspiratory pressures are generated

37. Talking at the nurses' station, ventilatory alarms, and the continuous lighting of the critical care unit can cause Mr. D. to experience:

A. Sensory monotony
B. Sensory deprivation
C. Sensory overload
D. Sleep deprivation

38. Pancuronium bromide (Pavulon) is ordered to block Mr. D.'s respiratory efforts through paralysis of his respiratory muscles. The following medication should be available if it becomes necessary to reverse the effects of Pavulon:

    A. Neostigmine
    B. Atropine
    C. Narcan
    D. Tubocurarine

39. Which of the following may prolong the effects of neuromuscular blockade on Mr. D.?

    A. Hyperthermia
    B. Administration of penicillin
    C. Blood administration
    D. A history of myasthenia gravis

40. Two days later, the pancuronium bromide has been discontinued and Mr. D. is assessed for ability to be weaned. Which criterion best predicts successful weaning?

    A. Vital capacity of 10 ml/kg
    B. Minute ventilation of 9 l/min
    C. Negative inspiratory force of 10 cms H_2O
    D. Tidal volume of 3 ml/kg

41. Which mode of ventilation is indicated for weaning?

    A. Assist control ventilation
    B. Inverse ratio ventilation
    C. High frequency jet ventilation
    D. Pressure support ventilation

42. Thirty minutes after the initiation of weaning, which assessment indicates potential weaning failure?

   A. O_2 saturation drops from 98% to 94%
   B. The respiratory rate increases by 8 breaths/minute
   C. The heart rate rises by 24 beats/minute
   D. Minute ventilation is 7 l/minute

Case Study
Questions 43-55 refer to the following case study:

Ms. B., a visitor in the cafeteria, suffers a cardiac arrest. As a member of the code team, you respond. Ms. B. is receiving cardiopulmonary resuscitation (CPR) with mouth-to-mouth resuscitation.

---

43. Your first action is to attempt to ventilate Ms. B. with a manual resuscitator bag attached to portable oxygen. You base this action on the knowledge that mouth-to-mouth ventilation during CPR delivers what percentage of oxygen?

   A. 9%
   B. 17%
   C. 21%
   D. 30%

---

44. After Ms. B. is successfully intubated, her breath sounds are assessed for possible right mainstem intubation. This is a concern because the left main bronchus bifurcates from the trachea at a more acute angle than the right because of the position of the:

   A. Stomach
   B. Heart
   C. Thyroid gland
   D. Liver

45. Ms. B. is successfully resuscitated from ventricular fibrillation and transported to the coronary care unit, where you are now her nurse. As part of your assessment, you measure the endotracheal tube cuff pressure because it should not exceed:

  A. Peak inspiratory pressure
  B. End expiratory pressure
  C. Tracheal capillary filling pressure
  D. Pulmonary capillary wedge pressure

46. The endotracheal cuff requires 60 mm Hg of pressure to maintain an adequate air seal. What is the probable cause for this?

  A. Endotracheal tube is in the right mainstem bronchus
  B. Endotracheal tube has a leaky cuff
  C. Patient has tracheal stenosis
  D. Patient needs a larger endotracheal tube

47. Later that shift, Ms. B. is awake and slightly restless. Arterial blood gases are drawn but cannot be sent to the laboratory immediately; they are placed on ice. What would happen if the samples are not placed on ice or analyzed immediately?

  A. The sample would clot
  B. The PCO_2 level would decrease
  C. The PO_2 level would decrease
  D. The HCO_3 level would decrease

48. Ms. B. is overriding her intermittent mandatory ventilation (IMV) rate of 8 with a respiratory rate of 40 breaths/minute. Her tidal volume is 850 ml and FIO_2 is 35%. Arterial blood gas values are as follows: pH = 754, PO_2 = 80 mm Hg, PCO_2 = 25 mm Hg, and HCO_3 = 23 mEq/liter. Match her acid-base status with its cause:

  A. Respiratory acidosis due to cardiac arrest
  B. Respiratory alkalosis due to cardiac arrest
  C. Respiratory acidosis due to hyperventilation
  D. Respiratory alkalosis due to hyperventilation

49. Ms. B.'s problem would most likely be corrected by:

A. Decreasing her IMV rate
B. Increasing her FIO_2
C. Decreasing her respiratory rate
D. Increasing her tidal volume

50. The physician considers placing Ms. B. on the assist mode of the mechanical ventilator. How does this mode differ from IMV?

A. Patient triggers respirator breaths at a set volume
B. Respiratory rate is fixed
C. Tidal volume varies
D. Patient is allowed to generate an inspiratory effort

51. Instead, Ms. B. is placed on pressure support ventilation (PSV) of 25 cms and 35% FIO_2. An important assessment to monitor while Ms. B. is on PSV is:

A. Peak inspiratory pressure
B. Negative inspiratory force
C. Minute ventilation
D. For the development of auto-PEEP

52. ABG's one hour after the change to PSV 25 cms H_2O and 35% FIO_2 are pH = 7.55, pO_2 = 100, pCO_2 = 24 and a respiratory rate of 16 breaths/minute. Measured tidal volume is 1100 ml. Ms. B weighs 58 kg. Which action is recommended?

A. Decrease PSV to reach a tidal volume of 800 ml
B. Switch back to IMV
C. Increase FIO_2 to 40%
D. Change to assist mode of ventilation

53. Inspiratory pressure is measured on Ms. B. as part of her respiratory assessment. Inspiratory pressure is:

   A. Desirable if between 0 and -10 cm H_2O
   B. An indication of inspiratory muscle strength
   C. Not a criterion for weaning from a ventilator
   D. Not affected by the addition of positive end-expiratory pressure

54. The next day Ms. B. is extubated. After extubation, Ms. B. is assessed for signs of upper airway obstruction, a concern because the narrowest part of the airway is the:

   A. Trachea
   B. Nares
   C. Larynx
   D. Bronchus

55. The sign of upper airway obstruction that Ms. B. should be assessed for after extubation is:

   A. Crackles
   B. Rhonchi
   C. Stridor
   D. Wheezing

Case Study
Questions 56-65 refer to the following case study:

Ms. F. is admitted to the intensive care unit (ICU) from a long-term care facility with a diagnosis of impending respiratory failure. She has had a decreased level of consciousness for 3 days and a chronic problem with thick mucus production.

56. Early signs of impending respiratory failure include:

   A. Cyanosis
   B. Wheezing and rhonchi
   C. Intercostal and substernal retractions
   D. Tachycardia and restlessness

57. Nursing care of the patient in impending respiratory failure is aimed toward:

   A. Sedation to ensure rest
   B. Drawing of arterial blood gases
   C. Preventative measures
   D. Suctioning

58. Acute respiratory failure in a patient with normal lung function is defined as:

   A. PCO_2 above 50 mm Hg, PO_2 below 60 mm Hg
   B. PCO_2 above 40 mm Hg, PO_2 below 40 mm Hg
   C. PCO_2 below 60 mm Hg, PO_2 below 70 mm Hg
   D. PCO_2 below 20 mm Hg, PO_2 below 60 mm Hg

59. The most common cause of airway obstruction is:

   A. Bronchospasm
   B. Aspiration
   C. Laryngeal edema
   D. Relaxation of the tongue

60. Which condition is associated with increased mucus production?

   A. Asthma
   B. Pulmonary emboli
   C. Emphysema
   D. Chronic bronchitis

61. Evaluation of Ms. F.'s chest X-ray reveals consolidation of the lower lung segments. The nursing plan includes promotion of respiratory effort, postural drainage, and suctioning of retained secretions. The best position for proper respiratory excursion and promotion of the patient's respiratory effort is:

A. Sitting in a chair
B. Lying flat
C. Left lateral decubitus
D. Semi-Fowler's

62. Postural drainage should be used for:

A. A patient with pneumonia who is 8 months pregnant
B. A postoperative craniotomy patient
C. A patient in the immediate postprandial period
D. A patient receiving aerosol therapy

63. The correct patient position for draining the anterior lower lung segments is:

A. Sitting upright or semireclining
B. Lying face down with the hips elevated
C. Lying on the back with the hips elevated
D. Lying on the right side with the head elevated

64. The correct patient position for nasotracheal suctioning is:

A. Leaning forward with the chin on the chest
B. Sitting up at a 45-degree angle, with the head turned toward the nares entered
C. Sitting up at a 45-degree angle, with the head turned away from the nares entered
D. Lying on the back with the head forward

65. When the catheter passes the vocal cords during nasotracheal suctioning, the nurse should:

A. Withdraw the catheter and apply suction for 20 seconds
B. Continue passing the catheter until resistance is met; then withdraw the catheter and apply suction for 10 seconds
C. Apply suction and continue passing the catheter until resistance is met; then withdraw the catheter and apply suction for 10 seconds
D. Stop passing the catheter, apply suction 10 seconds, then withdraw the catheter

Case Study
Questions 66-68 refer to the following case study:

Mr. Z. undergoes an open-lung biopsy complicated by massive pulmonary hemorrhage. An open thoracotomy is performed to stop the bleeding, and the patient returns to the intensive care unit (ICU) on a mechanical ventilator, with a chest tube draining about 50 ml/hr of bright red blood. Mr. Z.'s hemoglobin and hematocrit are 8.6 mg/dl and 29%, respectively. Ventilator settings are IMV of 10 breaths/minute, FIO_2 of .40%, tidal volume of 700ml and PSV of 5 cms H_2O.

66. The most appropriate nursing action at this point would be to notify Mr. Z.'s physician in order to:

A. Start a blood transfusion
B. Prepare the patient to return to surgery
C. Suggest an autotransfusion
D. Prepare the patient for a second chest tube insertion

67.   The use of PSV of 5 cms H₂O in this setting is utilized for which of the following reasons?

A.   To overcome resistance from ventilator tubing
B.   To increase functional residual capacity
C.   Weaning
D.   To decrease risk of barotrauma

68.   Three hours after surgery, the chest tube stops draining. The most appropriate nursing action at this time is to:

A.   Increase the suction
B.   Call the physician to remove the chest tube
C.   Assess for subcutaneous emphysema
D.   Assess for tracheal deviation

Case Study
Questions 69-86 continued from the previous case study:

The day after surgery, Mr. Z. is still on a volume mechanical ventilator. Arterial blood gas analysis reveals hypoxemia without hypercapnia. Mr. Z. also has an increasing alveolar-arterial oxygen gradient and a high peak inspiratory pressure.

69.   A high peak inspiratory pressure in a patient on a volume mechanical ventilator indicates that:

A.   Lung compliance is decreasing
B.   Lung compliance is increasing
C.   The patient is not receiving the full tidal volume
D.   The ventilator system is disconnected

70.   An increasing alveolar-arterial oxygen gradient indicates:

A.   Pulmonary embolism
B.   Eupnea
C.   Dead space
D.   Shunting

71. Which statement correctly described right-to-left shunting?

A. Normal physiologic shunting causes the alveolar PO_2 to drop from 104 to 95 mm Hg as it enters the arterial system
B. Breathing 100% oxygen will correct pathologic shunting
C. Normal physiologic shunting is 10% to 20% of cardiac output
D. Normal physiologic shunting is a result of bronchial and thebesian arterial blood flow

72. A diagnosis of adult respiratory distress syndrome (ARDS) is made for Mr. Z. ARDS is characterized by all of the following *except:*

A. High peak inspiratory pressures
B. Large alveolar-arterial oxygen gradient
C. Increased lung compliance
D. Pulmonary edema

73. The goal of treatment for ARDS is to:

A. Increase PCO_2 elimination
B. Decrease respiratory rate
C. Increase functional residual capacity
D. Increase tidal volume

74. Which of the following statements about ARDS is true?

A. It can be caused by hyperalbuminemia
B. On autopsy, the diseased lung looks like the intestine
C. It causes an increase in shunting
D. It results in an increase in lung compliance

75. ARDS is characterized by destruction of surfactant. Which of the following statements accurately describes surfactant?

A. It increases surface tension as alveolar volume decreases
B. Reduced surfactant increases compliance
C. It allows alveoli to collapse and re-expand during respiration
D. It is produced by alveolar epithelial cells

76. Pulmonary capillary leakage occurs in ARDS because of a decrease in:

A. Cardiac output
B. Blood pressure
C. Colloid osmotic pressure
D. Pulmonary capillary wedge pressure

77. Mr. Z. has hypoxemia without hypercapnia because carbon dioxide is:

A. Much more soluble than oxygen
B. Equally as soluble as oxygen
C. Much less soluble than oxygen
D. Retained because of obstructive processes

78. Most carbon dioxide in the blood is carried:

A. In combination with hemoglobin
B. As bicarbonate
C. Dissolved in plasma
D. As carbonic anhydrase

79. Before positive end-expiratory pressure (PEEP) is instituted for Mr. Z. he must be assessed for hypovolemia because PEEP can directly result in:

A. Dysrhythmias
B. A low cardiac output
C. Hypoxia
D. A high pulmonary capillary wedge pressure

114

80. Hemodynamically, PEEP causes an increase in:

A. Pulmonary vascular resistance
B. Blood pressure
C. Cardiac output
D. Preload

81. A complication of PEEP may be:

A. Atelectasis
B. Liver infarction
C. Pneumothorax
D. Hypertension

82. An increasingly higher FIO_2 is required in Mr. Z. to prevent hypoxemia. Oxygen toxicity is a concern. Signs and symptoms of oxygen toxicity include all of the following *except:*

A. Decreasing alveolar-arterial oxygen gradient
B. Dyspnea
C. Parasthesias in extremities
D. Decreasing lung compliance

83. To reduce the likelihood of oxygen toxicity, oxygen therapy that is to last longer than 48 hours should not exceed:

A. 28%
B. 35%
C. 40%
D. 50%

84. Complications of oxygen therapy include:

A. Pneumothorax
B. Hyperventilation
C. Atelectasis
D. Anemia

85. The physician decides to initiate inverse ratio ventilation to improve Mr. Z.'s respiratory status. A common complication that must be assessed for is:

    A. Mucus plugs
    B. Atelectasis
    C. Pneumothorax
    D. Air trapping

86. A potential nursing diagnosis appropriate for the patient receiving inverse ratio ventilation is:

    A. Anxiety related to altered breathing patterns
    B. Impaired gas exchange related to insufficient tidal volume
    C. Ineffective airway clearance related to thick secretions
    D. Impaired gas exchange related to lung collapse

87. A common respiratory complication in septic shock is:

    A. Pneumothorax
    B. Tension pneumothorax
    C. Adult respiratory distress syndrome (ARDS)
    D. Cor pulmonale

Case Study
Questions 88-104 refer to the following case study:

Mr. W., a postoperative GI patient, has returned from the operating room and has been placed on a mechanical ventilator. He was not weaned from the respirator in the recovery room because of long-standing cardiac and respiratory diseases. A chest X-ray reveals Kerley's B lines, especially in the hilar area. Arterial blood gas-studies reveal a shift to the right of the oxyhemoglobin dissociation curve.

88.   Kerley's B lines on chest X-ray indicate:

A.   Pneumothorax
B.   Pulmonary emboli
C.   Emphysema
D.   Pulmonary edema

89.   The hilar area of the lung is the:

A.   Bifurcation of the bronchi
B.   Apex of the lung
C.   Mediastinal surface where the blood vessels and bronchi
        enter the lung
D.   Base of the lung above the diaphragm

90.   A shift to the right of Mr. W.'s oxyhemoglobin dissociation curve
        may be due to:

A.   Hypothermia
B.   Hypocarbia
C.   Acidosis
D.   Decreased 2,3-diphosphoglycerate

91.   2,3-diphosphoglycerate:

A.   Is carried in plasma
B.   Is a metabolite of glucose
C.   Is decreased in anemia
D.   Impedes the dissociation of O_2 from hemoglobin

92.   The most common complication of intubation and mechanical
        ventilation is:

A.   Barotrauma
B.   Starvation
C.   Laryngeal edema
D.   Tracheoesophageal fistula

93. The low pressure alarm on Mr. W.'s ventilator is triggered. You cannot find a disconnection in the system. Your next action is to:

A. Bypass the alarm
B. Suction the patient
C. Reset the alarm limits
D. Manually aerate the patient until the cause is determined

94. Sighs are not a component of Mr. W.'s respiratory settings. The effect of sighs can be achieved in mechanical ventilation by:

A. Increasing the tidal volume
B. Increasing the respiratory rate
C. Instituting positive end-expiratory pressure
D. Increasing the percentage of inspired oxygen

95. Mr. W. cannot be weaned from the respiratory, and a tracheostomy is scheduled because his vital capacity is below normal. The vital capacity is the amount of air:

A. Breathed in and out for 1 minute
B. Breathed in and out in one breath
C. Remaining in the lungs after a maximal exhalation
D. Maximally exhaled after a maximal inhalation

96. Which is *not* an advantage of a tracheostomy?

A. It provides humidification to the airway
B. It decreases dead space
C. It bypasses narrowed airways
D. It is useful for long-term airway management

97. Which principle is true regarding care of the patient with a tracheostomy?

A. Humidification should always be used
B. The inner cannula should be removed only for cleaning
C. The cuff should always be kept inflated
D. A tracheostomy should never be capped unless the patient can talk

98.   Hemorrhage resulting from a tracheostomy is due to erosion of the:

A.   Innominate artery
B.   Subclavian artery
C.   Pulmonary artery
D.   Aorta

99.   Continuous positive airway pressure is ordered for Mr. W. This may be used to:

A.   Assist ventilations in an apneic patient
B.   Decrease lung compliance
C.   Wean a patient from positive end-expiratory pressure
D.   Reduce the need for a high FIO_2

100.   Mr. W. is weaned from the respirator. A fenestrated tracheostomy tube is inserted, and Mr. W. is receiving humidified O_2 at 35%. Which statement accurately describes humidification in respiratory therapy?

A.   All gases hold the same amount of water vapor
B.   Mechanical ventilation does not allow for exhalation of water vapor
C.   Inspired dry gas is irritating because it cannot add water vapor once it enters the airway
D.   The colder the air, the more water vapor it can hold

101.   During morning care, Mr. W.'s tracheostomy tube falls out of his trachea and he becomes cyanotic. Your action is to:

A.   Initiate mouth-to-stoma respiration
B.   Prepare for endotracheal intubation
C.   Reinsert the tube, using the obturator
D.   Call the physician to insert a new tracheostomy tube

102. Mr. W.'s cyanosis is a result of:

A. Unsaturated hemoglobin
B. Acidosis
C. CO_2 retention
D. Physiologic shunting

103. When capping a fenestrated, cuffed tracheostomy tube, you should:

A. Deflate the cuff
B. Tell the patient he won't be able to speak
C. Provide oxygen via a tracheostomy collar
D. Insert the inner cannula

104. You determine that Mr. W. has Cheyne-Stokes respirations. Which of the following is *not* true regarding this type of breathing?

A. It is characterized by alternation periods of hyperventilation and apnea
B. It is normal during sleep in children and the elderly
C. It is due to changing carbon dioxide levels in the blood
D. It is commonly seen in patients with chronic obstructive pulmonary disease

Case Study
Questions 105-113 refer to the following case study:

Ms. J. is admitted to the intensive care unit (ICU) on a mechanical ventilator after a motor vehicle accident in which she was the driver. She wasn't wearing a seatbelt. She is a long-term smoker with a past history of bleb formation. A diagnosis of flail chest is made.

105. In a flail chest, which of the following occurs during expiration?

A. The affected side becomes depressed
B. The mediastinum shifts to the unaffected side
C. The flail portion bulges out
D. Negative pressure decreases on the affected side

106. All of the following statements about blebs are true *except:*

A. They can be found within the lung tissue
B. They can cause a spontaneous pneumothorax
C. They usually are a result of diffuse emphysema
D. They are treated by surgical resection

107. Two hours after her admission, you assess subcutaneous emphysema over Ms. J.'s left lateral chest. Subcutaneous emphysema is a complication of:

A. Adult respiratory distress syndrome
B. Pneumothorax
C. Lung contusion
D. Atelectasis

108. The physician inserts a chest tube in Ms. J. When correctly placed, the lumen of the chest tube is situated in the:

A. Intercostal space
B. Intra-alveolar space
C. Pericardial space
D. Pleural space

109. Which of the following statements about chest tube therapy is accurate?

A. Chest tubes should be stripped toward the patient
B. In three-bottle suction, the first bottle is the water-seal bottle
C. The length of the glass tube below the water surface of the suction-control bottle determines the amount of suction
D. Oscillation of the underwater seal fluid with ventilation indicates lung reexpansion

110. Clamping of chest tube may cause:

A. Tension pneumothorax
B. Hemorrhage
C. Cardiac tamponade
D. Flail chest

111. Which assessment would be made on the affected side if the above complication occurred in Ms. J.?

A. Dull to percussion
B. Increased fremitus
C. Tracheal deviation toward the affected side
D. No adventitious breath sounds

112. Ms. J.'s chest tube is connected to a an underwater seal drainage system. Bubbling in the underwater seal area during expiration demonstrates that:

A. The suction is working properly
B. An air leak is present
C. The lung has reexpanded
D. Subcutaneous emphysema is present

113. Ms. J. begins to complain about puffiness of her face and neck. You assess the chest tube insertion site and palpate subcutaneous emphysema. This usually signifies that the:

A. Patient needs thoracic surgery
B. Chest tube needs repositioning
C. Lung is reexpanding as expected
D. Chest tube needs stripping

114.   The physician places Ms. J. on high-frequency ventilation. Which statement accurately describes this type of ventilation?

    A.   Tidal volumes are 5 to 10 ml/kg
    B.   Gas exchange occurs through osmosis
    C.   Respiratory rates are 100 to 200 breaths/minute
    D.   The low tidal volume increases atelectasis

115.   A potential nursing diagnosis appropriate for the patient receiving high frequency jet ventilation is:

    A.   Anxiety related to altered breathing patterns
    B.   Impaired gas exchange related to insufficient tidal volume
    C.   Ineffective airway clearance related to thick secretions
    D.   Impaired gas exchange related to lung collapse

116.   High frequency jet ventilation is indicated for the patient with a flail chest because this type of ventilation:

    A.   Stabilizes the chest wall
    B.   Improves oxygenation through increased tidal volumes
    C.   Lengthens inspiratory time
    D.   Promotes mobilization of secretions

117.   Which assessment is difficult for the nurse caring for a patient receiving high frequency jet ventilation?

    A.   Arterial blood gas interpretation
    B.   Pulse and blood pressure
    C.   Respiratory rate
    D.   Lung sounds

118.   Which diagnosis is most appropriate for a patient on a ventilator like Ms. J. who feels she cannot control her environment?

    A.   Social isolation
    B.   Powerlessness
    C.   Fear
    D.   Self-esteem disturbance

Questions 119-124 refer to the following case study:

Mrs. T., a l-day postoperative patient, had a Bilroth I surgery for gastric ulcer. She has a nasogastric tube attached to intermittent low suction, which is draining bile-colored secretions. Respiratory assessment indicates decreased breath sounds with an increase in fremitus over the upper and middle lobes and a decrease in fremitus at the bases. Arterial blood gas values are pH, 7.44; PO_2, 90 mm Hg; PCO_2, 46 mm Hg; and HCO_3, 32 mEq/liter. Chest X-ray demonstrates blunting of the costophrenic angles.

119. An increase in fremitus may be noted:

    A.   In atelectasis
    B.   In pneumothorax
    C.   In emphysema
    D.   Over pleural effusions

120. Sound is best conducted through:

    A.   Air
    B.   Water
    C.   Solid material
    D.   Both air and solid material

121. Correct interpretation of Mrs. T.'s arterial blood gas results is:

    A.   Compensated metabolic alkalosis
    B.   Compensated respiratory alkalosis
    C.   Uncompensated respiratory alkalosis
    D.   Uncompensated metabolic alkalosis

122. Causes of Mrs. T.'s acid-base imbalance include all of the following except:

A. Vomiting
B. Diarrhea
C. Diuretic treatment
D. Corticosteroid administration

123. A medication used to correct this acid-base imbalance is:

A. Acetazolamide
B. Sodium bicarbonate
C. Morphine sulfate
D. Oxygen

124. Blunting of the costophrenic angle on chest X-ray is most characteristic of:

A. Pulmonary embolism
B. Atelectasis
C. Pneumothorax
D. Pleural effusions

Case Study
Questions 125-132 refer to the following case study:

Mrs. J. is admitted to the intensive care unit (ICU) with a diagnosis of pulmonary embolism from deep vein thrombosis. A continuous heparin infusion is started.

125. The amount of Mrs. J.'s cardiac output that does not take part in gas exchange is called:

A. Dead space
B. Shunting
C. Residual volume
D. Stroke volume

126. The area from the nares to the bronchioles is called the:

    A.   Nasopharynx
    B.   Oropharynx
    C.   Anatomic dead space
    D.   Residual volume

127. Which of the following statements about the pulmonary circulatory system is true?

    A.   Five percent of the cardiac output is found in the pulmonary circulatory system at any time
    B.   Hypoxia causes a decrease in pulmonary vascular tone
    C.   Blood flow to the lung is greater at the apex than at the base
    D.   The average diameter of a pulmonary capillary is equal to the average diameter of an erythrocyte

128. Which of the following statements about ventilation and perfusion is true?

    A.   Normally, ventilation and perfusion are equally balanced throughout the lung
    B.   Normal ventilation-perfusion ratio is 0.8:1
    C.   Perfusion scans are performed by having the patient inhale a radioactive substance
    D.   Low ventilation-perfusion ratio occurs in pulmonary embolism

129. Which clinical finding is present in pulmonary embolism?

    A.   Vesicular breath sounds over most of the lung
    B.   Increased tactile fremitus
    C.   Hyperresonance to percussion
    D.   Pleural friction rub

130. Pathophysiologic factors predisposing Mrs. J. to pulmonary embolism include all of the following except:

A. Pre-existing pulmonary disease
B. Hypercoagulable state
C. Venous stasis
D. Trauma to vascular walls

131. Which statement is not true regarding pulmonary embolism?

A. It is usually characterized by a sudden onset of dyspnea
B. Chest X-rays are usually not diagnostic
C. Oxygen administration will significantly reverse hypoxemia
D. Therapy is aimed at preventing further emboli

132. A pulmonary embolism can be definitively diagnosed by:

A. Chest X-ray
B. Arterial blood gas studies
C. Lung scan
D. Pulmonary angiogram

Case Study
Questions 133-135 refer to the following case study:

Mr T., an automobile mechanic overcome by emission fumes, was admitted with a diagnosis of carbon monoxide poising.

133. The primary treatment for carbon monoxide poisoning is:

A. Having the patient breathe into a paper bag
B. Administering Mucomyst
C. Administering 100% oxygen
D. Suctioning

134. Care of the patient with carbon monoxide poisoning includes:

A. Continuous pulse oximetry monitoring
B. Monitoring carbon monoxide levels by co-oximetry
C. Diuretic administration
D. SvO_2 monitoring

127

135. All of the following are at increased risk of developing carbon monoxide poisoning *except* the person who:

A. Smokes
B. Has emphysema
C. Has diabetes
D. Has pre-existing cardiac disease

Mental Humor Break

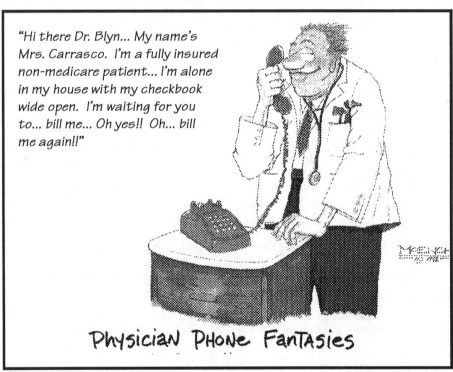

In Your Face
1-800-658-8508

1. **Correct answer - B**

The partial pressure of oxygen (PO2) in the air is 160 mm Hg. Atmospheric, or barometric, pressure is 760 mm Hg at sea level. The percentage of oxygen in room air is 21%; 21% of 760 mm Hg gives a room PO2 of 160 mm Hg. Alveolar PO2 is 105 mm Hg, and venous PO2, 40 mm Hg.

2. **Correct answer - C**

$$7.35 - 7.45 = pH$$
$$22 - 26 \; mEq/L = HCO_3$$

The arterial blood gas results indicate uncompensated metabolic acidosis. The pH of 7.31 (normal is 7.35 to 7.45) indicates acidosis. The HCO3 of 18 (normal range is 22 to 26 mEq/liter) reflects a metabolic imbalance. When either the PCO2 or the HCO3 value is abnormal and the pH also falls outside the normal range, the arterial blood gas result is considered uncompensated.

3. **Correct answer - A**

The patient compensating for metabolic acidosis would probably be hyperventilating. Metabolic acidosis results from decreased HCO3 causing a base deficit. Hyperventilation - the body's attempt to compensate for acidosis - decreases PCO2 an acid. Apnea and severe wheezing would most likely lead to respiratory acidosis. Cyanosis primarily results from oxygen imbalance rather than acid-base imbalance.

4. **Correct answer - C**

The most probable cause for metabolic acidosis is diabetic ketoacidosis, a condition in which increased fat metabolism (resulting from impaired glucose utilization) causes a buildup of ketones. Other causes include lactic acidosis, starvation ketosis, ethylene glycol and methanol poisoning, renal failure, diarrhea, drainage of pancreatic juices, and ingestion of acidic drugs, as in aspirin overdose. Diarrhea and drainage of pancreatic juices, however, will result in a non-anion gap acidosis. Nasogastric suction drains hydrochloric acid, causing metabolic alkalosis. Neuromuscular disease causes hypoventilation, manifested by respiratory acidosis. Anxiety causes respiratory alkalosis as a result of hyperventilation.

129

5. **Correct answer - B**

The PCO_2 is elevated (normal is 35 to 45 mm Hg), a condition seen in primary respiratory acidosis and as a compensatory response to metabolic alkalosis. HCO_3 is elevated (normal is 22 to 26 mEq/liter), a condition seen in primary metabolic alkalosis and as a compensatory response to respiratory acidosis. The pH determines the primary imbalance because when complete compensation occurs, the pH returns to near normal, never overcompensating. In this case, the pH is normal but tending toward acidosis. Thus, the correct interpretation is compensated respiratory acidosis.

6. **Correct answer - D**

The acid-base imbalance can be a chronic condition if the pH is normal. This physiologic, homeostatic mechanism attempts to maintain a normal pH by altering the acid-base component not primarily affected. Thus, the body compensates for metabolic alkalosis or acidosis by altering the rate of carbon dioxide removal from the lungs through hypoventilation or hyperventilation, respectively. In respiratory alkalosis or acidosis, the body stimulates the kidneys to excrete or retain bicarbonate, respectively. The body never overcompensates, so the pH will tend toward the primary abnormality. Abnormal blood gas results that remain unchanged after admission do not necessarily indicate a chronic condition.

7. **Correct answer - D**

Administration of 50% oxygen to the patient with chronic respiratory acidosis would probably cause hypoventilation. Patients with chronically high PCO_2 levels fail to respond to the powerful respiratory stimulant effects of PCO_2. Instead, they must rely on the less powerful respiratory stimulus of hypoxia, which increases tidal volume and respiratory rate. Administration of oxygen, especially at 50% reduces hypoxia and the stimulus to breathe, causing hypoventilation and possibly apnea.

8. **Correct answer - C**

The patient's respiratory control is most likely affected by a change in PO_2. Normally, however, a change in PCO_2 affects respiratory

130

control. Carbon dioxide is a powerful respiratory stimulant - directly affecting respiratory neurons in the lungs and indirectly increasing hydrogen-ion concentration in the cerebrospinal fluid, which stimulates respiratory centers in the brain stem. People with chronically high PCO_2 levels no longer respond to the PCO_2 stimulus; to breathe, they must rely on their hypoxic drive, normally a weak stimulant to respiration. Low PO_2 levels stimulate chemoreceptors of the carotid bodies and the aortic arch, causing increases in tidal volume and respiratory rate. Thus, raising the PO_2 with O_2 therapy in patients with chronic obstructive pulmonary disease (including emphysema and chronic bronchitis) will depress respiration and possibly result in respiratory arrest from hypoventilation. Through a change in hydrogen-ion concentration, pH has the second strongest effect on respiration. A pH below 7.41 stimulates respiration; a pH above 7.41 inhibits it. O_2 saturation, a measure of the percentage of hemoglobin saturated with O_2 does not affect respiration because hemoglobin has no direct influence on the respiratory centers in the brain stem.

9. **Correct answer - B**

The cortex can be a voluntary, regulator of respiration; for example, a person willfully holds his breath or hyperventilates. The respiratory center of the brain lies in the medulla and the pons and contains three parts: the medulla rhythmicity center, which provides the basic rhythmicity for respiration; the apneustic center, which provides deep and prolonged inspirations when stimulated; and the pneumotaxic center, which inhibits inspiration, allowing for expiration. Carbon dioxide levels, hydrogen-ion concentration, and oxygen levels involuntarily regulate respiration.

10. **Correct answer - A**

Barrel chest, usually a response to aging or increased air trapping, is an increase in anteroposterior chest diameter. Normally, the lateral chest diameter is larger than the anteroposterior chest diameter in adults, but the two are equal in barrel chest. Congenital chest deformities include kyphosis, scoliosis, pigeon chest, and funnel chest.

11. **Correct answer - B**

In emphysema, the thorax and lungs will sound hyperresonant. Percussion helps determine if an area is filled with air, fluids, or solids; as fluids and solids replace air, the lung becomes dull to percussion. Normally, the lung is resonant to percussion but becomes hyperresonant upon air trapping, as seen in emphysema. The liver and the lung over pleural effusions will be dull to percussion.

12. **Correct answer - A**

Functional residual capacity increases in emphysema. Air trapping causes the alveoli to be distended with air, leaving more air in the lungs after expiration.

13. **Correct answer - A**

Functional residual capacity is the volume of air remaining in the lungs after a normal expiration. It is a combination of the expiratory reserve volume (maximal exhalation after tidal volume is expired) and residual volume (volume of air remaining in the lungs after a maximal exhalation). Functional residual capacity cannot be easily measured at the bedside because residual volume cannot be directly measured by a spirometer. However, functional residual capacity can be measured, if necessary, by body plethysmography and helium dilution. Forced vital capacity is a maximal exhalation after a maximal inhalation.

14. **Correct answer - A**

Systemic responses to chronic obstructive pulmonary disease do not include splenomegaly. Pulmonary hypertension results from long-standing lung disease and can lead to right ventricular failure. Signs of right ventricular failure include distended neck veins and hepatomegaly. So that more oxygen can be carried to body tissues, polcythemia (increased production of red blood cells) occurs in response to chronic hypoxia. Clubbing of the fingers also results from chronic hypoxia, although the reason for this is unknown.

15. **Correct answer - D**

Chronic hypoxia causes increased erythropoiesis, the stimulation of red blood cell production, to compensate for chronically low PO_2 levels. The bone marrow is stimulated to produce more red blood cells, a condition known as secondary polycythemia. Chronic hypoxia also causes a compensatory increase in cardiac output. Central (not peripheral) cyanosis occurs in hypoxia. Peripheral cyanosis results from a lack of blood flow to an extremity. Anemia is important during acute hypoxic episodes because decreased red blood cell production reduces the blood's oxygen-carrying capacity, exacerbating hypoxia.

16. **Correct answer - A**

In clients with pulmonary disease and hypercapnea, a high fat, low carbohydrate diet is recommended. Carbon dioxide is produced from metabolism, especially from metabolism of carbohydrates, and may contribute to increase PCO_2 levels. Fats cause less CO_2 production than carbohydrates (and proteins as well) so a diet high in fat and low in carbohydrates is recommended in patients with COPD with CO_2 retention.

17. **Correct answer - C**

Pulmonary capillary wedge pressure reflects functioning of the left side of the heart, which is not usually impaired in pulmonary hypertension. Pulmonary hypertension increases pulmonary vascular resistance, the resistance to forward flow through the pulmonary blood vessels. Pulmonary hypertension also impedes ejection of blood from the right side of the heart into the pulmonary circulation and is reflected by hemodynamic changes - increases in right atrial, right ventricular, and pulmonary artery pressures.

18. **Correct answer - B**

Due to negative inspiratory effort, there is a decrease in waveform pressures during inspiration in the spontaneously breathing patient. During positive pressure mechanical ventilation, there is a rise in waveform pressures during mechanically ventilated inspiration. It is recommended that waveform pressures be measured during end expiration in both the spontaneously breathing and ventilated patients in order to obtain correct values.

19.   **Correct answer - A**

A mixed venous PO_2 of 35 mm Hg indicates adequate tissue perfusion (normal is 35 to 40 mm HG). This implies adequate ventilation and circulation. A low mixed venous PO_2 is due to ventilatory hypoxia (tissues extract their normal amount of oxygen, sending deoxygenated blood back to the right of the heart) or diminished cardiac output (blood flow is sluggish through the capillaries, allowing tissues to extract more than the normal amount of oxygen). Comparing the mixed venous sample with an arterial sample and determining cardiac output will indicate which problem is at fault. Blood gases, whether arterial or mixed venous, should always be interpreted in light of the patient's history and past blood gas readings to determine a chronic acidotic state.

20.   **Correct answer - C**

A mixed venous blood sample helps assess ventilation and circulation, whereas an arterial sample helps assess ventilation and the circulation to the extremity from which it was drawn. A mixed venous sample is drawn from the pulmonary artery (distal) port of a Swan-Ganz catheter and is a sample of deoxygenated blood. It is not drawn from the right atrial (proximal) port because the interior vena caval venous return enters the low right atrium and might be excluded from a right atrial sampling. A mixed venous sample does not replace the need for an arterial sample; rather, it should be used with an arterial sample for total assessment of cardiopulmonary functioning.

21.   **Correct answer - C**

Peaked P waves are a common ECG change in patients with chronic obstructive pulmonary disease. Pulmonary hypertension stresses the right side of the heart, causing right atrial enlargement and position change. Incomplete right bundle branch block (RBBB) commonly occurs because of these rotational changes and right ventricular hypertrophy; complete RBBB is rare. Pulmonary hypertension does not affect the left side of the heart, so left ventricular hypertrophy will not be observed. ST and T wave changes are rare, seen only with right ventricular hypertrophy in the early precordial leads.

22.   Correct answer - B

Serum alpha antitrypsin is an enzyme inhibitor; its deficiency is thought to cause enzymal destruction of lung tissue. It is an autosomal recessive trait, usually noted in whites of European descent, and its appearance can signal familial emphysema. Symptoms can occur from the teenage years until early middle age. Familial emphysema accounts for only 1% to 2% of all people with chronic obstructive pulmonary disease.

$NaCL \Rightarrow Na+HCO_3 \Rightarrow [Cl \text{ excreted}]$

23.   Correct answer - B

Electrolyte imbalances resulting from chronic hypoxia include low chloride levels. In response to chronic respiratory acidosis, the kidney acts to correct this imbalance by retaining the base bicarbonate (in the form of sodium bicarbonate) in exchange for the acid chloride (in the form of sodium chloride). Also, increased ammonia (an acid) excretion occurs in the form of ammonium chloride. Thus, in chronic respiratory acidosis, elevated bicarbonate levels and low chloride levels will be noted. Sodium ions are reabosorbed as hydrogen ions are secreted. This maintains an appropriate electrical balance between the anions and cations in the tubular and extracellular fluid. Acidosis does not affect calcium levels.

24.   Correct answer - C

Most people with chronic obstructive pulmonary disease (COPD) are current or former smokers. Smoking reduces the activity of cilia and macrophages and induces bronchoconstriction. This increases sputum production and the risk of respiratory infection and decreases pulmonary functions. Other causes of COPD include aging, pollution, long-term occupational exposure to dust or fumes, allergies, heredity, and frequent respiratory infections.

25.   Correct answer - A

Pursed-lip breathing prevents air trapping and airway collapse. In patients with COPD, diseased airways easily collapse on expiration from increased intrathoracic pressure, causing air trapping in the alveoli. Pursed-lip breathing allows air to be exhaled more slowly, because the lips partially obstruct the air. Airway pressure increases in relation to intrathoracic pressure, preventing airway collapse. Pursed-lip breathing does not affect surface tension, or surfactant.

26.   Correct answer - D

Atmospheric pressure decreases as altitude increases, so O_2 saturation is usually lower at higher altitudes. Because the percentage of oxygen in the air remains the same, the partial pressure of oxygen also drops. This lowers arterial PO_2 and, to a lesser extent, O_2 saturation. Later, PCO_2 levels drop - and the pH level may rise - as a result of hyperventilation, a response to hypoxia.

27.   Correct answer - B

Room air PO_2 drops from 160 mm Hg to 104 mm Hg and the PN_2 drops from 597 to 569 mm Hg in the alveolus to accommodate the addition of carbon dioxide and water vapor; atmospheric air contains little of either. By the time air reaches the alveolus, it is totally humidified with water vapor, which has a partial pressure of 47 mm Hg. Alveolar air contains about 40 mm Hg of carbon dioxide. This addition of water vapor and carbon dioxide dilutes the partial pressures of oxygen and nitrogen because the total pressure cannot rise above 760 mm Hg atmospheric pressure. The diffusion gradient and venous admixture from normal physiologic shunting cause the PO_2 to drop from 104 to 95 mm Hg as it crosses from the alveolus into the arterial system.

28.   Correct answer - A

The arterial blood gas results indicate uncompensated respiratory alkalosis. The pH is elevated (normal is 7.35 to 7.45), indicating an alkalotic state. HCO_3 is normal (22 to 26 mEq/liter), ruling out a metabolic component, either primary or compensatory. The PCO_2 is decreased (normal is 35 to 45 mm Hg), indicating respiratory alkalosis.

29.   Correct answer - B

The most probable cause is hyperventilation due to anxiety and bronchial constriction from asthma. Hypoventilation causes respiratory acidosis. A side effect of steroids, such as prednisone, is metabolic alkalosis. Side effects of theophylline toxicity do not include an acid-base imbalance.

30.   Correct answer - D

Associated symptoms likely for Mr. D are numbness, tingling to extremities, and perioral tingling. Headache and somnolence are symptoms of metabolic acidosis, nausea and vomiting are associated with metabolic alkalosis. Decreased ventilation and constricted pupils are symptoms of respiratory acidosis from narcotic overdose.

31.   Correct answer - A

Venturi oxygen therapy allows accurate oxygen concentration by mixing oxygen with entrained air; it cannot deliver oxygen concentrations higher than 40% to 50% depending on the mask, because the oxygen is diluted during mixing. Delivery of low concentrations of oxygen through Venturi oxygen therapy is especially useful in patients with chronic obstructive pulmonary disease (COPD). A partial rebreathing mask conserves oxygen through rebreathing one-third of expired air from a reservoir bag and can deliver up to 90% oxygen. Nasal cannulas, which deliver a low percentage of oxygen through two soft plastic tubes inserted into the nostrils, are useful to nose breathers and those with COPD.

32.   Correct answer - A

Vesicular breath sounds have a short expiration phase, are soft in nature, and are normally heard over most of the lung. Bronchial breath sounds have a long expiration phase, sound tubular, and are normally heard over the trachea. Bronchovesicular lung sounds are a combination of the above two and have equal inspiration and expiration phases. They are heard over large airways. Suspect consolidation, tumor, or atelectasis when bronchial or bronchovesicular breath sounds are heard where vesicular breath sounds are normally heard.

33.   Correct answer - A

Propranolol (Inderal) is contraindicated in asthma because it may cause bronchospasm. Propranolol blocks the beta-adrenergic effects of the sympathetic nervous system, such as increased heart rate and contractility, as well as bronchodilation. Newer beta-blocking agents, such as atenolol and metoprolol, are cardioselective, blocking the beta effects on the heart without inducing bronchoconstriction. These are considered safe, in low doses, for patients with asthma.

34.   Correct answer - A

A patient with extrinsic asthma may have status asthmaticus precipitated by hay fever. Extrinsic asthma is caused by allergens (including ragweed, shellfish, and drugs, such as penicillin) that release histamines, leading to increased mucus production and bronchoconstriction. Intrinsic asthma is nonallergic; attacks are precipitated by smoke, exercise, respiratory infection, or emotional distress. These factors induce bronchial irritation or bronchoconstriction.

35.   Correct answer - C

Hypercapnia associated with asthma occurs during severe airway obstruction. Asthma is characterized by increased responsiveness of the airway to stimuli that cause airway constriction. In less severe asthma attacks, the PCO_2 level is low because of hyperventilation, and the patient develops respiratory alkalosis. As airway obstruction increases, carbon dioxide is retained and respiratory acidosis ensues. Airway obstruction results from airway narrowing and mucous plugs; immediate therapy must be initiated to prevent the patient from developing respiratory arrest or status asthmaticus.

36.   Correct answer - D

A disadvantage of a volume ventilator is that it delivers the set tidal volume despite the possibility of generating high peak inspiratory pressures in the patient with decreased lung compliance. This increases the risk of barotrauma. Positive end-expiratory pressure can be initiated while the patient is on a volume ventilator. Some pressure ventilators lack an adequate alarm system. With all pressure ventilators, hypoventilation may ensue if set pressures are reached

138

early, as in the patient with decreased lung compliance.

37.   Correct answer - C

Talking at the nurses' station, ventilatory alarms, and continuous lighting of the critical care unit can cause the patient to experience sensory overload, a state that occurs from an increase in frequency of stimuli. Sensory deprivation is a decrease in such frequency. Sensory monotony, which can be either overload or deprivation, is simply monotonous stimuli: a windowless room or a continuous meaningless noise, such as the beeping of a heart monitor. Excessive noise or stimuli induce stress, depriving a compromised patient of much-needed sleep. The patient can become confused or hostile and may hallucinate. This response, along with medications that may alter perceptions, leads to ICU (intensive care unit) psychosis.

38.   Correct answer - A

Neostigmine, an anticholinesterase that prevents acetylcholine breakdown by its enzyme cholinesterase, thus improving impulse transmission, reverses the effects of pancuronium bromide (Pavulon). Atropine is not an antagonist of Pavulon but is administered with neostigmine to reduce the latter's side effects, such as decreased heart rate and increased bronchial secretions. Narcan is a narcotic antagonist that reverses the effects of morphine sulphate. Tubocurarine, also causing muscle paralysis, is an analog of Pavulon.

39.   Correct answer - D

The effects of neuromuscular blocking agents may be prolonged in patients with myasthenia gravis or hypothermia, and in those receiving large doses of aminoglycoside antibiotics. These agents interrupt impulses at the neuromuscular junction, where motor nerve meets muscle fiber. Patients with myasthenia gravis already have an impairment at the neuromuscular junction, due to accelerated breakdown of acetylcholine, which transmits the nervous impulses. Blood administration has no effect on the excretion of neuromuscular blocking agents.

40.   Correct answer - B

A minute ventilation between 5-10 1/minute is predictive of weaning success. Other such parameters include a vital capacity of 10-15 ml/kg, a negative inspiratory force of 20 - 30 cms H20 and a tidal volume of 4-5 ml/kg.

41.   Correct answer - D

Pressure support ventilation is a mode of ventilation useful in the weaning process because it reduces airway resistance and the work of breathing. Spontaneous breaths are supported during inspiration with a preset amount of pressure until a desired tidal volume is achieved. The amount of PSV can be decreased during weaning as the patient assumes more control over breathing.

42.   Correct answer - C

A rise in heart rate of 24 beats/minute may indicate weaning failure. Other indicators are a drop in O_2 saturation below 91%, a rise in minute ventilation above 10 1/minute and a rise in respiratory rate by 14 breaths/minute.

43.   Correct answer - B

Mouth-to-mouth ventilation during cardiopulmonary resuscitation (CPR) delivers 17% oxygen (expired air contains more carbon dioxide than room air). Artificial ventilations must be performed correctly to deliver the optimal amount of oxygen; it is most important to open the airway through forward movement of the tongue. This can be accomplished by the head-tilt, chin-lift maneuver, which lifts the chin forward and hyperextends the head. Two ventilations, lasting 1 to 1-1/2 seconds, are performed after opening the airway and before beginning cardiac compressions in a pulseless victim. As soon as possible during CPR, the nurse should switch from mouth-to-mouth resuscitation to ventilation with a manual resuscitation bag attached to high-flow oxygen.

44.   **Correct answer - B**

The left main bronchus bifurcates from the trachea at a more acute angle than the right because of the heart's position. Thus, an endotracheal tube enters the right main bronchus easier than the left. The heart's position also causes the left lung to be narrower than the right, with the left lung having only two lobes; the right has three. Because of the liver's position, the right hemidiaphragm is higher than the left, causing the right lung to be shorter. The thyroid gland and the stomach do not normally interfere with lung anatomy.

45.   **Correct answer - C**

Endotracheal tube cuff pressure should not exceed tracheal capillary filling pressure, the amount necessary to maintain an adequate blood flow to the trachea - about 15 to 25 mm Hg. If cuff pressure exceeds tracheal capillary filling pressure, tracheal ischemia, necrosis, or tracheoesophageal fistula can occur. Peak inspiratory pressure is the maximal pressure necessary to generate an inspiratory effort. End expiratory pressure is the pressure in the alveolus at the end of expiration. Pulmonary capillary wedge pressure is the vascular pressure in the pulmonary capillary bed, a direct reflection of venous return to the heart.

46.   **Correct answer - D**

If the cuff pressure in an endotracheally intubated patient requires 60 mm Hg to maintain an adequate seal, the patient probably needs a larger endotracheal tube because the cuff is overinflated on one side of the trachea and cannot adequately seal the other side. Most tracheas are oval rather than circular. A large diameter endotracheal tube (7.5 to 8 mm inner diameter for females and 8 mm or larger for males) should be inserted to ensure a proper seal. Cuff pressure does not reflect a right mainstem intubation. A leaky cuff registers low tracheal cuff pressures. High cuff pressure with a small amount of inserted air and adequate seal maintenance suggest tracheal stenosis.

47.   **Correct answer - C**

If an arterial blood gas sample is not immediately analyzed or placed on ice, the PO_2 level will decrease because blood will continue to

141

use O_2 and produce CO_2. The falsely elevated PCO_2 level will cause a falsely low pH reading. Placing the sample on ice retards this process. HCO_3 levels are usually not affected. Not using a heparinized syringe will cause the sample to clot.

48. **Correct answer - D**

The patient's pH is high (normal is 7.35 to 7.45) indicating an alkalotic state; HCO_3 is normal (22 to 26 mEq/liter), ruling out a metabolic component; and PCO_2 is low (normal is 35 to 45 mm Hg), indicating respiratory alkalosis. Respiratory alkalosis results from hyperventilation caused by nervousness, anxiety, pulmonary embolus, or too high a respiratory setting on a mechanical ventilator. Too low a setting causes the patient to override the respirator with an increased respiratory rate and, along with sepsis and liver disease, may also cause respiratory alkalosis. Cardiac arrest usually results in a mixed respiratory and metabolic acidosis due to hypoventilation and lactic acidosis.

49. **Correct answer - C**

Ms. B.'s problem would most likely be corrected by decreasing her respiratory rate, usually through sedation. Because she was overriding the ventilator with a respiratory rate of 40 breaths/minute, decreasing her intermittent mandatory ventilation (IMV) rate would not make sense. Ms. B.'s PO_2 level was satisfactory, so increasing her FIO_2 would not resolve her condition. The same holds true for the tidal volume, which would increase the PO_2 level and may further reduce the PCO_2 level.

50. **Correct answer - A**

The assist mode on a mechanical ventilator differs from IMV in that the patient triggers respiratory breaths at a set volume. Both allow the patient to generate an inspiratory effort. The assist mode allows the patient to set his own respiratory rate but, once initiated, establishes a set tidal volume. Intermittent mandatory ventilation delivers a set amount of respiratory breaths with a fixed tidal volume but also allows the patient to spontaneously breathe with a varied tidal volume.

51.   Correct answer - C

Since a patient does not receive a specific amount of tidal volume while on PSV, it is important to monitor minute ventilation and tidal volume during this mode of ventilation.

52.   Correct answer - A

This patient is receiving too much tidal volume, causing respiratory alkalosis. Reducing the amount of PSV will reduce her tidal volume and solve the problem. A patient weighing 58 kg. should have a desired tidal volume between 580 - 870 ml (10-15 ml/kg). She is not hypoxic or tachypneic so does not require a rise in FIO_2 or the institution of IMV or assist mode of ventilation.

53.   Correct Answer - B

Inspiratory pressure is an indication of inspiratory muscle strength. Measured by a pressure gauge, it is the amount of pressure needed to inflate the lungs and expand the thorax. The more negative the reading, the better the inspiratory effort. An inspiratory pressure lower than - 20 cm H_2O meets the criteria for weaning from a mechanical ventilator. The addition of positive end-expiratory pressure improves both inspiratory and expiratory pressures. Inspiratory muscles can fatigue when the work of breathing increases, as in neuromuscular disease, malnutrition, decreased compliance, hypoxia, cardiac arrest, anemia, and diminished cardiac output.

54.   Correct answer - C

The narrowest part of the airway is the larynx, specifically the vocal cords in adults and the cricoid cartilage in children. This eliminates the need for cuffed endotracheal tubes in children because the cricoid cartilage, the only complete ring of cartilage, provides a seal for the tube. Because of its narrowness, irritation or trauma to the layrnx can cause edema and airway obstruction, a true respiratory emergency. A sign of laryngeal edema is stridor, inspiratory crowing that can be audible, palpated, or auscultated over the neck.

55.   Correct answer - C

Stridor, the high-pitched crowing that is audible, palpable, or auscultated over the trachea during inspiration, is a sign of upper airway obstruction, usually indicating laryngeal edema. Crackles, rhonchi, and wheezing are signs of lower airway obstruction. Crackles are heard on inspiration in dependent areas of the lungs and usually indicate fluid in the alveoli. Rhonchi and wheezing occur when air passes through larger airways, such as the bronchi or bronchioles, that are narrowed by secretions or spasm. Rhonchi are low-pitched sounds, whereas wheezing has a much higher pitch.

56.   Correct answer - D

Tachycardia from carbon dioxide retention is an early sign of impending respiratory failure. Other early signs include restlessness, confusion, headache, somnolence, and papilledema. Cyanosis, wheezing, and intercostal retractions are late signs of respiratory failure and are not always present. For example, wheezing may occur only in bronchospasm, whereas cyanosis is a dependent characteristic that differs from patient to patient and from observer to observer.

57.   Correct answer - C

The patient in impending respiratory failure must be assessed to discover which preventative measures are needed. These measures may include opening the airway, suctioning, positioning, initiating aerosol therapy, and administering oxygen. Clinical findings, subjective information from the patient, arterial blood gas results, and chest X-rays may help in assessing the situation, but preventive care is the best way to avoid respiratory failure. Sedation, usually avoided because it can cause hypoventilation, may be necessary if mechanical ventilation is used.

58.   Correct answer - A

Acute respiratory failure in a patient with normal lung function is defined as a PCO_2 above 50 mm Hg and a PO_2 below 60 mm Hg. Hypoxia occurs with carbon dioxide retention to produce acute respiratory failure; thus, the PO_2 drops as the PCO_2 rises. When the PO_2 falls below 60 mm Hg, the percentage of saturated hemoglobin

144

dramatically drops off. The patient with chronic obstructive pulmonary disease (COPD) must be closely assessed because he lives with chronic hypoxia and hypercapnia, typically presenting with a PCO_2 of about 50 mm Hg and a PO_2 of about 60 mm Hg.

59.   Correct answer - D

Relaxation of the tongue is the most common cause of airway obstruction. This occurs in unconscious states, such as narcotic overdosage and neurologic disease, or as a result of muscle weakness secondary to neuromuscular disease. The tongue relaxes, falling back in the oral cavity and obstructing the airway. Hyperextending the neck with the patient in the supine position opens the airway and often returns spontaneous respirations in an apneic patient. Bronchospasm is a common cause of airway obstruction in patients with exacerbations of chronic obstructive pulmonary disease. Aspiration can obstruct the airway in comatose patients or in those who have lost the gag reflex. Laryngeal edema may cause airway obstruction in the postextubation period.

60.   Correct answer - D

Chronic bronchitis is associated with increased mucus production. Inflammation and hypertrophy of the mucous glands produce the typical cough and sputum production associated with chronic bronchitis. Mucus production is uncommon in primary asthma or emphysema unless chronic bronchitis or respiratory infection accompanies it. Hemoptysis (expectoration of blood) is a symptom of pulmonary emboli and chronic bronchitis.

61.   Correct answer - A

The best position for proper respiratory excursion is sitting in a chair, which allows for fuller diaphragm movement and more effective breathing and coughing while preventing atelectasis and muscle fatigue. Bed rest, including supine and semi-Fowler's positions, encourages physical inactivity, which results in muscle weakness, atelectasis and retained secretions. Most patients with chronic respiratory insufficiency cannot tolerate prolonged bed rest, especially lying flat, because they are in a state of general debilitation. The left lateral decubitus position may be used in the patient requiring bed rest, but only with the right lateral decubitus, prone and supine positions.

62.   Correct answer - D

Postural drainage should be used for the patient receiving aerosol therapy; the therapy loosens secretions, and postural drainage mobilizes them. To prevent nausea, vomiting, and aspiration, the nurse should never institute postural drainage immediately after the patient has eaten but should wait at least 1 hour. Certain patients are poor risks for postural drainage. Positioning the head lower than the body causes increased intracranial pressure, a damage to postoperative craniotomy patients. In advanced pregnancy, this position causes the fetus to move toward the lungs, impeding ventilation and possibly causing respiratory distress.

63.   Correct answer - C

During postural drainage of the anterior lower lung segments, the correct patient position is supine, with the hips elevated. Sitting upright or semireclining drains the upper lobes. Lying flat down with the hips elevated drains the posterior lower lobes. Lying on the right side with the head elevated drains the left lobe. Sitting upright and leaning forward while the nurse performs cupping and clapping above the patient's clavicles drains the apical lung segment.

64.   Correct answer - C

The correct patient position for nasotracheal suctioning is sitting up at a 45-degree angle, with the head turned away from the nares entered. This position straightens the trachea, aligns the airway, and eases entry into the bronchus. Hyperextending the head may curl the catheter at the back of the throat, and flexing the head could cause the catheter to enter the esophagus. Having the patient cough opens the epiglottis and vocal cords and may facilitate entry into the trachea.

65.   Correct answer - B

During nasotracheal suctioning, the nurse should pass the catheter until resistance is met, withdraw the catheter, and apply suction for 10 seconds. If the catheter is just passing the vocal cords, it has not yet entered the trachea or bronchus and should be advanced until resistance is met. Never advance the catheter while suctioning or after meeting resistance because trauma to the airway can ensue. To prevent hypoxia or a choking sensation, never apply suction for more than 10 seconds in a conscious patient.

66.   Correct answer - C

Immediately after an open thoracotomy, bloody drainage from the chest tube at 50 to 100 ml/hr is common. An autotransfusion would return lost blood to the patient, preventing hypovolemia from hemorrhage. An autotransfusion is possible if sterile blood is collected, as from chest drainage systems, and the procedure helps prevent risks of infection or blood incompatibilities than can occur with donated blood.

67.   Correct answer - A

A low PSV of 5 cms H_2O helps to reduce the workload of breathing during spontaneous breaths by overcoming the resistance to breathing caused by ventilatory tubing or small endotracheal tubes. Higher levels of PSV are required to overcome increased work of breathing due to disease processes or for the purpose of weaning.

68.   Correct answer - D

A chest tube should continue to drain for about 48 hours after surgery. If drainage stops in the immediate postoperative period, catheter occlusion has occurred. Fluid and air can build up in the pleural space of the affected lung, causing a tension pneumothorax. Signs of a tension pneumothorax include tracheal deviation, which should be assessed for immediately; deviation of the cardiac structures to the unaffected side; and hypotension. Notify the physician promptly if chest tube drainage stops in the immediate postoperative period.

69.   Correct answer - A

Decreasing lung compliance in a patient on a volume mechanical ventilator may be determined by a high peak inspiratory pressure.

147

Compliance helps determine lung expansibility; decreased compliance results in stiffened lungs that require more pressure to achieve the same ventilation. Peak inspiratory pressure is the amount necessary to deliver a set tidal volume in volume mechanical ventilators. In pressure ventilators, high inspiratory pressure causes a lower tidal volume to be delivered because the preset pressure is quickly reached, causing CO_2 retention. Because of this, pressure ventilators should not be used in patients at risk for decreased lung compliance. A decreasing alveolar-arterial oxygen gradient is a desired event; it will not be seen in decreased lung compliance.

70.   Correct answer - D

An increasing alveolar-arterial oxygen gradient indicates pathologic shunting due to underventilated alveoli caused by atelectasis, pulmonary edema, or pneumonia. In most cases, physiologic shunting causes an alveolar-arterial oxygen gradient of about 10 mm Hg on room air. Alveolar-arterial oxygen gradient is measured after the patient has received oxygen therapy at 100% for 15 minutes to wash out all nitrogen from the alveoli, after which all that remains in the alveolus is oxygen, water vapor (47 mm Hg), and carbon dioxide. Alveolar oxygen is measured by subtracting water vapor and the measured PCO_2 from atmospheric pressure (760 mm Hg), multiplying the result by the percentage of FIO_2 the patient is receiving, then subtracting the measured PO_2. The normal alveolar-arterial oxygen gradient on 100% oxygen is 30 to 50 mm Hg. Alveolar-arterial oxygen gradient is increased by uneven ventilation in relation to perfusion. In pulmonary embolism, perfusion is interrupted; thus, the alveolar-arterial oxygen gradient does not usually indicate pulmonary embolism. A small alveolar-arterial oxygen gradient is desired and will occur in eupnea, or normal breathing. Increased dead space, as in emphysema, may result in an increased alveolar-arterial oxygen gradient through hypoventilation and hypercapnia without a compensatory increase in minute ventilation.

71.   Correct answer - A

Normal physiologic shunting, about 2% to 5% of cardiac output, causes the alveolar PO_2 to drop from 104 to 95 mm Hg as it enters the arterial system. Venous return from the bronchial and thebesian

148

venous circulation delivers deoxygenated blood to the pulmonary veins and left side of the heart, respectively. Pathologic shunting occurs in states of decreased ventilation, when blood perfusing underventilated regions returns poorly oxygenated to the arterial system. Breathing 100% oxygen will not correct pathologic shunting because this does not open alveoli and blood remains poorly oxygenated.

72.   **Correct answer - C**

Adult respiratory distress syndrome (ARDS) is characterized by high peak inspiratory pressures, large alveolar-arterial oxygen gradient, pulmonary edema, and decreased lung compliance. For an unknown reason, damage to the alveolocapillary membrane occurs, causing pulmonary capillary fluid leakage and results in a diffusion defect and pulmonary edema. This fluid leakage decreases surfactant, which causes a stiffening of the lung, or decreased compliance. Higher pressures must be generated to do the same work of breathing to overcome the lung stiffness. Hypoxia and atelectasis result.

73.   **Correct answer - C**

The goal of treatment for ARDS is to increase functional residual capacity, the volume of air remaining in the lungs at the end of a normal expiration. Such an increase forces collapsed alveoli to open, an effect usually achieved by instituting positive end-expiratory pressure. Increasing PCO_2 elimination, decreasing respiratory rate, and increasing tidal volume help reduce respiratory insufficiency but do not reverse ARDS. Damage to the alveolocapillary membrane impairs oxygen rather than carbon dioxide diffusion, because carbon dioxide is 20 times more soluble than oxygen.

74.   **Correct answer - C**

ARDS causes increased shunting, the blood returning partially unoxygenated to the left side of the heart. The disease can be caused by hypoalbuminemia, in which osmotic pressure decreases, allowing fluid to leak in the pulmonary capillaries. This fluid leakage decreases surfactant, which stiffens the lung, thus decreasing lung compliance. On autopsy, the diseased lung looks like the liver, dark and tough; hence, some people use the term "liver lung" when referring to ARDS.

75.   Correct answer -D

Surfactant, produced by alveolar epithelial cells, alters surface tension with alveolar volume. As the volume in the alveolus decreases during expiration, surfactant concentrates and decreases surface tension, preventing alveolar collapse. During inspiration, surfactant spreads over a larger area, increasing surface tension. Reduced surfactant reduces compliance, stiffening the lung. This increases the work of breathing, creating hypoxia and respiratory acidosis. Atelectasis, ARDS, near-drowning, and oxygen toxicity are some causes of reduced surfactant.

76.   Correct answer - C

A decrease in the colloid osmotic pressure exerted by albumin and other proteins in the blood to keep fluid in the intravascular system may cause the pulmonary capillary leakage typical of ARDS. Normally, colloid osmotic pressure is 8 to 25 mm Hg higher than pulmonary capillary wedge pressure. If the wedge pressure rises or the colloid osmotic pressure drops, fluid leaks from the blood into the pulmonary interstitium, the hallmark of ARDS.

77.   Correct answer - A

Carbon dioxide is about 20 times more soluble than oxygen. As a result, if damage to the alveolocapillary membrane occurs, oxygen diffusion is more severely impaired than carbon dioxide diffusion. Gas solubility determines its rate of diffusion across the alveolocapillary membrane, a rate also affected by thickness and surface area of the membrane and pressure differences between the two sides of the membrane.

78.   Correct answer - B

Most carbon dioxide is carried in the blood as bicarbonate, through the conversion of carbon dioxide and water, with the assistance of the enzyme carbon anhydrase. From 60% to 70% of carbon dioxide is carried in this manner; 7% to 10% is physically dissolved as arterial PCO_2. The remainder is carried in chemical combination with hemoglobin as carbaminohemoglobin.

79.   Correct answer - B

Use of positive end-expiratory pressure (PEEP) in a patient with hypovolemia will most likely result in a low cardiac output. Hypovolemia is a decrease in circulating blood volume. Applying PEEP increases intrathoracic pressure, which may compress the heart and blood vessels, especially the low-pressure venous system. Venous return to the heart decreases, further exacerbating the hypovolemia. Since venous return to the heart is a major determinant of cardiac output, a decreased venous return accompanied by hypovolemia is certain to result in a low cardiac output and a low pulmonary capillary wedge pressure. Once the cardiac output drops, hypoxia and dysrhythmias may occur as a result of decreased tissue perfusion.

80.   Correct answer - A

Hemodynamically, PEEP causes an increase in pulmonary vascular resistance, the resistance to forward blood flow in the pulmonary vasculature. Applying pressure to the thorax, as occurs in PEEP, increases the resistance. PEEP decreases venous return to the heart (preload), which in turn decreases cardiac output. A drop in cardiac output may decrease blood pressure.

81.   Correct answer - C

Pneumothorax is a complication of PEEP. Applying positive pressure may cause barotrauma to weakened lung tissue, causing tearing and resulting in a tension pneumothorax. Air builds up in the pleural space because it has no avenue of escape. This may reduce cardiac output or cause compression of the mediastinum, heart, or trachea. The goal of PEEP is to prevent alveolar collapse, which can occur in pulmonary edema, atelectasis, ARDS, and respiratory failure. Decreased venous return to the heart can lead to liver congestion, decreased cardiac output, and hypotension.

82.   Correct answer - A

An increasing alveolar-arterial oxygen gradient is a sign of oxygen toxicity, along with dyspnea, decreased lung compliance, and

151

paresthesias in extremities. Long-term use of high percentages of oxygen reduces surfactant and destroys alveolar tissue. Oxygen toxicity can also result in central nervous system disturbances, such as paresthesias and seizures.

83.   Correct answer - C

A patient can develop oxygen toxicity after breathing 100% oxygen for 6 hours. To reduce the likelihood of oxygen toxicity, oxygen therapy should not exceed 40% if in use longer than 48 hours. This limitation can create a dilemma if the patient continues to have a low PO_2 after being treated with high FIO_2 although PEEP may resolve the low PO_2 and reduce the high FIO_2.

84.   Correct answer -C

Atelectasis is a complication of oxygen therapy. When high percentages of oxygen are delivered, the airways contain less nitrogen, a condition known as nitrogen washout. Subsequently, the alveolus contains only oxygen, carbon dioxide, and water vapor. If the airway becomes occluded by secretions, oxygen diffuses into the pulmonary capillary, leaving nothing in the alveolus, and it collapses.

85.   Correct answer - D

In inverse ratio ventilation, more time is spent in inspiration than expiration. A problem that may occur is air trapping, referred to as "auto-PEEP", which occurs if the next inspiration begins before the patient has completed expiration. Airway pressure should be monitored at the end of expiration by occluding the expiratory valve on the ventilator to determine the development of auto-PEEP.

86.   Correct answer - A

Since breathing patterns are reversed in inverse ratio ventilation with more time being spent in inspiration than expiration, patient discomfort and anxiety may result from the inability to exhale when desired. Patients may complain of a feeling of fullness or bloatedness and sedation may be required to reduce discomfort and anxiety.

87. **Correct answer - C**

A patient in septic shock should be assessed for adult respiratory distress syndrome (ARDS). Capillary leakage, the cause of ARDS, occurs as the late phase of septic shock develops, causing a relative fluid volume deficit.

88. **Correct answer - D**

Kerley's B lines on chest X-ray indicate pulmonary edema and mitral stenosis. Horizontal, linear shadows in the lower, peripheral lung fields, Kerley's B lines are thought to be caused by increased lymphatic drainage resulting from elevated pulmonary capillary wedge pressure. They appear most clearly during inspiration and usually disappear on resolution of pulmonary edema unless fibrosis has occurred. Vascular markings will not appear on the affected side of pneumothorax; a shift in the trachea and heart may occur. Chest X-rays are not usually diagnostic of pulmonary emboli. The chest X-ray of the patient with emphysema will reflect overinflation through a lowered diaphragm and flattened costophrenic angles.

89. **Correct answer - C**

The mediastinal surface where the pulmonary blood vessels and the bronchi enter the lung is called the hilar area, or hilus. It is visible on chest X-ray as the area on either side of the sternum with clear, light vascular markings. The hilar area is also where the visceral pleural folds back to become the parietal pleura.

90. **Correct answer - C**

A shift to the right of the oxyhemoglobin dissociation curve may be due to acidosis (see figure below). The oxyhemoglobin curve is a nonlinear, empirical description of the relationship between the partial pressure of oxygen in the blood and the actual amount of oxygen carried on the hemoglobin molecule (O_2 saturation). At the upper flat end of the curve, large changes in PO_2 are associated with small changes in O_2 saturation, but along the lower steep portion of the curve, small changes in PO_2 are associated with large changes in O_2 saturation. A shift of the curve to the right allows more O_2 to be released from hemoglobin for a given PO_2, and is caused by acidosis, CO_2 retention, hyperthermia, and increased 2,3-diphosphoglycerate (2,3-DPG). A shift of the curve to the left impairs the release of oxygen from hemoglobin for a given PO_2 and is caused by alkalosis, hypocarbia, hypothermia, and decreased 2,3-DPG.

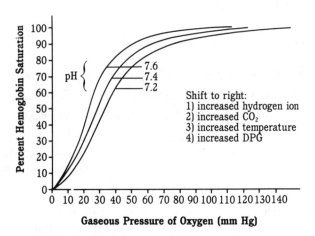

Figure 1. Shift of the oxygen-hemoglobin dissociation curve to the right by increases in (1) hydrogen ions, (2) CO_2, (3) temperature, or (4) DPG. Adapted from A. Guyton, *Textbook of Medical Physiology*, 7th ed. Philadelphia: W.B. Saunders, 1986, p. 498.

91. **Correct answer - B**

2,3-DPG, a metabolite of glucose that is contained in the red blood cell, decreases the affinity of hemoglobin for oxygen, thus increasing oxygen uptake at the cellular level. In other words, 2,3-DPG shifts the oxyhemoglobin dissociation curve to the right. Increased 2,3-DPG levels occur in anemia and hypoxia, compensating for the tissue hypoxia created by these conditions.

92. **Correct answer - C**

Laryngeal edema is the most common complication of intubation and mechanical ventilation. Because the larynx is the narrowest part of the airway, it is most at risk for edema. The patient must be closely watched in the postextubation period for signs of laryngeal edema, especially stridor. Aggressive therapy to avoid reintubation includes humidification of the airway and sympathomimetic aerosol therapy. However, reintubation and eventual tracheostomy may be necessary.

Barotrauma, or rupture of lung tissue, is a rare complication mostly associated with PEEP. Starvation is another infrequent complication indirectly related to mechanical ventilation; it occurs if a time lag exists between the institution of mechanical ventilation and the institution of an alternate means of proper nutrition. Tracheosophageal fistula is a rare, late complication that results from tracheal damage and may not occur until the postextubation period.

93.   Correct answer - D

If a mechanical ventilator's low pressure alarm is triggered and you have checked the system for a disconnection, your next action should be to aerate the patient manually until the cause is determined. A low-pressure alarm indicates that the patient is disconnected from the ventilator and is not receiving the desired tidal volume. In many cases, the disconnection is not readily apparent; manual aeration prevents hypoxia until the problem has been rectified. A high-pressure alarm indicates rising pressures within the system from water obstructing the tubing, secretions obstructing the airway, or decreased lung compliance. Never bypass the alarm or reset the alarm limits

94.   Correct answer - A

The effect of sighs can be achieved in mechanical ventilation by increasing the tidal volume. A healthy person sighs every few minutes to reexpand alveoli when breathing at a normal tidal volume of 5 ml/kg. When mechanical ventilation was first instituted, therapy mimicked normal breathing. Later, it was found that increasing the tidal volume on mechanical ventilators to 10 to 15 ml/kg obviated the need for sighs.

95.   Correct answer - D

Vital capacity is the amount of air that can be maximally exhaled after a maximal inhalation. It is decreased by conditions that reduce thoracic expansion, such as muscle weakness, pleural effusions, pneumothorax, incisional pain, and abdominal distention. Minute ventilation is the amount of air breathed in and out in 1 minute; tidal volume is the amount of air breathed in and out in one breath. Residual volume is the amount of air remaining in the lungs after a maximal exhalation.

96. **Correct answer - A**

A tracheostomy does not provide humidification to the airway; it bypasses the upper airways where humidification occurs. Thus, humidification must always be provided artificially. A tracheostomy decreases dead space (the amount of tidal volume that does not take part in gas exchange), bypasses narrowed upper airways if laryngeal stenosis occurs, and proves effective in long-term airway management.

97. **Correct answer - A**

Always use humidification with a tracheostomy to prevent airway obstruction by dried secretions because a tracheostomy decreases the dead space that permits natural airway humidification. The inner cannula can be removed for cleaning and when capping a fenestrated tracheostomy tube. The cuff must be kept inflated only if the patient is on a mechanical ventilator or has no gag reflex. Otherwise, it may be deflated to increase airway size and prevent impinging on the esophagus. Ensuring that the patient can talk is unnecessary before capping a tracheostomy tube. Alternate means of communication, such as writing paper or an alphabet board, can suffice.

98. **Correct answer - A**

Hemorrhage resulting from a tracheostomy is due to erosion of the innominate artery, also known as the brachiocephalic artery, which arises off the aortic arch and lies alongside the trachea to the right. Later, it divides into the right subclavian and right carotid arteries. Initial treatment of such a hemorrhage includes slowly pulling the tracheostomy tube out, with the cuff inflated, until the cuff is against the hemorrhage site and hemostasis can occur. In most cases, the artery must then be repaired surgically.

99. **Correct answer - C**

Continuous positive airway pressure may be used to wean a patient on positive end-expiratory pressure (PEEP). The former uses positive pressure without machine-assisted breaths; the latter uses both. Continuous positive airway pressure provides increased intrathoracic pressure during expiration of spontaneous breaths; therefore, it is contraindicated in apneic patients. As spontaneous breathing increases, machine-delivered breaths can be reduced and positive pressure can still be maintained during expiration to prevent alveolar collapse. However, extubating a patient who requires positive pressure is not recommended because hypoxia quickly returns. Using continuous positive airway pressure in a patient who requires high FIO2 is also not recommended. Such a patient needs ventilatory assistance from PEEP.

100. Correct answer - B

Mechanical ventilation, by nature a closed system, does not allow for exhalation of water vapor. This can lead to overhydration, hyponatremia, and weight gain. Factors that determine the amount of water vapor a gas can hold include the temperature, partial pressure, and solubility of the gas. Inspired dry gas is irritating because it pulls moisture from the airway to become fully saturated by the time it reaches the alveoli. The warmer a gas is, the more water vapor it can hold.

101. Correct answer - C

If your patient's tracheostomy tube falls out, reinsert it using the obturator. The obturator is a rounded-end stylet that prevents the blunt end of the tracheostomy tube from causing trauma to the trachea during insertion. This should always be kept near the patient's bedside in case of such an occurrence. After inserting the obturator into the tracheostomy tube, make sure the cuff is deflated, and then insert the tube through the stoma. Usually, insertion is easier if the patient's head is hyperextended.

102. Correct answer - A

Cyanosis, a bluish tinge to the skin, is a result of unsaturated hemoglobin; poorly oxygenated blood is bluish purple. Cyanosis usually is not evident until the arterial oxygen saturation level drops to about 80% or unless the blood contains nonfunctional hemoglobin (as in methemglobinemia) or at least 5 mg of unsaturated hemoglobin per 100 ml. Cyanosis is a relatively late sign of hypoxia. Patients with anemia will not demonstrate cyanosis as a result of low hemoglobin levels.

103. Correct answer - A

When capping a fenestrated, cuffed tracheostomy tube, you should deflate the cuff. The patient is no longer aerating through the tracheostomy when it is capped and must breathe around it. Deflating the cuff increases the airway's diameter, most likely preventing partial airway obstruction. The cap is inserted after removing the inner cannula. Oxygen must then be provided through a face mask or nasal cannula. The patient will then be able to speak because expired air passes through the larynx instead of the stoma.

104. Correct answer - D

Patients with chronic obstructive pulmonary disease usually do not develop Cheyne-Stokes respirations, which are characterized by alternating periods of hyperventilation and apnea. They are thought to be due to changing carbon dioxide levels in the blood. As respirations increase, carbon dioxide levels decrease, which suppresses the respiratory center's drive to breathe. Then, as respirations decrease, carbon dioxide levels increase, causing hyperventilation and further perpetuating the cycle. Cheyne-Stokes respirations are normal during sleep in children and the elderly. They are also seen in congestive heart failure and brain damage.

105. Correct answer - C

In a flail chest, the flail portion bulges out during expiration, pulling the mediastinum toward the affected side. This depresses ventilation and cardiac performance. During inspiration, air is sucked in from the flail portion because of the negative intrathoracic pressure depressing it, shifting the mediastinum to the unaffected side.

106. Correct answer - A

Blebs are pockets of air found within the pleural space, whereas bullae are found within lung tissue. When blebs rupture, they usually cause a spontaneous pneumothorax. Both blebs and bullae can result from chronic, long-standing air trapping, as seen in emphysema. When they become too large and impinge on normal lung tissue or cause multiple spontaneous pneumothoraxes, they are surgically resected.

158

107. Correct answer - B

A complication of pneumothorax, subcutaneous emphysema (also known as crepitus) is the accumulation of air in the subcutaneous portions of the skin. The air has escaped from the lung and may travel up the neck or down the abdomen. Treatment is aimed at removing the cause, and skin maybe incised to release air if it causes too much discomfort.

108. Correct answer - D

When correctly placed, the lumen of a chest tube is situated in the pleural space, thus allowing for air or fluid drainage and lung reexpansion. Usually, the chest tubes pass through the intercostal spaces to reach the pleural space. If chest tubes were placed in the intra-alveolar space, they would be within the lung, which would, in essence, be a pneumothorax. If chest tubes are in the pericardial space, they would be situated in the lining of the heart.

109. Correct answer - C

In chest tube therapy, the length of the glass tube below the water surface of the suction-control bottle determines the amount of suction. Usually, this length is between 10 to 20 cm. Each centimeter the glass tube is submerged equals 1 cm of suction. Chest tubes should not be routinely stripped. If there is an obstruction by a blood clot, however, the chest tube should always be stripped away from the patient to prevent obstruction of the tubes by blood clots. In three-bottle suction, the first bottle is the drainage bottle, the second is the water-seal bottle, and the third is the suction-control bottle. Oscillation of the underwater seal fluid with ventilation indicates that the lung has not yet reexpanded.

110. Correct answer - A

Clamping a chest tube may cause tension pneumothorax. Clamping prevents air or fluid escape from the pleural space and, if dangerous buildup occurs, tension pneumothorax can ensue. Therefore, the nurse should never clamp a chest tube for more than a few seconds, except in the event of tube disconnection or bottle breakage or when changing or removing the system.

111. **Correct answer - D**

No adventitious breath sounds are present on the affected side in a tension pneumothorax because the lung has collapsed and no air movement occurs. The trachea may deviate to the unaffected side because of air buildup in the affected pleura. Because the pleura is filled with air, the affected side of hyperresonant to percussion with decreased fremitus, breath sounds, and heart sounds. Other symptoms include pleuritic chest pain, dyspnea, and hemoptysis.

112. **Correct answer - B**

If the patient's chest tube is connected to an underwater seal drainage system, bubbling in the under water seal area during expiration demonstrates that an air leak exists and that the lung has still not fully reexpanded. Constant bubbling during inspiration and expiration in the suction control manometer indicates the application of suction. Subcutaneous emphysema is usually noted by palpating the patient's skin along the insertion site for crackles.

113. **Correct answer - B**

Progressive subcutaneous emphysema in the patient with a chest tube usually signifies that the chest tube needs repositioning. Subcutaneous emphysema is the collection of air under the skin; in the patient with a chest tube, this indicates that the lumen of the tube is not totally in the pleural space or that the seal around the exit of the chest tube from the pleural space is not tight enough. Progressive subcutaneous emphysema can be uncomfortable and unsightly for the patient.

114. **Correct answer - C**

In high-frequency jet ventilation, respiratory rates are 100 to 200 breaths/minute. Under low pressure, small jets of entrained air enter the airway through an additional catheter or port on the endotracheal tube. This ventilation method, which enhances diffusion of oxygen and carbon dioxide across the alveolocapillary membrane, is useful in atelectasis and ARDS, presumably because it protects surfactant. Low tidal volumes of 2.5 to 3.5 ml/kg help prevent the barotrauma and decreased cardiac output associated with PEEP.

115. **Correct answer - C** "ATELECTASIS
AIRWAY
COLLAPS-

Insufficient humidification may result in high frequency jet ventilation, resulting in thick secretions and possible mucus plugs. Frequent suctioning may be required. Amount and consistency of secretions should be frequently assessed.

116. **Correct answer - A**

High frequency jet ventilation is indicated in patients with flail chest because it aids in stabilization of the chest wall. Since small tidal volumes are used in this mode of ventilation, chest excursion is minimized. This aids in preventing paradoxical respirations and allows the flail chest to heal.

117. **Correct answer - D**

Because of the constant flow of gas and small tidal volumes produced, lung sounds are difficult to assess in the patient receiving high frequency jet ventilation. Use of the manual resuscitation bag to augment lung sounds may be necessary.

118. **Correct answer - B**

A patient on a ventilator who feels unable to control her environment is experiencing powerlessness. The critical care environment reinforces this feeling by curtailing the patient's activity, taking away familiar aspects of her environment, and frightening her about the tenuousness of her mortality. The patient's family may also feel powerless because they can see their loved one only during prescribed hours and cannot always get information about her condition. The nurse can alleviate this powerlessness by acting as a patient-family advocate - supplying needed information, allowing the patient to make some decisions about her care and environment, and involving the family in the patient's care.

119. **Correct answer - A**

An increase in fremitus (the vibrations that reflect voice transmission through the lungs onto the chest wall, palpated by an examiner's hands when the patient speaks) may be noted in atelectasis.

161

120. Correct answer - C

Sound, as in fremitus, is best conducted through solid material, less through fluids, and least through air. Fremitus is increased when solid material replaces air in lung tissue, such as in pneumonia, atelectasis, tumors, and pulmonary fibrosis. Fremitus is decreased when fluid or increased air accumulation prevents sound transmission, such as in pleural effusions, emphysema, and pneumothorax. In the normal lung, fremitus is felt as soft vibrations on speaking that diminish toward the lower lobes.

121. Correct answer - A

The acid-base imbalance is compensated metabolic alkalosis. The pH is normal, indicating a compensated state but tending toward the alkalotic state. The bicarbonate is high, matching the alkalosis and indicating that the primary event is metabolic. The PCO_2 is high, indicating compensatory respiratory acidosis.

122. Correct answer - B

Causes of metabolic alkalosis include vomiting, diuretic treatment, corticosteroid administration, Cushing's disease, aldosteronism, and nasogastric suction. These cause either gastric acid loss or increased renal acid excretion. With diarrhea, the patient loses large amounts of bicarbonate, which results in metabolic acidosis.

123. Correct answer - A

Acetazolamide (Diamox) is used to correct metabolic alkalosis, a condition characterized by excess bicarbonate. Bicarbonate is formed through the conversion of carbon dioxide and water with the assistance of the enzyme carbonic anhydrase. Acetazolamide is a potent carbonic anhydrase inhibitor, promoting diuresis and excretion of HCO3. Overuse of acetazolamide can lead to metabolic acidosis.

124. Correct answer - D

Blunting on a chest X-ray of the costophrenic angle, the area where

162

the diaphragm meets the rib cage at the lower, lateral aspects of the lung fields, is most characteristic of pleural effusions. Normally, this angle should be clearly visualized. Blunting indicates pleural effusions because fluid is gravity-dependent, accumulating in the lower lung fields when the patient sits upright. Pulmonary embolism does not usually produce changes on the chest X-ray, although changes in vascular markings occasionally occur. Pneumothorax may be suspected if a dark area appears between the ribs and the lung fields at the outer border of the lung fields, or if the trachea, mediastinum, and heart are shifted abnormally. Atelectasis may produce areas of increased density on chest X-ray, where white replaces black.

125. Correct answer - B

The amount of cardiac output that does not take part in gas exchange is called shunting. Physiologic shunting, normally 2% to 5% of the cardiac output, is a result of the venous return of the bronchial circulation to the pulmonary veins and thebesian venous return to the left side of the heart. Pathologic shunting occurs when ventilation to a portion of the lung ceases while perfusion continues. The most common causes of pathologic shunting are atelectasis, pneumonia, and pulmonary edema. Dead space is the portion of the tidal volume that does not participate in gas exchange. The residual volume is the volume of gas remaining in lungs after a maximal exhalation. The stroke volume is the amount of blood ejected from the left ventricle in one contraction.

126. Correct answer - C

The area from the nares to the bronchioles is called the anatomic dead space - the portion of the tidal volume that does not take part in gas exchange, which is the sole function of the alveoli. Normally, dead space is about one-third of the tidal volume. Underperfused or underventilated alveoli do not take part in gas exchange, thereby increasing dead space. Mechanical ventilatory tubing lengthens the airway and also increases dead space. The nasopharynx lies immediately behind the nasal cavity, and the oropharynx is the posterior of the mouth.

127. Correct answer - D

The average diameter of a pulmonary capillary is equal to the average diameter of an erythrocyte, about 8 to 10 microns. Thus, the red blood cell must actually squeeze through the capillary, in effect touching the capillary wall. This increases the rapidity of oxygen and carbon dioxide diffusion across the alveolocapillary membrane. 10% and 20% of the cardiac output (about 1 liter) is in the pulmonary circulatory system at any one time, although only about 100 ml is in the pulmonary capillaries. Hypoxia increases pulmonary vascular tone, right ventricular pressures, pulmonary vascular resistance, and cardiac output. Because of the effects of gravity, blood flow is greater at the base of the lungs than at the apex.

128. Correct answer - B

Normally, the ventilation-perfusion ratio is 0.8:1, with 4 liters/minute of ventilation of 5 liters/minute of perfusion. Because of gravity and pleural pressure, ventilation and perfusion are weakest at the apex and strongest at the base, although the difference is smaller for ventilation. Anything that interferes with ventilation, such as bronchospasm, lowers the ratio. Anything that interferes with perfusion, such as a pulmonary embolism, increases the ratio. A ventilation-perfusion lung scan detects abnormalities. Ventilation scans are performed by having the patient inhale a radioactive substance; perfusion scans are performed by I.V. injection of a radioactive substance. A scanner then detects chest radiation.

129. Correct answer - A

Clinical changes in lung assessment are characteristically vague in pulmonary embolism. Vesicular breath sounds heard over most of the lung are a normal finding. Pulmonary embolism is assessed through significant patient history and diagnostic procedures.

130. Correct answer - A

Factors predisposing a patient to pulmonary embolism do not include pre-existing pulmonary disease. The three conditions, known as Virchow's triad, that predispose one to pulmonary embolism are venous stasis, hypercoagulability, and trauma to vascular walls. Venous stasis is a result of bed rest and immobilization; most pulmonary embolisms are due to thrombus formation in the deep veins of the legs. Hypercoagulability occurs after surgery or pregnancy and with oral contraceptive use. Patients who need multiple intravenous insertions are at risk for trauma to vascular walls. Thus, many hospitalized patients are at risk for pulmonary embolism.

131.   Correct answer - C

In pulmonary embolism, oxygen administration will not significantly reverse hypoxemia. The embolism blocks blood flow to the lungs, so hemoglobin cannot combine with oxygen. This is usually characterized by a sudden onset of dyspnea. Oxygen still diffuses across the alveolocapillary membrane, but the area is not perfused by blood and the blood returns, unoxygenated, to the left side of the heart. Because the defect is one of perfusion and not ventilation, chest X-rays are not usually diagnostic of pulmonary embolism. Treatment is aimed at preventing further pulmonary emboli through anticoagulation or surgical interruption, such as inferior caval umbrella or ligation. Newer treatment is under study to dissolve existing emboli through streptokinase administration.

132.   Correct answer - D

A pulmonary embolism can be definitively diagnosed by a pulmonary angiogram. A chest X-ray is not diagnostic of pulmonary embolism because changes are rare and could be confused with those of an infection. Arterial blood gas analysis will show a decrease in PO_2 which has many etiologies. Lung scans are helpful in the diagnosis of pulmonary embolism, but changes are similar to those of emphysema. Only pulmonary angiographic evidence of clots or embolism can definitively diagnose pulmonary embolism.

133.   Correct answer - C

Administration of 100% oxygen is the primary treatment of carbon monoxide poisoning. Carbon monoxide's affinity for hemoglobin is 200 times greater than oxygen's and quickly binds to it; forming carboxyhemoglobin. High percentages of oxygen speed the release of the carbon monoxide from the hemoglobin. Administering

165

Mucomyst, a mucolytic, is useful in bronchitis and also reverses an acetaminophen overdose. Breathing into a paper bag assists in CO_2 retention and is the treatment for hyperventilation caused by anxiety. Suctioning is helpful in clearing the airway of secretions.

134.   Correct answer - B

Carboxyhemoglobin levels must be monitored in a patient with carbon monoxide poisoning. Co-oximetry measures this level, whereas standard blood gas analysis does not. The PO_2 and O_2 saturations will be normal in a person with carbon monoxide poisoning, making pulse oximetry and SvO_2 monitoring unreliable. Diuretic administration has no benefit in the treatment of carbon monoxide poisoning.

135.   Correct answer - C

Diabetes does not increase the risk of carbon monoxide poisoning. A smoker has an increased risk of carbon monoxide poisoning because he already has detectable levels of carbon monoxide in the blood from smoking. Diseases that interfere with the oxygen-carrying capacity of the blood, such as chronic lung or cardiac diseases, also increase the risk of carbon monoxide poisoning.

Mental Humor Break

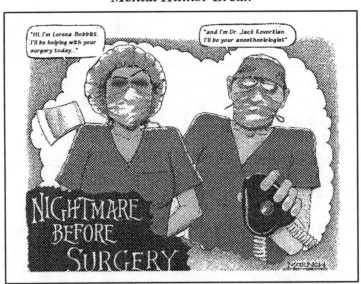

In Your Face
1-800-658-8508

CHAPTER 3

NEUROLOGIC SYSTEM

Case Study

Questions 1-19 refer to the following case study:

Mr. R. age 25, is admitted to the intensive care unit (ICU). He is disoriented to time and place. A co-worker reported that Mr. R. had been hit on the head with a beam 3 hours earlier, causing momentary unconsciousness, but appeared fine until an hour ago, when he became tired and "wasn't making any sense." Physical examination detects a dilated, nonreactive left pupil. The patient's blood pressure is 160/80 mm Hg, his pulse is 80 beats/ minute, and his respiratory rate is 16 breaths/minute.

1. Which diagnostic test should have been performed in the emergency department before Mr. R. was transported to the ICU?

   A. Lumbar puncture
   B. Computed tomography (CT) scan
   C. Cervical spine and skull X-rays
   D. Cerebral angiography

2. Mr. R.'s history and physical examination suggest which neurologic problem?

   A. Cerebral concussion
   B. Expanding lesion on the right side of the brain
   C. Expanding lesion on the left side of the brain
   D. Meningeal irritation

3. Diagnostic studies reveal a temporal fracture with a pineal shift. This finding is typically associated with:

   A. Subdural hematoma
   B. Epidural hematoma
   C. Subarachnoid hemorrhage
   D. Intracerebral hemorrhage

4. The ICU nurse should prepare Mr. R. for which treatment?

    A. Direct intracranial pressure (ICP) monitoring
    B. Pharmacologic management
    C. Lumbar puncture
    D. Surgical evacuation of clot

5. Which method of determining ICP in a patient with a head injury is unsafe?

    A. Lumbar puncture
    B. Epidural monitoring
    C. Intraventricular catheter
    D. Subarachnoid screw

6. Mr. R. is examined for signs of increased ICP. Which cranial nerve is surrounded by cerebrospinal fluid, providing information about pressure within the brain?

    A. Optic nerve
    B. Vagus nerve
    C. Oculomotor nerve
    D. Trigeminal nerve

7. An intraventricular catheter is inserted for direct ICP monitoring the next day. An advantage of this monitor is that:

    A. Infection risk is lessened
    B. It is easily inserted
    C. Cerebrospinal fluid (CSF) drainage can occur
    D. It has the least risk of complications

8. Intracranial pressure is:

    A. The difference between systolic and diastolic blood pressures
    B. Increased in hypoxic states
    C. Normally between 50 and 100 mm Hg
    D. Decreased while the patient is in the supine position

9. A goal of ICP therapy is to maintain:

   A. Cerebral perfusion pressure above 50 mm Hg
   B. Mean arterial pressure above 120 mm Hg
   C. Intracranial pressure below 40 mm Hg
   D. Diastolic blood pressure below 90 mm Hg

10. In ICP monitoring, the transducer should be level with the:

    A. Right atrium
    B. Foramen magnum
    C. Foramen of Monro
    D. Nuchal area

11. The ICP monitor waveform becomes progressively elevated. The first-line treatment in acute increased ICP is to administer:

    A. Aminocaproic acid (Amicar)
    B. Glucose
    C. Mannitol
    D. Barbiturates

12. Increased ICP is best relieved by which nursing intervention?

    A. Elevating the head of the bed 30 degrees
    B. Providing auditory stimulation to decrease sensory deprivation
    C. Increasing oxygenation through postural drainage and suctioning
    D. Sedating the patient with morphine sulfate, as needed

13. Cushing's reflex is a:

    A. Stress ulcer caused by vagal stimulation
    B. Cardiovascular response to increased ICP
    C. Compression of the respiratory centers
    D. Facial grimace in response to tapping the nose

14. Conditions that further increase ICP include:

    A. Hypoxemia, hypercapnia, and alkalosis
    B. Hypoxemia, hypercapnia, and acidosis
    C. Hypoxemia, hypocapnia, and alkalosis
    D. Hypoxemia, hypocapnia, and acidosis

15. Mr. R. develops a fever that, after negative culture reports, is diagnosed as a central fever. The brain area that regulates body temperature is the:

    A. Reticular activating system
    B. Hippocampus
    C. Hypothalamus
    D. Thalamus

16. During a neurologic assessment, a reliable early indicator of the patient's level of consciousness is his ability to:

    A. Think abstractly
    B. Open his eyes when addressed
    C. Squeeze the nurse's fingers tightly
    D. Name objects correctly

17. Two days after admission, the patient suffers a generalized (grand mal) seizure. The seizure phase characterized by contraction and apnea lasting about 1 minute is called the:

    A. Aura phase
    B. Tonic phase
    C. Clonic phase
    D. Postictal phase

18. Nursing interventions during a generalized seizure include:

    A. Securing physical restraints
    B. Maintaining the patient in a supine position
    C. Inserting an artificial airway
    D. Observing seizure activity

19. After the intraventricular catheter is removed, which finding may indicate chronic increased ICP?

A. Hypercapnia
B. Nystagmus
C. Hypotension
D. Widening pulse pressure

Case Study

Questions 20-34 refer to the following case study:

Mr. J., a 23-year-old man who had been weight lifting at a health spa, is admitted to the ICU with complaints of a sudden, explosive headache.

20. The presenting history and symptoms indicate:

A. Subarachnoid hemorrhage
B. Epidural hematoma
C. Basal skull fracture
D. Brain stem contusion

21. A lumbar puncture is performed. Mr. J is placed in a side-lying, knee-chest position to:

A. Prevent further headaches
B. Avoid spinal cord injury
C. Afford easier access to the spinal canal
D. Prevent accidental injury to nearby organs

22. Cerebrospinal fluid (CSF) is formed by the:

A. Aqueduct of Sylvius
B. Choroid plexus
C. Arachnoid mater
D. Nodes of Ranvier

23. Which statement accurately describes characteristics of CSF?

A. It is normally yellow
B. It is contained in the subdural space
C. Its glucose is 60% of blood glucose
D. A major portion is distributed in the brain

24. A cerebral angiogram is performed on Mr. J. Potential postprocedure nursing diagnoses include:

A. Pain related to postprocedure headache
B. Sensory-perceptual alteration related to photophobia
C. Altered tissue perfusion related to interruption of arterial flow
D. Fluid volume deficit related to contrast medium administration

25. The angiogram reveals rupture of an intracranial aneurysm in the parietal area. Blood is delivered to that area by the:

A. Vertebral arteries
B. Internal carotid arteries
C. Cerebeller arteries
D. Basilar arteries

26. Intracranial aneurysms most commonly develop in the:

A. Vertebral artery
B. Circle of Willis
C. Subarachnoid space
D. Pituitary gland

27. Venous blood leaves the brain through the:

A. Foramen of Monro
B. Aqueduct of Sylvius
C. Spinal cord
D. Superior sagittal sinus

28. The parietal lobe is the brain area responsible for:

A. Sensory interpretation
B. Speech
C. Vision
D. Emotional responses

29. Mr. J. is checked for stereognosis, which is an assessment of:

A. Vision and depth perception
B. Hearing
C. Muscle strength
D. Tactile discrimination

30. Animocaproic acid (Amicar) is ordered for Mr. J. An appropriate nursing diagnosis to monitor for while infusing this medication would be:

A. Decreased cardiac output related to altered cardiac electrical conduction
B. Fluid volume deficit related to active gastrointestinal blood loss
C. Decreased cardiac output related to allergic reaction
D. Impaired gas exchange related to disruption in pulmonary perfusion

31. An ECG shows T-wave inversion. ECG changes accompanying such a neurological disease as Mr. J. has are thought to be caused by:

A. Microemboli formation
B. Autonomic discharge
C. Inflammation
D. Coincident heart disease

32. This patient should be assessed for:

A. Battle's sign
B. Brudzinski's sign
C. Cullen's sign
D. Cushing's reflex

33. The nurse notes that the patient is in a state of extreme extension, with the neck and back arched. This is documented as:

    A.   Decorticate posturing
    B.   Decerebrate posturing
    C.   Opisthotonos
    D.   Nuchal rigidity

34. In a subarchnoid hemorrhage, immediately after initial bleeding or surgical repair, the patient is *most* at risk for:

    A.   Rebleeding
    B.   Vasospasm
    C.   Diabetes insipidus
    D.   Pulmonary emboli

Case Study
Questions 35-43 refer to the following case study.

Mr. V. is admitted to the ICU after a motor vehicle accident in which the right side of his head hit the windshield. A basal skull fracture with right middle meningeal artery damage and a left temporal lobe contusion are detected.

35. Mr. V. is likely to develop which condition?

    A.   Subdural hematoma
    B.   Subarachnoid hemorrhage
    C.   Epidural hematoma
    D.   Aneurysm

36. Mr. V. should be assessed for Battle's sign, which is:

    A.   A postconcussion syndrome
    B.   An ecchymosis over the mastoid bone
    C.   Black-and-blue discoloration around the eyes
    D.   A superficial hematoma on the skull

37. This patient may have injured the:

A. Oculomotor nerve
B. Olfactory nerve
C. Optic nerve
D. Ophthalmic nerve

38. Further assessment may also reveal:

A. Otorrhea
B. Meningism
C. Positive Kernig's sign
D. Hemianopia

39. A nurse caring for a patient with a basal skull fracture should:

A. Instruct him to blow his nose gently
B. Prevent the patient from performing Valsalva's maneuver
C. Promote coughing and deep breathing
D. Institute nasogastric suctioning to prevent vomiting

40. Injury to the brain area opposite the area of impact in a closed-head injury is:

A. Ipsilateral injury
B. Contrecoup injury
C. Battle's sign
D. Epidural hematoma

41. Appearance of "Raccoon's eyes" indicates:

A. A subarchnoid hemorrhage
B. An anterior fossa fracture
C. An epidural hematoma
D. Meningitis

42. Mr. V. is *least* likely to lose awareness of:

A. Person
B. Place
C. Time
D. Memory

43. While assessing Mr. V.'s pupillary response, the nurse detects nystagmus. Which of the following statements about nystagmus is *true?*

A. It is always an abnormal finding
B. It suggests a spinal cord lesion
C. It is analogous to a body tremor
D. It refers to unequal pupil size

Case Study
Questions 44-55 refer to the following case study:

Mr. D is admitted to the ICU after a motor vehicle accident. Spinal X-rays confirm a lesion at C5 to C6.

44. The nurse suspects that Mr. D. has:
A. Quadriplegia with intact triceps and biceps and intercostal breathing
B. Quadriplegia with gross arm movements and diaphragmatic breathing
C. Paraplegia with diaphragmatic breathing
D. Diaphragmatic and intercostal breathing with loss of intrinsic hand-muscle power

45. Motor neurons arising from which tract control gross motor movements?

A. Pyramidal tract
B. Extrapyramidal tract
C. Lateral spinothalamic tract
D. Posterior tract

46.   Functioning of the spinothalamic tract is determined by:

A.   Applying a tuning fork to a bony prominence and asking the patient to identify the vibration
B.   Asking the patient to close both eyes and touch the nose with a finger
C.   Asking the patient to identify areas stimulated by a pinprick
D.   Testing the patient's position sense

47.   Spinal reflexes in this patient indicate an intact:

A.   Upper motor neuron
B.   Lower motor neuron
C.   Brainstem
D.   Thalamus

48.   A functioning reflex arc requires all of the following to be intact *except* the:

A.   Sensory nerve
B.   Cortex
C.   Motor nerve
D.   Muscle

49.   Sensory impulses are relayed to the appropriate brain area by the:

A.   Cerebrum
B.   Medulla
C.   Thalamus
D.   Corpus callosum

50.   Which finding indicates the development of ineffective airway clearance in this patient?

A.   pH of 7.28, PCO_2 of 36 mm Hg, HCO_3 of 18 mEq, and PO_2 of 86 mm Hg
B.   Inspiratory force of - 20 cm
C.   Measured tidal volume of 500 ml
D.   Bronchial breath sounds over the lung lobes

51. In spinal cord injury, early hypoventilation is best manifested by:

A. Poor respiratory exchange
B. Development of cyanosis
C. Shortness of breath while talking
D. Arterial blood gas (ABG) values

52. Acute spinal cord injury will cause respiratory paralysis at and above which level?

A. C4
B. C6
C. C7
D. T1

53. During the first hours after admission, Mr. D. develops spinal shock. Physical examination would then detect:

A. Spasticity
B. Hypertension
C. Tachycardia
D. Areflexia

54. Which is *true* regarding autonomic dysreflexia in the spinal cord-injured patient?

A. This syndrome typically occurs in patients with lumbar lesions
B. It is caused by stimulation above the level of the lesion
C. It shows initial hypotension caused by vagal stimulation
D. Treatment includes atropine sulfate administration

55. Which statement describes the autonomic nervous system?

A. The vagus nerve is the only cranial nerve controlled by the parasympathetic nervous system
B. Sympathetic fibers exit the spinal cord from the cranial and sacral areas
C. Postganglionic, adrenergic, and sympathetic neurons release the neurotransmitter acetylcholine
D. The parasympathetic nervous system has long, preganglionic fibers that reach the innervated organ

Case Study
Questions 56-68 refer to the following case study:

Mrs. G., age 67, is admitted with a diagnosis of glioblastoma-type brain tumor. During the physical assessment, she is obtunded. Neurologic assessment reveals pinpoint pupils and an absent corneal reflex. Her serum sodium level is 120 mEq/liter; a secondary diagnosis of syndrome of inappropriate anti-diuretic hormone (SIADH) secretion also is made.

56. Which part of the brain controls sleep and wakefulness?

A. Reticular activating system
B. Cerebral cortex
C. Limbic system
D. Basal ganglia

57. The neuroglial cells known as oligodendroglia are:

A. Found along peripheral nerves
B. Star-shaped in nature
C. Responsible for myelin formation
D. Macrophages

58. Pinpoint pupils in an obtunded patient may indicate a lesion in the:

A. Pituitary gland
B. Hypothalamus
C. Cerebellum
D. Pons

59. With a lesion in this area, the nurse would most likely assess Mrs. G. for the development of which respiratory pattern?

A. Regular, rapid, deep ventilations
B. Irregular deep and shallow breathing with irregular periods of apnea
C. Regular breathing at a rate of 6/minute
D. Cyclical deep rapid and slow shallow breathing followed by periods of apnea

60. In a neurologic assessment, the nurse should expect which patient to have a decreased or absent corneal reflex?

A. The patient who also has normally unequal pupils
B. The patient who has had recent eye surgery
C. The patient with trigeminal neuralgia
D. The patient who wears contact lenses

61. The brain tumor with the best prognosis is a:

A. Meningioma
B. Glioblastoma
C. Astrocytoma
D. Pituitary adenoma

62. Which hormone is secreted from the posterior pituitary gland?

A. Antidiuretic hormone
B. Follicle-stimulating hormone
C. Thyroid-stimulating hormone
D. Adrenocorticotropic hormone

63. Which statement is *true* about SIADH?

A. Treatment is usually with vasopressin tannate in oil
B. It results in hypernatremia
C. Pulmonary tumors may be the precipitating cause
D. It can result in dehydration, particularly in elderly or unconscious persons

64. Mrs. G.'s neurologic status deteriorates and she begins to have seizures characterized by repetition of inappropriate acts (automatisms). This seizure type is known as:

A. Partial complex
B. Absence
C. Partial motor
D. Myoclonic

65. Mrs. G. also begins to exhibit altered respiratory patterns from depression of the respiratory center, and is placed on a ventilator. The respiratory center in the brain is located in the:

A. Cortex
B. Hypothalamus
C. Cerebellum
D. Medulla

66. The physician assesses the oculocephalic reflex and performs the caloric test. The oculocephalic reflex is:

A. An abnormal reflex when present
B. Absent in severe brain stem involvement
C. The movement of eyes in the direction the head turned
D. An indication of first cranial nerve function

67. The caloric test:

   A. Assesses vestibular nerve function
   B. Is also called the oculocephalic reflex
   C. Is abnormal if nystagmus is elicited
   D. Assesses the hunger and satiety centers of the hypothalamus

68. The most appropriate basis for discontinuing life support in a comatose patient like Mrs. G. with no hope of meaningful recovery is:

   A. An agreement reached by the health team and family
   B. Two flat EEGs
   C. State law on discontinuing life support
   D. Physician's order of "no code"

Case Study
Questions 69-77 refer to the following case study:

Mr. H., age 55, is admitted to the ICU after suffering a right hemispheric cerebrovascular accident.

69. Damage to the right cerebral hemisphere may exhibit:

   A. Right hemiparesis
   B. Left homonymous hemianopia
   C. Deviation of the eyes to the left
   D. Right hemiplegia

70. Loss of motor function in the left arm and leg may indicate a lesion in the:

   A. Pyramidal tract of the right hemisphere
   B. Spinocerebellar tract
   C. Motor nerve fibers in the anterior horn of the spinal cord
   D. Spinal cord at C7

71. Mr. H. develops a left field visual loss, indicating damage to the:

   A. Optic nerve
   B. Oculomotor nerve
   C. Trigeminal nerve
   D. Acoustic nerve

72. During a neurologic assessment, the nurse watches for signs of uncal-herniation. An early indication of this condition is:

   A. Absent doll's eyes reflex
   B. Ipsilateral dilated pupil
   C. Ataxic breathing
   D. Impaired motor function

73. The nurse also assesses the function of the ninth cranial nerve. This nerve is:

   A. A nerve associated with taste sensation
   B. A motor nerve only
   C. The hypoglossal nerve
   D. The innervator of the trapezius muscle

74. Assessing extraocular movements determines the function of all the following cranial nerves *except* the:

   A. Oculomotor nerve
   B. Trochlear nerve
   C. Trigeminal nerve
   D. Abducens nerve

75. In assessing consciousness, the nurse begins by using:

   A. Auditory stimulation
   B. Tactile stimulation
   C. Light pain
   D. Deep pain

76. The Glasgow Coma Scale, used to assess neurologic status, measures:

A. Pupillary reaction, motor response, and verbal response
B. Eye opening, motor response, and verbal response
C. Eye opening, vital signs, and verbal response
D. Pupillary reaction, motor response, and vital signs

77. Mr. H. exhibits decerebrate (extensor) posturing. Which areas of the brain have been injured?

A. The cerebrum and cerebellum
B. The cerebrum and brain stem
C. The hypothalamus and brain stem
D. The cerebellum and hypothalamus

Case Study
Questions 78-79 refer to the following case study:

Mr. L., age 32, is admitted to the ICU after a fall off a ladder. A myelogram reveals right hemisection of the spinal cord.

78. Mr. L.'s myelogram suggests:

A. Brown-Sequard syndrome
B. Anterior cord syndrome
C. Partial cord syndrome
D. Central cord syndrome

79. Which of the following clinical findings would be detected in this patient?

A. Complete motor, pain, and sensation loss below the level of the lesion
B. Greater loss of motor function in the arms than in the legs
C. Motor loss on the right side and loss of pain and temperature sensation on the left side below the level of the lesion
D. Spastic paralysis below the level of the lesion

Ms. C., age 31, is admitted to the ICU with a diagnosis of suspected meningitis. She complains of a headache and photophobia. A lumbar puncture has been performed, but the causative organism has not been isolated.

80. The meningeal layer that adheres to the sulci and gyri of the brain is the:

A. Pia mater
B. Sella turcica
C. Arachnoid mater
D. Dura mater

81. The blood-brain barrier:

A. Exists throughout the capillary bed of the brain and choroid plexus
B. Is impermeable to carbon dioxide
C. Is caused by the fusion of endothelial capillary cells
D. Attempts to maintain sterility of the brain

82. The organism that most frequently causes meningitis in young adults is the:

A. Hemophilus influenzae
B. Pneumococcus
C. Meningococcus
D. Streptococcus

83. The best method to assess Ms. C. for meningeal irritation is to:
A. Flex the leg at the hip and knee; then straighten the knee and watch for pain and resistance
B. Stroke the side of the sole and watch for dorsiflexion of the great toe
C. Check the temperature; a reading of 102°F. (38.9° C.) indicates meningeal irritation
D. Check for papilledema

84. Which assessment finding is *not* associated with meningeal irritation?

  A. Babinski's reflex
  B. Brudzinski's sign
  C. Kernig's sign
  D. Nuchal rigidity

85. Which nursing action is *not* implemented for a patient who has just been diagnosed as having viral meningitis?

  A. Instituting seizure precautions
  B. Instituting isolation precautions
  C. Monitoring temperature frequently
  D. Controlling increased intracranial pressure

86. Patients with bacterial meningococcal meningitis commonly exhibit:

  A. Petechiae
  B. Hypothermia
  C. Nystagmus
  D. Hypertensive crises

Case Study

Questions 87-90 refer to the following case study:

Ms. O., a 23-year-old woman with myasthenia gravis, is admitted with pneumonia, increasing weakness, and respiratory insufficiency.

87. The neurotransmitter acetylcholine, which is impaired in myasthenia gravis, normally carries the nervous impulse:

  A. Up the spinal cord
  B. Along the muscle
  C. Across the synapse
  D. Into the cerebral cortex

88. Neurophysiologically, summation causes:

A. Saltatory conduction
B. Neurotransmitter secretion
C. An action potential
D. Myelin formation

89. Care of Ms. O. includes:

A. Withholding anticholinesterase agents if muscle weakness occurs
B. Administering quinine for leg cramps
C. Assessing forced vital capacity before and after each dose of an anticholinesterase agent
D. Scheduling activities for the afternoon to avoid muscle fatigue

90. Which statement about myasthenia gravis is *true?*

A. Treatment may include immunosuppressive therapy
B. Cholinergic crisis is precipitated by infection, trauma, stress, or surgery
C. Myasthenia gravis results from decreased cholinesterase
D. Diagnosis is made if improvement occurs after I.V. administration of atropine sulfate

Case Study

Questions 91-100 refer to the following case study:

Mr. M., age 55, is admitted to the ICU for ascending weakness of the legs. His past medical history is insignificant except for a recent upper respiratory infection. A demyelinating disease is suspected.

91. Which statement about gray or white matter is most accurate?

    A.   White matter contains myelinated fibers
    B.   Gray matter is outside white matter in the spinal cord
    C.   White matter in the spinal cord contains preganglionic fibers of the autonomic nervous system
    D.   White matter forms an "H" pattern in the spinal cord

92. High-speed impulse transmission in myelinated fibers occurs because of the:

    A.   Nissl bodies
    B.   Myelin sheath
    C.   Schwann's cells
    D.   Nodes of Ranvier

93. Ascending muscle weakness in the legs would suggest:

    A.   Peripheral neuropathy
    B.   Parkinson's disease
    C.   Myasthenia gravis
    D.   Guillain-Barre syndrome

94. Observing Mr. M.'s ability to stand steadily with open eyes assesses:

    A.   Cerebellar function
    B.   Proprioceptive function
    C.   Cranial nerve function
    D.   Motor strength

95. The nurse assesses for motor impairment in Mr. M.'s arms. The most reliable technique for testing arm motor strength is to:

    A.   Observe for spontaneous movement
    B.   Test the bicep and tricep reflexes
    C.   Have the patient close his eyes; then ask him to identify whether you've moved his finger up or down
    D.   Have the patient close his eyes and raise his arms straight in front of him

96. The cremasteric reflex is absent in Mr. M. This reflex:

A. Is a deep tendon reflex
B. Is found only in men
C. Assesses level of consciousness
D. Indicates autonomic dysfunction

97. Mr. M. has a negative Babinski's reflex. A positive reflex would indicate:

A. An upper motor neuron lesion
B. A lower motor neuron lesion
C. Meningeal irritation
D. Peripheral neuropathy

98. Electromyography is performed on Mr. M. This may be useful in diagnosing:

A. Upper motor neuron lesions
B. Parkinson's disease
C. Seizure disorder
D. Lower motor neuron disease

99. Which statement describes lower motor neuron disease?

A. Deep tendon reflexes are present
B. It is associated with spastic paralysis
C. It is a neuron disease originating in the spinal cord and ending in the brain
D. It causes degenerative skin and nail changes

100. A high priority nursing diagnosis to assess Mr. M. for now would be:

A. Fluid volume excess
B. Sensory-perceptual deficit
C. Ineffective breathing pattern
D. Impaired tissue perfusion

Questions 101-109 refer to the following case study:

Mrs. G., age 44, is admitted to the ICU with a diagnosis of left frontoparietal astrocytoma. Preparations are made for a craniotomy and excision of the tumor.

101. Which of the following is the *most* important information for the physician to obtain before surgery?

   A. The dominant hemisphere
   B. The integrity of the corpus callosum
   C. The function of the upper motor neuron
   D. The function of the lower motor neuron

102. The corpus callosum:

   A. Maintains the structural integrity of the frontal lobe
   B. Provides communication between the hemispheres
   C. Provides communication from the cortex to the thalamus
   D. Forms the cerebrospinal fluid

103. Preoperative preparation for Mrs. G. would include:

   A. Initiating a continuous heparin infusion
   B. Putting on thigh-high, antiembolism stockings
   C. Administering 0.9% normal saline solution intravenously at 150 ml/hour
   D. Inserting a nasogastric tube

104. During surgery, the anesthesiologist hyperventilates the patient to decrease intracranial pressure. What is the rationale for this action?

   A. The fast respiratory rate depresses the respiratory center
   B. Antidiuretic hormone is inhibited to increase diuresis
   C. Hypocarbia causes vasoconstriction
   D. Alkalosis stimulates the blood-brain barrier to decrease blood flow to the brain

105. Postoperatively, the nurse evaluates which finding as evidence that Mrs. G. is developing a complication of surgery?

A. Serum osmolarity of 295 mOsm/liter
B. Urine specific gravity of 1.00
C. Urine output of 100 ml/hour
D. Serum sodium of 134 mEq/liter

106. The most reliable index of Mrs. G.'s neurologic condition is:

A. Level of consciousness
B. Pupillary responses
C. Nystagmus
D. Inward deviation of the eyes

107. If damage occurred to the sixth cranial nerve during surgery, the nurse would observe which condition?

A. Absent gag reflex
B. Fixed and dilated pupils
C. Nystagmus
D. Inward deviation of the eyes

108. The evening after surgery, Mrs. G. develops tonic-clonic movements of the right arm and leg, a seizure type called:

A. Generalized motor
B. Generalized myoclonic
C. Partial motor
D. Partial complex

109. The nurse should expect which postictal problem?

A. Right side paralysis
B. Loss of consciousness
C. Incontinence
D. Left side seizure activity

Case Study

Questions 110-115 refer to the following case study:

Mr. P., a 45-year-old man with a history of seizure disorders, is admitted to the ICU after having a seizure 30 minutes earlier. His family states he takes phenytoin (Dilantin) and phenobarbital at home. His vital signs are stable, but he grimaces only in response to tactile stimuli.

---

110. Which statement describes the pathology of seizures?

    A.   The abnormal excessive firing of brain cells causes the clinical signs and symptoms of a seizure

    B.   The entire brain is involved in a seizure

    C.   The metabolism of the involved cells is greatly decreased during a seizure

    D.   The abnormal firing of the neurons, once initiated, is perpetuated indefinitely until therapy is instituted

---

111. Which nursing action has the highest priority for Mr. P. in a postictal state?

    A.   Obtaining a complete history from the family

    B.   Administering 0.9% normal saline solution intravenously

    C.   Placing the patient on his side and inserting an I.V. line

    D.   Calling the physician and obtaining a suction apparatus at the bedside

---

112. Mr. P. develops a continuous generalized seizure, and the physician diagnoses status epilepticus. The drug of choice to control status epilepticus is:

    A.   Pentobarbital

    B.   Diazepam

    C.   Phenobarbital

    D.   Pavulon

113. The seizures continue, so the physician administers phenytoin inravenously. Which of the following actions is essential?

    A.   Placing the patient on a cardiac monitor during administration
    B.   Obtaining serum phenytoin levels immediately after administration
    C.   Administering the drug in a dextrose solution
    D.   Administering the drug at a rate no faster than 500 mg/minute

114. Which situation can occur if I.V. phenytoin is administered by a rapid bolus?

    A.   Ventricular tachycardia
    B.   Supraventricular tachycardia
    C.   Third-degree heart block
    D.   Electromechanical dissociation

115. After discharge teaching with Mr. P. regarding phenytoin therapy the nurse evaluates that he correctly understand his medication by which of the following statements?

    A.   "I should avoid alcohol because it makes the dilantin build up in my body"
    B.   "I can take the dilantin in the morning or in the afternoon"
    C.   "I should not make up missed doses"
    D.   "I should take aspirin, rather than actaminophen, for head-aches"

Case Study
Questions 116-120 refer to the following case study:

Mr. S., age 67, is discharged from the hospital after treatment for a subarachnoid hemorrhage. He is readmitted 2 weeks later with increasing dementia and ataxia. Hydrocephalus is suspected.

116. Which type of hydrocephalus is suspected in Mr. S?

   A.   Communicating
   B.   Noncommunicating
   C.   Normal-pressure
   D.   Excessive cerebrospinal fluid (CSF) production

117. Which diagnostic tool is used to document hydrocephalus?

   A.   Lumbar puncture
   B.   Craniotomy
   C.   Angiogram
   D.   Computed tomography (CT) scan

118. Which type of hydrocephalus does *not* warrant a shunt implant?

   A.   Communicating
   B.   Noncommunicating
   C.   Normal-pressure
   D.   Excessive CSF production

119. A ventriculoperitoneal shunt is implanted in Mr. S. Which is a common postoperative nursing diagnosis?

   A.   Decreased cardiac output related to altered cardiac conduction
   B.   Constipation related to lack of peristalsis
   C.   Fluid volume deficit related to active gastrointestinal blood loss
   D.   Fluid volume excess related to hormonal imbalances

120. Postoperative care of Mr. S. includes:

   A.   Maintaining high Fowler's position
   B.   Promoting a high-fiber diet the day after surgery
   C.   Repositioning on alternate sides every 2 hours
   D.   Assessing for subdural hematoma

1. **Correct answer - C**

Once the patient's vital signs are stabilized in the emergency department, cervical spine and skull X-rays must be evaluated for a cervical spinal cord injury before transporting the patient to the intensive care unit (ICU) or beginning further diagnostic procedures, such as a computed tomography (CT) scan (to pinpoint the area of damage). Cerebral angiography is not indicated because the origin of the problem was trauma rather than a vascular incident. A lumbar puncture is contraindicated in expanding cerebral lesions because the test may cause a brainstem herniation from pressure shifts.

2. **Correct answer - C**

The history and physical examination suggest an expanding lesion on the left side of the brain; the increasing confusion suggests neurologic impairment. However, if an expanding lesion is developing, the ipsilateral (same side) pupil will dilate because the oculomotor nerve is compressed.

3. **Correct answer - B**

The temporal fracture, development of a hematoma (which causes a contralateral pineal shift), the ipsilateral fixed pupil, and a deteriorating level of consciousness indicate an epidural hematoma.

4. **Correct answer - D**

Epidural hematomas are treated by surgically evacuating the hematoma and ligating the damaged vessel. Early diagnosis and immediate surgical treatment improve the patient's prognosis.

5. **Correct answer - A**

Although a means of measuring intracranial pressure (ICP), lumbar puncture is contraindicated if an expanding cerebral mass exists. A lumbar puncture gives accurate pressure readings only if cerebrospinal fluid (CSF) is flowing freely within the subarachnoid space. An expanding lesion, adhesions, or constrictions will alter CSF flow, causing an inaccurate pressure reading. Also, with increased ICP, lumbar puncture may reduce spinal pressure, causing brain stem herniation. Epidural monitoring, intraventricular catheters, and sub-arachnoid screws accurately and safely measure ICP in patients with head injury.

6.   **Correct answer - A**

The optic (second cranial) nerve is bathed in CSF and contains arteries and veins. Thus, funduscopic retina examination reveals much about pressure within the brain, because the retina is the optic nerve ending. Congestion of retinal blood vessels and swelling of the optic head are signs of increased ICP

7.   **Correct answer - C**

Three frequently used devices measure ICP: intraventricular catheter, epidural sensor, and subarachnoid screw. The intraventricular catheter, inserted directly into the lateral ventricle, also allows drainage and sampling of CSF. Although reliable, it is the most difficult to insert and has the most complications - infection and the risk of excess CSF drainage. An epidural sensor sits atop the dura, is easily inserted, and carries less infection risk because it doesn't penetrate the meninges. However, CSF sampling cannot be performed. A subarachnoid screw is easily inserted under the dura into the space and carries less infection risk than the intraventricular catheter. It allows sampling, but not drainage, of CSF.

8.   **Correct answer B**

ICP, the difference between mean arterial pressure (MAP) and cerebral perfusion pressure (CPP), increases in hypoxic states. The cerebral blood vessels dilate when the arterial PO_2 drops below 50 mm Hg and when carbon dioxide is retained. A normal CPP is between 50 and 130 mm Hg, while a normal ICP is between 0 and 15 mm Hg. ICP is decreased with the head elevated 10 to 20 degrees, so CSP drains more easily.

9.   **Correct answer - A**

A goal of therapy in ICP monitoring is to maintain CPP, the difference between MAP and ICP, above 50 mm Hg. Below that level, impaired cerebral perfusion occurs.

10.   Correct answer - C

In ICP monitoring, the transducer should be level with the foramen of Monro - the interventricular foramen connecting the lateral and third ventricles. When the patient is supine, the external landmark for this foramen is midway between the eyebrow's end and the tragus of the ear. Successive readings should be taken with the transducer and the patient in the same position.

11.   Correct answer - C

First-line treatment for acute increased ICP is administration of mannitol, an osmotic diuretic that reduces cerebral edema by increasing blood osmolarity. Interstitial fluid shifts into the blood interstitial fluid to decrease osmolarity. Mannitol begins acting rapidly and lasts several hours. If given in concentrations above 20% it must be administered via an in-line I.V. filter because of possible crystallization.

12.   Correct answer - A

Elevating the head of the bed 30 degrees enhances venous drainage by gravity, reducing ICP. Auditory stimuli, postural drainage, and suctioning should be avoided because they increase ICP. Morphine sulfate should not be used for sedation because it causes respiratory depression, which raises ICP if hypoxemia and hypercapnia result.

13.   Correct answer - B

Cushing's reflex, a cardiovascular response to increased ICP, includes widening pulse pressure, increasing systolic blood pressure, and bradycardia. Blood pressure is controlled in the medulla; as this is compressed, systolic blood pressure rises, widening the pulse pressure. The rising systolic blood pressure stimulates baroreceptors in the aortic arch and carotid sinus to lower the heart rate through vagal stimulation. A stress ulcer caused by vagal stimulation is called

Cushing's ulcer and typically presents with acute spinal cord injury. Compression of the respiratory centers occurs in brainstem herniation. A facial grimace in response to tapping the nose is called the stout reflex.

14.   Correct answer - B

Hypoxemia, hypercapnia, and acidosis are potent vasodilators as the body attempts to increase oxygen supply to the brain. Cerebral vasodilation causes an increase in brain blood volume and a subsequent rise in ICP.

15.   Correct answer - C

The hypothalamus regulates body temperature and water retention and excretion. In its preoptic and anterior areas, heat-sensitive neurons are stimulated to cause heat loss when body temperature rises. When body temperature falls, these neurons are inhibited, and cold-sensitive neurons in the hypothalamus and midbrain are stimulated to initiate shivering. The hypothalamus regulates body water by stimulating thirst and secreting antidiuretic hormone (ADH). When electrolytes become concentrated in the thirst center (the lateral hypothalamus), thirst is stimulated. The hypothalamus also stimulates or inhibits secretion of ADH stored in the posterior pituitary gland in response to dehydration or fluid excess.

16.   Correct answer - B

The patient's ability to open his eyes when addressed is a reliable early indicator of his level of consciousness. A response to verbal stimuli indicates intactness of higher cortical areas, such as the reticular activating system, responsible for wakefulness via the arousal mechanism. An inability to open the eyes when addressed indicates brain stem involvement, hearing loss, or facial paralysis.

17.   Correct answer - B

The tonic phase of a generalized seizure, characterized by contraction and apnea, usually begins with a shrill cry as the vocal cords contract with air passing through them. This phase follows the preictal (aura) phase, characterized by a seizure prodome, such as irritability, blurred vision, confusion, or focal seizures. The clonic phase follows the tonic phase and is characterized by rhythmic, jerking movements and loud hyperventilations, lasting 2 to 5 minutes. The postictal phase, characterized by a few hours of sleepiness and lethargy, occurs after the seizure ends.

18. **Correct answer - D**

Nursing interventions during a generalized seizure include observing seizure activity. Noting length of seizure, time of day, presence of an aura or cry, characteristics of seizure activity, incontinence, and postictal activity may assist the physician in diagnosing the seizure and its possible cause. Assessing the pulse may help rule out a primary dysrhythmia as the seizure's cause. Physical restraint may cause an injury, such as a fracture, to the patient. The patient's head should be turned to the side to prevent aspiration of secretions. Once seizure activity has begun, the nurse should not attempt to insert an artificial airway; it may injure the patient's teeth if they are clenched, or the nurse's fingers may be bitten.

19. **Correct answer - D**

A widening pulse pressure may indicate chronic increased ICP. Considered a part of Cushing's reflex, the systolic pressure rises as the medulla is compressed. In patients with more chronic intracranial diseases, such as hydrocephalus, monitoring the pulse pressure for an increase may give a clue to slowly rising ICP.

20. **Correct answer - A**

The patient is most likely experiencing a subarachnoid hemorrhage caused by an arteriovenous malformation brought on by strenuous activity. Epidural hematoma, basal skull fracture, and brain stem contusion are caused by traumatic injuries.

21. **Correct answer - C**

Placing the patient in a side-lying, knee-chest position provides easier access to the spinal canal. This position separates the vertebrae in the lumbar region, widening the intervertebral spaces. A lumbar puncture is usually performed in the intervertebral space between L4 and L5.

22.   Correct answer - B

Cerebrospinal fluid (CSF) is formed by the choroid plexus, a network of capillaries in the pia mater covered by epithelial cells in the brain's lateral, third, and fourth ventricles. Most CSF is formed in the lateral ventricles; a small amount is formed by the regular capillary beds that supply the arachnoid meningeal layer.

23.   Correct answer - C

The glucose of CSF is 60% of the blood glucose. A high cerebral glucose level is needed to maintain proper neurologic functioning, which is why hypoglycemia can cause permanent brain damage. CSF is normally clear; yellow CSF indicates the presence of old blood - a condition termed xanthochromia - caused by degradation of red blood cells. Although some CSF is contained in the subarachnoid space and four ventricles of the brain, most is contained in the spinal cord.

24.   Correct answer - C

A potential nursing diagnosis following a cerebral angiogram is altered tissue perfusion related to interruption of arterial flow. Femoral arterial occlusion can result following this study. Hence, distal pulses should be frequently assessed and the leg kept straight for 12 hours. High-Fowler's position should be avoided as this position can compress the femoral artery. This procedure should not routinely cause a headache or photophobia. An adverse renal reaction to contrast medium may result in kidney failure with the development of fluid volume excess.

25.   Correct answer - B

About 75% of blood to the brain is supplied by the internal carotid arteries, which supply the anterior portion of the brain (the frontal, temporal, and parietal areas). The vertebral arteries, which originate off the subclavian artery, supply the posterior portion of the brain (the occipital area), dividing into two branches and then later reuniting to form the basilar artery.

26.   **Correct answer - B**

About 60% of intracranial aneurysms develop in the circle of Willis, which is formed by the anastomosis of the internal carotid artery, anterior and posterior cerebral arteries, and anterior and posterior communicating arteries. About 50% of the population has congenital abnormalities at the circle of Willis, with 8% of this population developing intracranial aneurysms because of the many bifurcations of arteries occurring within the circle. These congenital defects usually do not appear until midlife, when hypertension and arteriosclerosis have taken their toll on the weakened artery, causing it to balloon or rupture.

27.   **Correct answer - D**

Venous blood leaves the brain through the superior sagittal sinus in the dura mater. The dura mater consists of an outer layer adhered to the cranial bone and an inner layer adhered to the brain. Sinuses are formed between these two layers, which drain venous blood from the brain. The blood then enters the internal jugular vein to return to the superior vena cava.

28.   **Correct answer - A**

The parietal lobe, the area of the brain controlling sensory interpretation, is at the top posterior portion of the head, between the frontal and occipital lobes. Each hemisphere receives sensory impulses from the opposite side of the body. These sensations include pain; proprioception; heat; cold; recognition of qualities of objects, such as size, shape, and texture, and interpretation of the written word.

29.   **Correct answer - D**

Stereognosis is an assessment of tactile discrimination. With the eyes closed, the patient is asked to identify an object by touch. This assesses intact sensory pathways and a functioning parietal lobe. Inability to identify the object is called astereognosis.

30. Correct answer - D

Aminocaproic acid (Amicar) is an antithrombolytic drug used to prevent lysis of a clot after cerebral bleeding in an attempt to prevent rebleeding that may take place 7 to 10 days later. The drug may predispose a patient to greater risk of a thromboembolism or pulmonary embolism.

31. Correct answer - B

ECG changes (such as ventricular dysrhythmias, ST-segment and T-wave changes, and bradycardia) that accompany subarachnoid hemorrhage or cerebrovascular accident may be caused by autonomic discharge. A sympathetic or parasympathetic discharge is thought to occur, although the exact mechanism is unknown. On autopsy, some patients with these diagnoses have myocardial damage that may be caused by autonomic discharge.

32. Correct answer - B

Brudzinski's sign may occur in the patient with subarachnoid hemorrhage. A sign of meningeal irritation, it is elicited by flexing the patient's head onto the chest and watching for hip and knee flexion, an abnormal response. Meningeal irritation occurs in meningitis and subarachnoid hemorrhage.

33. Correct answer - C

Opisthotonos, extreme extension of the body with the neck and back arched, occurs in patients with tetany or brain stem damage. Decorticate posturing (flexor posturing) occurs in patients with damage to the cortex, thalamus, internal capsule, or basal ganglia; it consists of arm flexion and leg extension. Decerebrate posturing (extensor posturing), seen in brain stem damage, exhibits extension of all extremities, with outward pronation of the wrists and hands. Nuchal rigidity occurs in meningeal irritation and produces pain and stiffness when the patient's head is flexed toward the chest.

34. **Correct answer - B**

In a subarachnoid hemorrhage, immediately after initial bleeding or surgical repair, the patient is most at risk for vasospasm, or constriction of cerebral arteries. Its cause is unknown but may be irritation or sympathetic discharge. Symptoms include hemiparesis, visual disturbances, seizure activity, decreasing level of consciousness and, if severe enough, cerebral ischemia or infarction. Rebleeding from clot dissolution typically occurs 7 to 10 days after the initial insult.

35. **Correct answer - C**

The patient is likely to develop an epidural hematoma, which is caused by arterial bleeding. A subdural hematoma results from venous bleeding. A subarachnoid hemorrhage is caused by a ruptured aneurysm, which is a weakening of a vessel wall.

36. **Correct answer - B**

Battle's sign, bleeding with resultant ecchymosis over the mastoid bone, may take up to 24 hours to develop. It is commonly seen in basal skull fractures involving the middle fossae. A basal skull fracture may involve the anterior, middle, or posterior fossae at the base of the skull.

37. **Correct answer - B**

Basal skull fractures may cause nerve injuries. Injury to the olfactory (first cranial) nerve is common, causing loss of the sense of smell (anosmia). Other cranial nerve injuries include those to the facial nerve (seventh), causing ipsilateral facial paralysis, and the acoustic nerve (eighth), leading to hearing or equilibrium disturbances.

38. **Correct answer - A**

Further assessment of a basal skull fracture may reveal otorrhea or rhinorrhea of CSF. Otorrhea occurs if the dura mater is torn and the tympanic membrane is ruptured, whereas rhinorrhea results if the tympanic membrane is intact. Drainage samples from either site will test positive for glucose.

39.   Correct answer - B

The patient with a basal skull fracture should avoid further tearing of the dura by preventing transient increases in ICP; therefore, he must be instructed to avoid coughing and performing Valsalva's maneuver. Also, he should be told to allow fluid to drain freely from the nose rather than blowing it. If rhinorrhea is significant, then a small loose dressing may be applied. Nasogastric tubes, suction catheters, and other objects should not be put into the nose or ears.

40.   Correct answer - B

Injury to the brain area opposite the impact in a closed-head injury is called a contrecoup injury. A coup injury occurs at the impact site because of the object's impact. A contrecoup injury occurs as brain tissue rebounds from the impact, hitting the opposite side of the brain. Thus, two sites of the brain are injured.

41.   Correct answer - B

"Racoon's eyes", accumulation of blood with edema formation around the eyes, results from blood leaking into the orbital cavity and indicates an anterior fossa basal skull fracture.

42.   Correct answer - A

In neurologic disease, the patient is least likely to lose awareness of person, which usually indicates psychosis. Even in the most severe neurologic diseases, the patient who is conscious retains knowledge of the self.

43.   Correct answer - C

Analogous to a body tremor, nystagmus is a rhythmic tremor of the eyeball, normally elicited when the patient watches a rapidly moving object, such as a train. It occurs in damage to the vestibular portion of the eighth cranial nerve, in cerebeller dysfunction, and in drug toxicity. The tremor is usually faster in one direction than the other and is defined by the faster direction, either right or left.

44.   Correct answer - B

A lesion of C5 to C6 would cause paralysis of intercostal respiration, but diaphragmatic respiration would continue without abdominal muscle action because the diaphragm is innervated by C2, C3 and C4. Complete loss of motor power in the trunk and legs (quadriplegia) and bladder and bowel retention occur.

45.   Correct answer - B

Motor neurons arising from the extrapyramidal tract control gross motor movements and posture. These upper motor neurons course from the cortex to the spinal cord but are mediated by the cerebellum, basal ganglia, thalamus, and reticular formation. Impulses are transmitted to the rubrospinal, vestibulospinal, reticulospinal, and tectospinal tracts in the spinal cord. Upper motor neurons of the pyramidal tract course from the cortex to the internal capsule, then to the pyramids of the medulla, where some fibers cross, and down to the spinal cord. These control fine, skilled motor movements.

46.   Correct answer - C

To assess spinothalamic tract function, the nurse asks the patient to close both eyes and identify areas stimulated by pinprick. The lateral spinothalamic tract conveys pain and temperature sensation; the anterior spinothalamic tract conveys these as well as light touch and pressure. Identifying vibration and position assesses proprioreceptive sensation; point-to-point testing assesses coordination.

47.   Correct answer - B

Spinal reflexes indicate an intact lower motor neuron, which originates in the spinal cord's anterior horn and ends in a specific muscle fiber. A simple reflex arc occurs when a receptor, such as the patellar tendon, is stimulated, and the impulse is transmitted via a sensory neuron to the spinal cord's anterior horn. The impulse then exits the spinal cord via the lower motor neuron to the muscle, eliciting a knee jerk. The reflex does not travel up the spinal cord, so the functioning of the upper motor neuron or the thalamus as a relay station cannot be established. The brainstem does not transmit motor reflexes.

48.   Correct answer - B

A functioning reflex arc does not require an intact cortex. A reflex arc consists of a sensory receptor, a sensory neuron, the spinal cord's anterior horn, the motor nerve, and the muscle or organ responding to the reflex. Because the reflex does not travel up the spinal cord into the brain, reflexes are still present after damage to the cortex.

49.   Correct answer - C

The thalamus relays sensory impulses to the appropriate brain area, conveying all but olfactory impulses to the correct area of the cerebral cortex. Located on either side of the brain's third ventricle, the thalamus also coordinates motor responses and controls brain rhythmicity and emotional affect.

50.   Correct answer - D

Bronchial breath sounds over the patient's lung lobes indicate developing pneumonia, most likely caused by immobility, an ineffective cough, and a decreased vital capacity. The arterial blood gas (ABG) results indicate metabolic acidosis. An inspiratory force of - 20 cm and a tidal volume of 500 ml are normal values.

51.   Correct answer -D

In spinal cord injury, early hypoventilation is best manifested by ABG values. Poor values indicate inadequate oxygenation and ventilation. Cyanosis, a late sign of hypoventilation, is not an accurate indicator because anemic patients may never develop this sign. Cyanosis is also difficult to assess in dark-skinned persons. Poor respiratory exchange and shortness of breath while talking are symptoms related to the level of spinal cord injury and may not differentiate proper ventilation from hypoventilation.

52.   Correct answer - A

Acute spinal cord injury will cause respiratory paralysis at and above the level of C4; diaphragmatic and intercostal innervation occurs at this level. Mechanical ventilation or pacing of the phrenic nerve, which innervates the diaphragm and intercostal muscles, will be necessary.

53.   Correct answer - D

Areflexia (a loss of reflexes, sensation, and movement below the level of the lesion, lasting from minutes to weeks) occurs in acute spinal shock, which results from trauma to the spinal cord. Associated symptoms include flaccid paralysis, hypotension, and bradycardia. Paralysis becomes spastic when the patient is no longer in spinal shock. Hypotension results from loss of vascular tone below the lesion, leading to venous pooling of blood, and is usually orthostatic. Bradycardia results from loss of sympathetic activity with a relative increase in parasympathetic activity.

54.   Correct answer - D

Treatment of autonomic dysreflexia in the spinal cord-injured patient includes administration of atropine sulfate. Characterized by exaggerated autonomic reaction, this syndrome occurs in patients with cervical or high thoracic lesions and in response to stimuli below the level of the lesion, such as a distended bowel or bladder or an erection. The initial response is sympathetic stimulation, causing flushed skin, headache, and severe hypertension. Then, as baroreceptors are stimulated by the hypertension, parasympathetic discharge causes bradycardia. Usually, removing the stimulus may reverse the dysreflexia. If not, atropine may be administered, because it is a sympathetic, posganglionic blocking agent and a vagolytic agent. It will block sympathetic impulses to the arterioles, reversing the hypertension, and will inhibit vagal action, raising the heart rate. Antihypertensives may also be used.

55.   Correct answer - D

The parasympathetic nervous system has long, preganglionic fibers that reach the innervated organ. These exit from the spinal cord's cranial and sacral areas. The short postganglionic fibers of the para-sympathetic nervous system, called cholinergic fibers, secrete acetycholine. The oculomotor, facial, glossopharyngeal, and vagus nerves have parasympathetic activity. Sympathetic fibers exit from the thoracolumbar areas of the spinal cord and consist of short pregan-glionic fibers and long postganglionic fibers. The latter, called adr-energic fibers, secrete noradrenalin.

56.   Correct answer - A

The reticular activating system (RAS) controls sleep and wakeful-ness. A diffuse network of neurons in the medulla, pons, and mid-brain, it controls the state of consciousness. During sleep, RAS ac-tivity is diminished, whereas its stimulation causes wakefulness. Almost any sensory impulse can stimulate wakefulness through the arousal reaction.

57.   Correct answer - C

The neuroglial cells known as oligodendroglia are responsible for myelin formation. Neuroglial cells are the supportive tissue of the nervous system and are classified as astrocytes, oligodendroglia, or microglia. Astrocytes are star-shaped in nature; their function is unknown but may be part of the blood-brain barrier. Oligodendro-glia take part in myelin formation only in the central nervous sys-tem; their counterparts, the Schwann cells, perform that function in the peripheral nervous system. Microglia are phagocytes.

58.   Correct answer - D

A lesion or hemorrhage compressing the pons also compresses the oculomotor nerve, constricting the pupils to pinpoint size. Opiate usage may also cause pinpoint pupils from overstimulation of the oculomotor nerve, which controls pupillary constriction. This nerve originates in the midbrain and passes from the brain stem at the up-per pons.

59. **Correct answer - A**

Central neurogenic hyperventilation, which are regular rapid, deep ventilations, may be assessed in the patient with a lesion of the pons. Biot's respirations, also known as ataxic breathing, is regular deep and shallow breathing with irregular periods of apnea. This pattern of breathing is associated with brainstem compression. Bradypnea, or slow breathing, usually occurs with an abrupt increase in intracranial pressure or narcotic overdosage. Cheyne-Stokes respiration, or cyclical deep rapid and slow shallow breathing followed by periods of apnea, is associated with lesions of the cerebral hemispheres.

60. **Correct answer - D**

The patient wearing contact lenses typically has a decreased or absent corneal reflex. This reflex helps assess the trigeminal nerve's sensory function and the facial nerve's motor function of blinking. The reflex is tested by brushing the cornea with cotton, which normally results in blinking. However, people with contact lenses accommodate to having something in their eye and respond weakly, if at all, to the corneal reflex. Otherwise, absence of this reflex indicates brain stem damage.

61. **Correct answer - D**

A pituitary adenoma is the brain tumor with the best prognosis because it is benign, is easily accessible through transphenoidal surgery, and rarely recurs. Meningiomas, although also benign, are less accessible and have a recurrence rate of 25% to 75% within several years. Astrocytomas and glioblastomas are malignant tumors of the glial cells. An astrocytoma's prognosis depends on its grade (I to III) and accessibility. A glioblastoma, sometimes called a grade IV astrocytoma, has the worst prognosis - a 0% survival within 5 years.

62. **Correct answer A**

Antidiuretic hormone (ADH) is secreted from and stored in the posterior pituitary gland, or neurophypophysis, which also secretes oxytocin. Its secretion is controlled by the hypothalamus. The anterior pituitary gland, or adenohypophysis, secretes growth hormone, prolactin, adrenocorticotropic hormone, thyroid-stimulating hormone, follicle-stimulating hormone, luteinizing hormone, and melanin-stimulating hormone.

63.   Correct answer - C

Pulmonary tumors may precipitate SIADH. Oat cell carcinomas, a type of pulmonary tumor, may inappropriately produce ADH. Other causes of SIADH include cerebrovascular accident, cranial surgery, and intracranial tumors. In these situations, the posterior pituitary gland is stimulated by the hypothalamus to produce excessive ADH and water is reabsorbed, causing hyponatremia. This can result in fluid overload in someone prone to congestive heart failure (CHF). Treatment includes fluid restriction, diuretics, saline replacement, and administration of demeclocycline (Declomycin), an antibiotic that impairs antidiuretic secretion. Diabetes insipidus (DI), causes by a deficiency of ADH, results in hypernatremia and dehydration. Vasopressin tannate in oil, a form of ADH, may be used to treat DI.

64.   Correct answer - A

Partial complex seizures (also called psychomotor or temporal lobe seizures) are characterized by repetition of inappropriate acts. These acts - called automatisms - may include lip smacking, grimacing, or chewing and are sometimes mistaken for psychotic behaviors. Absence (petit mal) seizures are more likely to occur in childhood and consist of a sudden loss of awareness, but consciousness is retained. Partial motor (Jacksonian) seizures are focal seizures characterized by jerking movements up or down on extremity. Myoclonic seizures, brief contractions of certain muscles, are similar to the jerking movements that occur during sleep.

65.   Correct answer - D

The brain's respiratory center is in the medulla, the brain portion extending to the beginning of the spinal cord. The respiratory center has three major areas: the medullary rhythmicity, apneustic, and pneumotaxic centers. The medullary rhythmicity, or respiratory, center controls the basic rhythmicity of respiration and is affected by impulses from the spinal cord, cerebrum, pneumotaxic center, and apneustic center. The apneustic center influences depth of respirations; the pneumotaxic center influences their rate.

66.   Correct answer - B

The oculocephalic reflex (doll's eyes), absent in severe brain stem involvement, normally is elicited by turning the head from side to side with the eyes opened. The eyes move in the direction opposite to which the head is turned. If brain stem damage occurs, the eyes do not move or move in any combination of ways. The reflex may also be abnormal in third cranial nerve dysfunction, which involves external eye movements.

67.   Correct answer - A

The caloric test assesses vestibular function of the eighth nerve. Also known as the oculovestibular reflex, it is performed by instilling ice water into the ear canal. A normal response is nystagmus and vertigo. An abnormal response is conjugate deviation of the eyes to the irrigated ear, indicating brain stem compression.

68.   Correct answer - A

An agreement between the health team and family is the most appropriate basis for stopping life support in a comatose patient with no hope of meaningful recovery. Discontinuing life support has legal, ethical, and psychosocial implications that can never be fully resolved by legal or procedural methods. Making an informed decision after carefully considering the facts prepares the family for death, reduces needless suffering and cost, diminishes the ambiguity surrounding verbal "no code"orders, and decreases the risk of legal action. The agreement should be carefully documented in the patient's chart and made known to all concerned.

69.   Correct answer - B

Left homonymous hemianopia, or blindness of the left visual field, may occur in right cerebral hemisphere damage. The optic tracts to the right half of each eye, which relay vision from the left visual field, may be damaged. Avoidance of the left visual field may occur, causing the eyes to deviate to the right. Contralateral motor weakness or loss also may occur, resulting in left hemiparesis or hemiplegia.

70.   Correct answer - A

Loss of left arm, and leg motor function may indicate a lesion in the pyramidal tract of the right hemisphere. The lateral corticospinal (pyramidal) tract is the most important upper motor neuron tract. Damage to it causes contralateral motor loss.

71.   Correct answer - A

Left homonymous hemianopia indicates damage to the optic, or second, cranial nerve, specifically to the right optic tract. The optic nerve, which controls vision, originates from the retina of each eye; as it courses near the pituitary gland, half of the fibers from the nerve cross at the optic chiasm going to the opposite side of the brain, while the other half continue on the same side of the brain. The tracts then continue to the occipital lobe, where interpretation of vision occurs. Damage to the right optic tract between the optic chiasm and the occipital lobe causes loss of left-sided vision in each eye as the optic tracts reflect vision coming in from the opposite field.

72.   Correct answer - B

Ipsilateral pupil dilation is an early sign of uncal herniation. An expanding lesion of the lateral middle fossa, most often the temporal lobe, causes shifting of the inner basal temporal lobe. This area contains the uncus, which is forced through the tentorium as pressure builds. The third cranial nerve and the posterior cerebral artery on the same side of the expanding temporal lobe lesion commonly are caught between the uncus and the tentorium. Ataxic or irregular respirations occur in later stages of herniation. Absence of doll's eyes reflex, a late sign of herniation, indicates brain stem dysfunction. Impaired motor function is a common sign in various neurologic and neuromuscular diseases, such as cerebrovascular accident, multiple sclerosis, and myasthenia gravis.

73.   Correct answer - A

.Associated with taste sensation, the ninth cranial (glossopharyngeal) nerve has sensory, motor, and parasympathetic functions. The nerve's sensory aspect controls taste sensation and sensation within the phyarynx, which elicits the gag reflex. The nerve's motor portion controls swallowing and movement of the pharynx during phonation. Parasympathetic activities of this nerve include salivation from stimulation of the parotid glands.

74.   Correct answer - C

The fifth, or trigeminal, nerve is a sensory and motor nerve controlling sensation of the fact and innervation of the jaw muscles - not extraocular eye movements. The third, fourth, and sixth cranial nerves, known as the oculomotor system, are the oculomotor, trochlear, and abducens nerves, respectively - all motor nerves.

75.   Correct answer - A

In assessing consciousness, the nurse begins by using auditory stimuli, usually by speaking to the patient, and evaluates level of consciousness by observing the response. When any stimulation is provided, one should begin with the minimal amount necessary to evoke a response.

76.   Correct answer - B

The Glasgow Coma Scale assigns a numeric value to the patient's ability to open the eyes, respond verbally, and demonstrate motor response to different kinds of stimuli. For a possible total of 15, the points are distributed as follows: eye opening = 1 to 4; motor response = 1 to 6; verbal response = 1 to 5.

77.   Correct answer - B

The cerebrum and brain stem have been damaged if decerebrate posturing is evident. Both control motor function. The cerebellum coordinates muscle tone with movement and maintains equilibrium. The hypothalamus does not regulate motor function.

78.   **Correct answer - A**

In Brown - Sequard syndrome, damage is located on one side of the spinal cord. As a result, complete motor paralysis occurs on the same (ipsilateral) side, with nearly complete loss of pain and temperature sensations on the opposite (contralateral) side below the lesion. In anterior cord syndrome, damage caused by a forward dislocation or compression injury is mainly concentrated in the cord's anterior aspect. Complete motor paralysis usually occurs below the lesion with complete loss of pain and temperature sensations. In central cord syndrome, injury usually is caused by hyperextension of the cervical spine with compression, resulting in greater motor loss to the arms than to the legs. Partial cord syndrome does not exist.

79.   **Correct answer - C**

Brown - Sequard syndrome results from trauma or tumor and causes an incomplete transection of the spinal cord. On the side of the transection below the lesion, motor paralysis and sensory loss of vibration and position occur. The corticospinal and posterior column tracts carrying those impulses cross at the level of the medulla, so the loss is on the same (ipsilateral) side. The spinothalamic tract crosses soon after it enters the spinal cord, carrying sensations of pain and temperature. In Brown - Sequard syndrome, loss of pain and temperature sensation occurs on the opposite (contralateral) side. As a result, the side of the body with motor paralysis retains pain and temperature sensations, and the other side retains movement.

80.   **Correct answer - A**

The pia mater, the meningeal layer that adheres to the sulci and gyri of the brain, is rich in blood, which it provides to the brain. Its folds form the choroid plexus that produce cerebrospinal fluid (CSF), and it also nourishes the spinal cord cells. The arachnoid layer is the meninges' middle layer, which is in contact with venous blood. Arachnoid villi, finger-like projections of arachnoid mater through the dura mater and into the venous sinuses, regulate resorption of CSF into the venous system. The outer, or dura, layer controls venous drainage by forming venous sinuses. The dura mater also supports structures of the brain. The sella turcica is a bone in the frontal area, not a meningeal layer.

81.   Correct answer - C

The blood-brain barrier is produced by fusion of endothelial cells, which causes "tight junctions" at the site of brain capillaries and a relative impermeability to certain substances. The mechanism for determining this impermeability is unknown. The blood-brain barrier exists throughout the choroid plexus and the brain except in the hypothalamus, because it is so involved in water regulation that it must come in contact with more solutes. The blood-brain barrier is most permeable to water, oxygen, and carbon dioxide.

82.   Correct answer - C

Meningococcus most commonly causes meningitis in young adults. Meningococcal meningitis, which spreads via the nasopharynx by intimate contact or droplets, is the most contagious form of the disease and causes the highest mortality. Penicillin is the drug of choice. Hemophilus influenzae is the most common cause of meningitis in children, and pneumococcus, the most common cause in adults over age 40.

83.   Correct answer - A

Kernig's and Brudzinski's signs indicate meningeal irritation. Kernig's sign is elicited by flexing the upper leg at the hip to a 90-degree angle and then attempting to extend the knee. With meningitis, pain and spasm of the hamstrings occur when an attempt is made to extend the knee. Brudzinski's sign is positive when both legs flex at the hip and knees after passive flexion of the head and neck onto the chest. A stiff neck (nuchal rigidity) and photophobia are other symptoms of meningeal irritation.

84.   Correct answer - A

Babinski's reflex, which is not associated with meningeal irritation, indicates pyramidal tract damage, an alteration in the motor tracts of the brain.

85.   **Correct answer - B**

Isolating the patient with viral meningitis is unnecessary. Correct nursing interventions include frequent temperature monitoring, because fever increases ICP, and maintaining the patient on seizure precautions, because seizure activity is common in central nervous system infection. Monitoring and managing increased ICP are also critical.

86.   **Correct answer - A**

Petechiae commonly appear in bacterial meningococcal meningitis. Petechiae, rash, purpuric lesions, or ecchymoses develop in about 50% of patients. Also common are symptoms of fever, headache, lethargy, confusion, irritability, and stiff neck.

87.   **Correct answer - C**

Neurotransmitters, such as acetylcholine, carry an impulse across the synapse - the junction between two nerves or between nerve and muscle. When the impulse reaches the synapse, an excitatory neurotransmitter is secreted, increasing the receptivity of the synapse to the impulse. Inhibitory neurotransmitters decrease the receptivity of the synapse for the impulse, preventing the impulse from crossing the synapse.

88.   **Correct answer - C**

Neurophysiologically, summation is the stimulation of many nerve fibers at one time, which increases the change of creating an action potential, or impulse. The nodes of Ranvier and the myelin sheath control saltatory conduction. Arrival of an impulse at a synapse creates neurotransmitter secretion. Schwann's cells and oligodendroglia control myelin formation in the peripheral and central nervous systems, respectively.

89.   **Correct answer - C**

Care in myasthenia gravis includes assessing forced vital capacity before and after each dose of an anticholinesterase. Because this disease is characterized by weakness of skeletal muscles, respiratory muscle strength is a reliable indication of proper medication dosage. Anticholinesterase medication should be given promptly and should not be withheld because of muscle weakness. Muscle weakness from an overdose of anticholinesterase medication can be reversed by administering atropine. The patient should not be given medications that may precipitate severe muscle weakness, such as quinidine, quinine (and tonic water, which contains quinine), procainamide, aminoglycosides, and curare. Activities should be performed in the morning, with rest periods in the afternoon to avoid fatigue.

90.   Correct answer - A

Treatment of myasthenia gravis may include immunosuppresive drugs, such as steroids, or experimental use of cytotoxic drugs, such as Imuran and Cytoxan. An autoimmune disease, myasthenia gravis is characterized by development of antiacetylcholine receptor antibodies that destroy acetylcholine and cause muscle weakness. Therapy is aimed at breaking down cholinesterase - the enzyme that eliminates acetylcholine - by administering an anticholinesterase such as Mestinon or at suppressing receptor antibody formation (immunosuppression). Diagnosis is made if symptoms temporarily improve after intra-venous injection of Tensilon, a rapid-acting anticholinesterase. Excessive amounts of anticholinesterase may precipitate cholinergic crisis, causing muscle weakness and respiratory paralysis. This is reversed by administering atropine - the antidote for an anticholinesterase. Myasthenic crisis, treated by an anticholinesterase, also induces muscle weakness, but this is a result of too little anticholinesterase or of stress, trauma, infection, surgery, or pregnancy.

91.   Correct answer - A

White matter contains both myelinated and unmyelinated fibers, with the myelin giving white matter its color. In the cerebrum, the white matter forms the inner layer, and the gray matter forms the outer layer. White matter consists of the association and projection pathways, and gray matter consists of unmyelinated fibers, cell bodies, and the nuclei of the thalamus, hypothalamus, and basal ganglia. However, in the spinal cord, white matter becomes the outer layer, while the gray matter is an H-, or butterfly-shaped, inner layer. White matter in the spinal cord consists of three tracts or pathways. The posterior tract conducts the sensation of pressure, touch, and body position from the same side of the body (it later crosses over in the brain); the anterolateral, or spinothalamic, tract, whose fibers immediately cross over to the opposite side, conducts pain and temperature sensations; and the lateral, or pyramidal, tract transmits motor impulses from the opposite side of the brain. Gray matter of the spinal cord contains motor nerves for voluntary and reflex activity, sensory nerves, and preganglionic fibers of the autonomic nervous system.

92. Correct answer - D

The nodes of Ranvier enable high-speed impulse transmission in myelinated fibers. The myelin sheath results from the presence of Schwann's cells or oligodendroglia; the interruption of this insulation is called a node of Ranvier. This node is highly responsive to impulse reception, and the impulse swiftly jumps from node to node, a condition known as saltatory conduction. It is actually the myelin that causes the fast conduction, with the impulse slowing at the node. Saltatory conduction prevents fatigue of the myelinated fiber, since only the node is depolarized.

93. Correct answer - D

Ascending muscle weakness in the legs suggests Guillain-Barr syndrome. Abnormal sensations may also be felt. Peripheral neuropathy would be suggested by bilateral sensory loss in distal extremities. Tremors, rigidity, and slow movement characterize Parkinson's disease. Muscle weakness, especially of the face and respiratory musculature, suggests myasthenia gravis.

94. Correct answer - A

An inability to stand steadily with the eyes open indicates cerebellar dysfunction. Romberg's test, of the ability to stand steadily with the eyes closed, assesses both proprioceptive ability (the awareness of body parts) and cerebellar function. A positive Romberg's test due to proprioceptive problems indicates dysfunction of the posterior ascending column of the spinal cord, which transmits sensory and proprioceptive information to the brain.

95. Correct answer - D

The most reliable test of arm motor strength is to have the patient close his eyes and raise his arms straight in front of him, palms up. The nurse should watch how well this position is maintained. Observing for spontaneous movement does not assess strength. Testing reflexes assesses the intactness of the reflex arcs. Asking the patient to close his eyes and identify if you've moved his finger up or down assesses proprioceptive function.

96. Correct answer - B

Found only in men, the cremasteric reflex is a superficial, cutaneous reflex elicited by stroking the inner thigh. The reflex is present if the scrotum elevates on the same (ipsilateral) side. Damage to either the upper or lower motor neuron is suspected if this reflex is absent.

97. Correct answer - A

A positive Babinski's reflex indicates an upper motor neuron lesion. Also called the plantar reflex, it is elicited by stroking the sole with a key or pen up the outer aspect of the foot, curving medially when reaching the ball of the foot. A normal response, or negative Babinski's reflex, is plantar flexion of the large toe or all toes. A positive response is fanning of the toes with dorsiflexion of the large toe, indicating upper motor neuron lesions of the pyramidal tract. A positive response may be normal in children under age 2.

98. Correct answer - D

Electromyography may aid in diagnosing lower motor neuron lesions and diseases of the muscle and myoneural junction, such as myasthenia gravis, amyotrophic lateral sclerosis, and muscular dystrophy. Electromyography records electrical activity along the muscle, which reflects its nervous innervation from the lower motor neuron. An electromyogram may be abnormal if spinal cord compression results from a herniated disk or spinal cord tumor, but these are best diagnosed by a myelogram - a radiographic study of the spinal cord after the injection of dye.

99. **Correct answer - D**

Lower motor neuron diseases are characterized by degenerative changes of the skin and nails along the lesion and by flaccid paralysis and absent reflexes. The lower motor neuron originates in the muscle and ends in the spinal cord.

100. **Correct answer - C**

If the ascending muscle weakness continues, Mr. M. is at risk for the development of ineffective breathing patterns as respiratory muscles weaken. Assess for hypoventilation and decreased respiratory excursion.

101. **Correct answer - A**

Before surgery, the physician should determine which hemisphere is dominant. Because the speech centers are in the dominant hemisphere's frontal and parietal areas, speech loss may occur if the surgical site is the dominant hemisphere. The physician can detect which hemisphere is dominant by injecting a small amount of a barbiturate (usually amobarbital sodium) into one internal carotid artery. If temporary aphasia results, that side is the dominant speech center.

102. **Correct answer - B**

The corpus callosum provides communication between the brain's right and left lobes. The largest of the commissures - bands of fibers that interconnect the hemispheres - it allows the two hemispheres to function as a whole, exchanging sensory information, memory, and discrimination. Cutting the corpus callosum blocks information transmission from the dominant hemisphere to the nondominant motor cortex and prevents transmission of visual and proprioceptive information from the nondominant to the dominant hemisphere.

103. **Correct answer - B**

Thigh-high, antiembolism stockings are used preoperatively, and up to 2 days postoperatively, to reduce venous stasis and prevent emboli formation. Anticoagulants, such as heparin, are contraindicated because they increase the risk of bleeding. The patient is kept dehydrated to reduce risk of increased intracranial pressure (ICP). a nasogastric tube is not indicated because the patient should be able to resume oral feedings soon after surgery.

104. Correct answer - C

Hypocarbia, a reduced PCO2 from hyperventilation, causes vasoconstriction, thereby reducing blood volume to the brain, and assists in decreasing ICP.

105. Correct answer - B

Postoperatively, the patient should be assessed for complications of diabetes insipidus caused by interruption of the nerve fibers connecting the hypothalamus and pituitary gland. Antidiuretic hormone is not secreted, resulting in the production of dilute urine. Up to 15 liters of urine per day may be lost. A low specific gravity will be noted, along with signs of fluid volume deficit, such as increased serum osmolarity and increased serum sodium.

106. Correct answer - A

Level of consciousness is the most important factor in neurologic assessment of a patient. It is the earliest and most sensitive of indicators, providing information about changes in neurologic status.

107. Correct answer - D

Inward deviation of the eyes would indicate damage to the sixth cranial nerve, the abducens. The gag reflex is controlled by the ninth and tenth cranial nerves, the glossopharyngeal and vagus nerves, respectively. The third cranial nerve, the oculomotor, controls pupillary constriction and dilation. Interruption of cerebellar function causes nystagmus.

108.   **Correct answer - C**

Partial motor seizures are characterized by tonic-clonic movement limited to one side of the body. Generalized motor, or grand mal, seizures produce tonic-clonic movement of the entire body and loss of consciousness, followed by a postictal state of drowsiness. Jerking motions occur in generalized myoclonic seizures. Partial complex seizures are characterized by bizarre behavior with no loss of consciousness, followed by postictal drowsiness and amnesia about the episode.

109.   **Correct answer - A**

A person with partial motor seizures develops paralysis of the affected side postictally. This transient paralysis, called Todd's paralysis, does not always occur after a partial motor seizure. Unconsciousness and incontinence are associated with generalized motor seizures.

110.   **Correct answer - A**

The abnormal excessive firing of cells in a portion of all of the brain causes the clinical signs and symptoms of a seizure. The metabolism of the involved cells is greatly increased during seizure activity. The abnormal firing of the neurons can terminate as abruptly as it begins.

111.   **Correct answer - C**

Patent airway maintenance is the foremost nursing goal. Placing the patient in a side-lying position with the head in alignment with the body helps to prevent aspiration. An I.V. line may then be established to administer anticonvulsants.

112.   **Correct answer - B**

The drug of choice to manage status epilepticus is diazepam, a rapid-acting anticonvulsant with less tendency than other anticonvulsants to produce hypotension.

113. Correct answer - A

The patient should be placed on a cardiac monitor and carefully observed. Rapid administration of phenytoin depresses the myocardium and can cause cardiac arrest. Obtaining a level before administration - because the patient was taking this medication at home - provides the physician with baseline levels and prevents possible toxicity. I.V. phenytoin must be given in a saline solution no faster than 50 mg/minute.

114. Correct answer - C

Because phenytoin is a myocardial depressant, third-degree heart block and cardiac arrest are most likely to occur if excessive or rapid doses of I.V. phenytoin are administered.

115. Correct answer - B

Because phenytoin is absorbed slowly from the gastrointestinal tract, timing of the daily dose can vary, according to patient convenience, and missed doses can be made up. Alcohol inhibits the action of phenytoin, while aspirin potentiates its effects.

116. Correct answer - A

Communicating hydrocephalus occurs from an obstruction outside the ventricles, such as decreased absorption in the subarachnoid space. Noncommunicating or obstructive hydrocephalus occurs from an obstruction within the ventricular system. Excessive cerebrospinal fluid production may occur with a tumor of the choroid plexus. Dilated ventricles with an unknown cause occurs in normal-pressure hydrocephalus.

117. Correct answer - D

A computed tomography (CT) scan is used to document hydrocephalus because it visualizes the dilated ventricles.

118. Correct answer - C

Normal-pressure hydrocephalus does not increase ICP. This results from dilation of the ventricles from an unknown cause.

119. Correct answer - B

Paralytic ileus may occur postoperatively from manipulation of the bowel when inserting the shunt into the peritoneum. Postoperatively, the patient is given nothing by mouth for a few days, then is started on clear liquids, and bowel status is frequently assessed.

120. Correct answer - D

Rapid reduction of ventricular size postoperatively may pull the dura away from the cerebrum, causing a subdural hematoma; the nurse must watch for signs of this. A headache may also follow rapid reduction in ventricular size, especially if the patient is in the upright position. The patient should be kept flat postoperatively, with the head of the bed slowly raised over a period of time, and should be kept off the operative side to avoid impeding functioning of the shunt. Usually the patient is given nothing by mouth, then started on clear liquids, to prevent complications if a paralytic ileus results.

Mental Humor Break

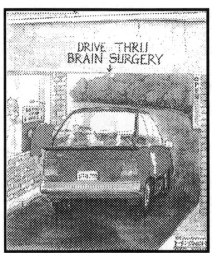

In Your Face
1-800-658-8508

CHAPTER 4

RENAL SYSTEM

---

1. Hypocalcemia may develop in a patient with which condition?

A. Chronic renal failure
B. Hyperparathyroidism
C. Thiazide therapy
D. Vitamin D overdose

---

2. Hypocalcemia also may occur in which of the following circumstances?

A. Renal trauma
B. Multiple transfusions
C. Metabolic acidosis
D. Multiple myeloma

Case Study
Questions 3-8 refer to the following case study:

Mrs. C., age 65 is admitted to your unit with a chief complaint of muscle cramps. She has had bouts of diarrhea over the last week. Abnormal laboratory values include a calcium level of 6.2 mg/dl.

---

3. In assessing for hypocalcemia, you would elicit Chvostek's sign by:

A. Applying a blood pressure (BP) cuff to the upper arm, inflating it, and observing for carpopedal spasm
B. Tapping a finger on the skin above the supramandibular portion of the parotid gland and observing for twitching of the upper lip on the side opposite the stimulation
C. Tapping a finger on the skin above the supramandibular portion of the parotid gland and observing for twitching of the upper lip on the same side as the stimulation
D. Having the patient hyperventilate (breathe more than 30 breaths/minute) to produce carpopedal from respiratory alkalosis

225

4. You can elicit Trousseau's sign in Mrs. C. by:

    A. Applying a BP cuff to her upper arm, inflating it, and observing for carpopedal spasm

    B. Tapping a finger on the supramandibular portion of the parotid gland and observing for twitching of the upper lip on the side opposite the stimulation

    C. Tapping a finger on the supramandibular portion of the parotid gland and observing for twitching of the upper lip on the same side as the stimulation

    D. Having the patient hyperventilate (breath more than 30 breaths/minute) to produce carpopedal spasm resulting from respiratory acidosis

5. Patients with hypocalcemia should demonstrate which ECG change:

    A. Shortened PR interval
    B. Prolonged PR interval
    C. Prolonged QT interval
    D. U wave

6. Complications that may develop for Mrs. C include all of the following *except:*

    A. Seizures and twitching
    B. Oliguria or anuria
    C. Laryngeal stridor
    D. Bleeding abnormalities

7. Which of the following would you expect Mrs. C. to exhibit?

    A. Neuromuscular irritability and bronchospasm
    B. Neuromuscular weakness and flaccidity
    C. Polydipsia and polyuria
    D. Personality changes followed by coma

8. Calcium chloride has been ordered for Mrs. C. Which solution would *not* be appropriate for administering this medication?

    A. Dextrose 5% in water
    B. Lactated Ringer's
    C. Normal saline
    D. Dextrose 2.5% in water

Case Study

Questions 9-12 refer to the following case study:

Mrs. H., age 78, enters the emergency department (ED) with a chief complaint of abdominal cramping. She has a history of diabetes mellitus and chronic renal failure. An I.V. line is established and blood is drawn for laboratory studies. Her serum potassium level is 6 mEq/liter. Hyperkalemia is diagnosed.

9. Pharmacologic management of Mrs. H.'s hyperkalemia should include all of the following *except:*

   A. Lactulose enemas
   B. 50% glucose and regular insulin
   C. Sodium bicarbonate
   D. Calcium chloride

10. Patients with hyperkalemia must be monitored for which of the following ECG changes?

    A. Prolonged QT interval
    B. Peaked T waves
    C. Prominent U waves
    D. Shortened PR interval

11. In a physical assessment of Mrs. H., which of the following signs and symptoms would be expected?

    A. Apathy, oliguria and absent bowel sounds
    B. Ascending muscle weakness and bradycardia
    C. Descending muscle weakness and tachycardia
    D. Hyperactive bowel sounds and polyuria

12. Which acid-base imbalance is commonly associated with hyperkalemia?

    A. Respiratory acidosis
    B. Metabolic alkalosis
    C. Respiratory alkalosis
    D. Metabolic acidosis

Case Study

Questions 13-15 refer to the following case study:

Mr. J., age 24, boxes on the weekends. He has sustained blunt trauma to the left kidney during a boxing match. His chief complaint is flank tenderness. Urinalysis reveals microscopic hematuria. All other laboratory data are within normal limits.

13. Which manifestations by Mr. J. indicate renal trauma?

   A. Severe, colicky flank pain and diaphoresis
   B. Hematuria and flank tenderness
   C. Urethral bleeding and severe flank pain
   D. Severe flank pain and no urine output

14. Ecchymosis around the area of the left flank can indicate:

   A. Pulled muscles in the flank area
   B. Fractured iliac bone
   C. Retroperitoneal bleeding
   D. All of the above

15. If Mr. J. experiences increased pain, the nurse should first:

   A. Administer narcotics
   B. Draw a serum electrolyte level
   C. Take a hematocrit sample
   D. Take his blood pressure

16. The nurse would suspect renal trauma if a patient exhibits which finding?

   A. Positive Chvostek's sign
   B. Oliguria
   C. Hematoma in flank area
   D. Dysuria

17. The nurse would suspect renal trauma in the patient with which injury?

   A. Chest trauma
   B. Pelvic fracture
   C. Deceleration injury
   D. All of the above

18. Renal trauma is best diagnosed by which test?

   A. KUB (X-ray of kidneys, ureters, and bladder)
   B. Abdominal computed tomography (CT) scan
   C. IVP (intravenous pyelogram)
   D. Peritoneal tap

Questions 19-24 refer to the following case study:

Mr. T. is admitted to the coronary care unit (CCU) with complaints of vague chest pain and abdominal cramping. ECG findings include a prolonged QT interval. Serum phosphate level is 4.9 mg/dl. Hyperphosphatemia is diagnosed.

19. All of the following may be precipitating factors in the development of Mr. T.'s hyperphosphatemia *except?*

   A. Acute renal failure
   B. Chronic renal failure
   C. Hypoparathyroidism
   D. Overadministration of phospahte-binding gels

20. In assessing Mr. T., the nurse would anticipate which of the following findings:

   A. Cramps and possible tetany
   B. Shortening of the ST segment
   C. Muscle wasting and weakness
   D. Diminished neuromuscular activity

21. Which electrolyte must be present in the proximal tubule for phosphate reabsorption?

   A. Sodium
   B. Potassium
   C. Chloride
   D. Calcium

22. Which condition would *not* result in hypophosphatemia?

   A. Chronic alcoholism
   B. Hyperalimentation
   C. Chronic renal failure
   D. Hyperparathyroidism

23. Clinical manifestations of hypophosphatemia include:

   A. Chvostek's sign
   B. Seizure activity
   C. Trousseau's sign
   D. Muscle weakness

24. Which nursing intervention would *not* be appropriate in hypophosphatemia?

A. Monitoring complete blood count (CBC) and arterial blood gases (ABGs)
B. Administering phosphate-binding medications
C. Monitoring calcium levels closely
D. Providing frequent rest periods and small, frequent meals

Case Study
Questions 25-29 refer to the following case study:

Mr. L., a 50-year-old hemodialysis patient, is admitted to the intensive care unit (ICU) with a potassium level of 7.2 mEq/ liter. Ten units of regular insulin and 50 ml of a 50% dextrose solution IVP have been ordered.

25. Which of the following diuretics would *not* precipitate hyperkalemia?

A. Spironolactone
B. Mannitol
C. Aldactone
D. An aldosterone antagonist

26. Mr. L. has ECG changes indicating severe hyperkalemia. Which drug would *not* be appropriate to administer?

A. Plicamycin
B. I.V. glucose, insulin, sodium bicarbonate
C. I.V. calcium chloride or calcium gluconate
D. Sodium polystyrene sulfonate (Kayexalate) and Sorbitol

27. A weight gain by Mr. L. of one kilogram in 24 hours may indicate fluid retention of at least:

A. 250 ml
B. 500 ml
C. 1,000 ml
D. 2,000 ml

28. Hyperkalemia may occur in the patient with:

A. Alkalosis
B. Renal tubular acidosis
C. Adrenal insufficiency
D. Diuretic therapy in progress

230

29. Which of the following symptoms would *not* be consistent with hyperkalemia?

   A. Numbness and tingling
   B. Hyperactive bowel sounds and abdominal cramps
   C. Lethargy and nausea
   D. Paralytic ileus and dysrhythmias

30. The electrolyte abnormality that produces peaked T waves, a widened QRS complex, and impaired atrioventricular conduction is:

   A. Hypokalemia
   B. Hyperkalemia
   C. Hypercalcemia
   D. Hypocalcemia

31. Which of the following would *not* influence the amount of potassium excreted in the urine?

   A. Antidiuretic hormone (ADH) secretion
   B. The volume of urine excreted
   C. Acid-base status
   D. Serum potassium levels

32. Hyperparathyroidism, metastatic carcinoma, excessive doses of vitamin D, and chronic thiazide therapy can cause which electrolyte imbalance?

   A. Hypercalcemia
   B. Hypokalemia
   C. Hyponatremia
   D. Hyperphosphatemia

Case Study
Questions 33-37 refer to the following case study:

Mr. D., a 52-year-old man with newly diagnosed multiple myeloma, is admitted to the emergency department with back pain after falling against a bookcase at home. X-rays reveal a rib fracture. Electrolytes reveal a serum calcium level of 12.7 mg/dl. Hypercalcemia is diagnosed.

33. Hypercalcemia occurs in multiple myeloma as a result of:

A. Calcium being mobilized from the intestines, teeth, and bones
B. Lesions releasing calcium into plasma
C. Increased tubular reabsorption of calcium
D. Increased intestinal reabsorption of calcium secondary to excessive vitamin D intake

34. Complications of Mr. D.'s hypercalcemia may include:

A. Flank or thigh pain and polyuria
B. Anuria or oliguria and constipation
C. Diarrhea and metabolic alkalosis
D. Constipation and metabolic acidosis

35. Which ECG change occurs in hypercalcemia?

A. Prolonged PR interval
B. Prolonged QT interval
C. Shortened ST segment
D. U waves

36. With a serum calcium level of 12.7 mg/dl, Mr. D. is likely to exhibit which of the following signs and symptoms?

A. Anxiety, restlessness, and irritability
B. Diarrhea and hyperactive bowel sounds
C. Rigidity and neuromuscular irritability
D. Polyuria, nausea, and vomiting

37. Therapies to correct hypercalcemia include:

A. Normal saline infusion and loop diuretics
B. Normal saline infusion and thiazide diuretics
C. Sodium polystyrene sulfonate (Kayexalate) enemas
D. Hemodialysis, glucose, and insulin

38. Plicamycin may be used in treating:

A. Hyperkalemia
B. Hypercalcemia
C. Hyperchloremic acidosis
D. Hyperphosphatemia

Case Study

Questions 39-41 refer to the following case study:

Mr. P. is a patient admitted several days ago with a diagnosis of bowel obstruction. Vital signs are a blood pressure of 90/60, a pulse of 110 beats/minute, and a respiratory rate of 22 breaths/minute. Urine output has been steadily decreasing. Prerenal failure is diagnosed.

39. Oliguria is defined as urine output of less than:

   A.   400 ml/day
   B.   600 ml/day
   C.   60 ml/hour
   D.   40 ml/hour

40. Which condition would cause prerenal failure?

   A.   Nephrotoxicity
   B.   Glomerulonephritis
   C.   Acute tubular necrosis
   D.   Hypovolemia

41. Mr. P. has a urine output of 200 ml in the last 24 hours, with a urine sodium level of less than 10 mEq/liter. Which of the following would *not* cause these findings?

   A.   Decreased circulating fluid volume
   B.   Prerenal failure
   C.   Acute tubular necrosis
   D.   Diminished renal perfusion

42. A patient has a urine output of 1,000 ml/24 hours, with a urine sodium level of 26 mEq/liter. These findings suggest that:

   A.   The patient is probably on a salt-free diet
   B.   The patient's kidneys have a decreased blood perfusion
   C.   The patient is in the beginning of renal failure
   D.   The patient is progressing to the prerenal phase

43. After what time would a patient be at risk for intrarenal failure if compromised renal perfusion occurred with a mean systolic pressure below 60 mm Hg.

A. 40 minutes
B. 4 hours
C. 12 hours
D. 24 hours

44. The urine sodium level of an oliguric patient is 60 mEq/liter. Conditions that cause this finding include all of the following *except:*

A. Severe dehydration
B. Acute tubular necrosis
C. Glomerulonephritis
D. Nephrotoxicity

45. A patient has a urine output of 200 ml in the last 24 hours, with a specific gravity of 1.008. These findings suggest that:

A. Specific gravity is normal, but low urine output is a concern
B. Specific gravity is low; possible renal damage should be investigated
C. Specific gravity is high, possibly from severe dehydration
D. Specific gravity is low, probably from hypovolemia

46. Four abnormal serum laboratory findings common to patients with acute renal failure are:

A. ↑ Na, ↑ K ↑ BUN ↓ creatinine
B. ↑ Na, ↑ K ↑ BUN ↓ creatinine
C. ↓ Na, ↓ K ↑ BUN ↑ creatinine
D. ↓ Na, ↑ K ↑ BUN ↑ creatinine

47. In acute tubular necrosis caused by nephrotoxic drugs, furosemide (Lasix):

A. Increases toxicity
B. Causes diuresis, thus correcting oliguria
C. Increases blood flow to the kidneys, thus reversing tubular damage
D. Improves the patient's renal status

48. Which of the following electrolyte imbalances may develop as a result of diuretic therapy?

A. Hyponatremia, hypokalemia, and hyperuricemia
B. Hyponatremia, metabolic acidosis, and hyperchloremia
C. Hypokalemia, hypouremia and Hyponatremia
D. Metabolic alkalosis, hypernatremia, and hypokalemia

49. The primary site for the action of furosemide (Lasix) is the:

A. Distal and convoluted tubule
B. Proximal tubule
C. Descending loop of Henle
D. Ascending loop of Henle

50. In the diuretic phase of acute tubular necrosis, for which complication must the nurse be alert?

A. Fluid overload
B. Hypokalemia
C. Hypertension
D. Hypernatremia

51. All of the following herald recovery from acute tubular necrosis *except:*

A. Decreasing blood urea nitrogen (BUN)
B. Normalizing creatinine level
C. Increasing serum creatinine
D. Specific urine gravity of 1.020

52. Patients with acute renal failure may have all of the following cardiac complications *except:*

A. Peaked T waves ECG and pericarditis
B. Sinus tachycardia and ST elevations
C. Heart failure and friction rub
D. Mitral insufficiency and Mobitz Type II heart block

Case Study
Questions 53-57 refer to the following case study:

Mr. R., age 45, is admitted to the ICU with a diagnosis of chronic renal failure. His chief complaint is indigestion.

235

53. Which of the following may safely be given to Mr. R. for his indigestion?

A. Mylanta
B. Maalox
C. Amphojel or Basaljel
D. All of the above

54. Mr. R. must have a protein-restricted diet to:

A. Maintain a negative nitrogen balance
B. Prevent overburdening of kidney function
C. Decrease urea production
D. Allow for protein synthesis

55. Patients with chronic renal failure are given phosphate binders to:

A. Prevent ulcers caused by increased stimulation of hydro-chloric acid
B. Increase serum magnesium levels
C. Lower serum calcium levels
D. Reduce serum phosphorus levels

56. The primary acid-base disorder associated with renal failure is:

A. Respiratory acidosis
B. Metabolic acidosis
C. Respiratory alkalosis
D. Metabolic alkalosis

57. Complications of renal failure that Mr. R. could face include all of the following *except:*

A. Clotting dyscrasias and anemia
B. Metabolic acidosis
C. Hypertension and susceptibility to infection
D. Respiratory acidosis

58. Which structure is located within Bowman's capsule?

A. Loop of Henle
B. Glomerulus
C. Proximal tubule
D. Juxtaglomerular apparatus

59. The functional segments of the nephron include:

A. Bowman's capsule, juxtaglomerular apparatus, and ascending and descending loops of Henle
B. Glomerulus, Bowman's capsule, and renal tubules
C. Bowman's capsule, renal pyramids, and collecting tubules
D. Juxtaglomerular apparatus, glomerulus, and distal convoluted tubule

60. In which order does the glomerular filtrate flow?

A. Collecting duct, loop of Henle, proximal tubule, and distal tubule
B. Collecting duct, proximal tubule, loop of Henle, and distal tubule
C. Proximal tubule, collecting duct, distal tubule, and loop of Henle
D. Proximal tubule, loop of Henle, distal tubule, and collecting duct

61. An abnormal characteristic of the glomerular filtrate is that:

A. It has a specific gravity of 1.010 and a plasma-like quality
B. It is protein-free with few red blood cells (RBCs)
C. It contains glucose and sodium
D. It contains urea and creatinine

62. Glomerular filtration rate (GFR) can be measured by evaluating the patient's:

A. Serum creatinine
B. Blood urea nitrogen (BUN)
C. Serum osmolality
D. Creatinine clearance

63. What percentage of the glomerular filtrate do the renal tubules normally reabsorb?

A. Over 50%
B. Over 75%
C. Over 85%
D. Over 99%

64. Which of the following will reduce the GFR?

   A. Hypoproteinemia
   B. Serum albumin level of 4
   C. Cardiac output of 6 liters/minute
   D. Overhydration

65. Which of the following would *not* influence the GFR?

   A. Alterations in the pressure of Bowman's capsule
   B. Hypertrophy of the renal calices
   C. Alterations in oncotic pressure
   D. Changes in glomerular hydrostatic pressure

66. About 60% to 80% of the glomerular filtrate is reabsorbed in the:

   A. Bowman's capsule
   B. Glomerulus
   C. Proximal tubule
   D. Loop of Henle

67. The loop of Henle is primarily concerned with:

   A. Concentration or dilution of urine
   B. Reabsorption of HCO_3 and secretion of H^+
   C. Active reabsorption of NaCl with passive reabsorption of water
   D. Secretion of organic acids and foreign substances

68. Which of the following does *not* occur at the distal convoluted tubule?

   A. Water reabsorption under antidiuretic hormone (ADH) control
   B. Sodium reabosorption by aldosterone secretion
   C. Reabsorption of potassium, ammonia, and hydrogen
   D. Reabsorption of water, sodium chloride, and sodium bicarbonate

69. Normal serum osmolality is between:

   A. 250 and 275 mOsm/liter
   B. 285 and 295 mOsm/liter
   C. 275 and 325 mOsm/liter
   D. 325 and 350 mOsm/liter

70. If a patient's serum electrolytes are within normal limits, which of the following primarily influences serum osmolality?

   A. Sodium
   B. Glucose
   C. BUN
   D. Potassium

71. Sodium reabsorption increases in the renal tubules during all of the following conditions *except:*

   A. ADH release
   B. GFR decrease
   C. Aldosterone secretion
   D. Renal hypoperfusion

72. The substance directly responsible for peripheral vasoconstriction and increased aldosterone secretion is:

   A. Angiotensinogen
   B. Angiotensin I
   C. Angiotensin II
   D. Renin

73. All of the following conditions may precipitate hypernatremia *except:*

   A. Lack of ADH
   B. Hypercalcemia
   C. Uncontrolled diabetes mellitus with osmotic diuresis
   D. Hypoaldosteronism

74. Nursing implications in hypernatremia include all of the following *except:*

   A. Monitoring serum sodium levels, serum osmolality, and urine osmolality
   B. Performing neurologic assessments and correlating them with serum sodium levels
   C. Administering normal saline or dextrose 5% in normal saline solution to maintain blood pressure
   D. Knowing that rapid correction of sodium levels can cause cerebral edema

75. Serum sodium levels below 120 mEq/liter may be associated with:

   A. Seizures
   B. Neuromuscular rigidity
   C. Positive Chvostek's sign
   D. Hypertension

76. Which set of symptoms characterizes dilutional hyponatremia as a result of water intoxication?

   A. Good skin turgor and weight gain
   B. Increased BUN and serum osmolality
   C. Orthostatic pressures and tachycardia
   D. Increased hematocrit and flat neck veins

77. A commonly used glucose concentration of peritoneal dialysate is:

   A. 1.5%
   B. 4.25%
   C. 5%
   D. 25%

78. Normal peritoneal dialysate drainage should be:

   A. Clear and pinkish
   B. Clear and colorless
   C. Opaque beige
   D. Clear and straw-colored

79. Which of the following techniques may be used to facilitate peritoneal dialysate drainage?

   A. Turning the patient from side to side and elevating the head of the bed
   B. Introducing the stylet into the catheter as ordered by the physician, using sterile technique
   C. Massaging the abdomen
   D. All of the above

80. Principles underlying dialysis include:

   A. Diffusion
   B. Osmosis
   C. Filtration
   D. All of the above

81. Whenever 4.25% dialysate solution is used in peritoneal dialysis, the diabetic patient should be closely monitored for:

A. Fluid overload
B. Hyperglycemia
C. Congestive heart failure
D. Hypertension

82. Complications of peritoneal dialysis include:

A. Pneumonia and atelectasis
B. Bowel perforation and peritonitis
C. Hypoproteinemia
D. All of the above

Case Study
Questions 83-84 refer to the following case study:

Mr. K. is returned to the ICU from the operating room. He has received a kidney transplant.

83. Which of the following studies would *not* be essential in determining tissue compatibility between donor and recipient during the pretransplant phase of organ transplantation?

A. Sulkowitch's test
B. ABO blood typing
C. White cell crossmatching
D. Human leukocyte antigen (HLA) typing

84. Which of the following signs and symptoms may indicate acute organ rejection postoperatively in Mr. K?

A. BUN of 30 mg/dl and a serum creatinine level of 1mg/dl
B. Fever over 100° F. (37.8° C.) and a transplanted kidney that is swollen, soft, and tender on palpation
C. Urine output of 100 ml/hour with a specific gravity of 1.014
D. Renogram showing increased uptake of dye

85. Renal regulation of bicarbonate concentration includes all of the following *except:*

A. Secretion of hydrogen ions
B. Synthesis of ammonium
C. Reabsorption of bicarbonate
D. Reabsorption of hydrogen ions

86. With a disease that contributes to chloride loss, a patient is prone to:

A. Metabolic alkalosis
B. Respiratory alkalosis
C. Hyperkalemia
D. Hypernatremia

87. Severe diarrhea and intestinal fistulas may cause:

A. Metabolic alkalosis
B. Hypochloremia
C. Metabolic acidosis
D. Respiratory acidosis

88. Signs and symptoms of rapidly developing alkalosis may include all of the following *except:*

A. Obtundation
B. Nervous irritability
C. Muscle tremors
D. Seizures

89. The body compensates for metabolic alkalosis through:

A. Hypoventilation
B. Increased $PaCO_2$
C. Increased carbonic acid formation
D. All of the above

90. Which of the following symptoms do *not* usually indicate metabolic acidosis?

A. Hypoventilation and paresthesias
B. Headache and confusion
C. Central nervous system (CNS) depression and cardiac dysrhythmias
D. Hypotension and decreased myocardial contractility

91. Which of the following will contribute to metabolic acidosis?

A. Hypoxia
B. Diuretic abuse
C. Hypokalemia
D. Vomiting

92. Acidosis affects electrolyte balance by:

A. Shifting potassium from the cell into the intravascular space without affecting calcium

B. Translocating potassium into the interstitial space and lowering serum calcium levels

C. Having no effect on potassium and, when severe, causing hypocalcemia

D. Driving potassium out of the cell and decreasing the amount of binding between calcium and albumin

---

Case Study
Questions 93-98 refer to the following case study:

Mr. S., age 24, is admitted to the ICU after an automobile accident. The dashboard and steering wheel were pinned against his abdomen and legs for 1 hour before rescue workers freed him. He is conscious and in severe abdominal and pelvic pain. His vital signs are stable: blood pressure is 120/70 mm Hg; pulse is 86 beats/minute; respirations are 22 breaths/minute. His penis and testes are swollen and painful. Blood is oozing from his urethra. Pelvic fracture with genitourinary trauma is diagnosed. A urologist is scheduled to see the patient.

---

93. Which statement about urethral trauma is *true?*

A. The patient should be encouraged to void to prevent urinary retention

B. The nurse should insert an indwelling urinary drainage catheter as soon as possible to maintain a patent urethra

C. A suprapubic catheter may be inserted by the urologist to divert urine

D. The patient is usually incontinent because the sphincter is damaged

---

94. Which symptom will be present in Mr. S. if his urethra is completely transected?

A. Hematuria
B. Extravasation of urine from the bladder
C. Urethral bleeding
D. Severe, colicky pain

95. Rupture of the bladder is more likely to occur:

    A. When the bladder is full
    B. In women
    C. In straddle injuries
    D. In injuries to the lower chest

96. If Mr. S. has a ruptured bladder, he should also be assessed for:

    A. Ruptured spleen
    B. Pancreatitis
    C. Rectal injury
    D. Spinal cord injury

97. The patient with a ruptured bladder will probably exhibit which of the following signs and symptoms?

    A. Pyuria and fever
    B. Hematuria and fever
    C. Pyuria and severe pelvic pain
    D. Hematuria, pelvic discomfort, and difficulty in voiding

98. Besides pain relief, which nursing actions are indicated in caring for a patient after trauma to the testes?

    A. Applying ice packs and elevating the testes
    B. Applying heat packs and elevating the testes
    C. Applying heat packs and leaving the testes in their natural position to avoid further trauma
    D. Applying ice packs and leaving the testes in their natural position to avoid further trauma

1. **Correct answer - A**

Hypocalcemia may develop in a patient with chronic renal failure, in which the kidney cannot hydroxylate vitamin D into its final form. Vitamin D is necessary for calcium absorption from the small intestine. In addition, hyperphosphatemia from chronic renal failure potentiates peripheral deposition of calcium. Hyperparathyroidism, or increased levels of parathormone, causes excessive mobilization of calcium from bone. Vitamin D overdose causes an increased intestinal reabsorption of calcium. Thiazide diuretic therapy inhibits calcium excretion, thus producing hypercalcemia. Hypocalcemia may also occur in patients with excessive gastrointestinal losses secondary to diarrhea.

2. **Correct answer - B**

Hypocalcemia may develop in a patient who has received multiple transfusions. Banked blood contains sodium citrate, which binds with the calcium in stored blood. Multiple myeloma produces hypercalcemia. Renal trauma and metabolic acidosis do not affect calcium levels.

3. **Correct answer - C**

A decrease in ionized calcium increases neuromuscular excitability. Tapping over a branch of the facial nerve and observing for twitching of the upper lip on the ipsilateral (same) side as stimulation is considered a positive Chvostek's sign. Inflating a blood pressure cuff on the upper arm or having the patient hyperventilate will produce carpopoedal spasm; these measures are used to elicit Trousseau's sign.

4. **Correct answer - A**

Trousseau's sign is elicited by applying a blood pressure cuff to the patient's arm, inflating it to the patient's systolic pressure, and observing for carpopedal spasm. Another method for producing this phenomenon is hyperventilation, in which the alkalotic state decreases serum calcium levels.

5. **Correct answer - C**

Hypocalcemia impairs cardiac contractility (demonstrated on the ECG as a prolonged QT interval), which predisposes the patient to a polymorphous ventricular tachycardia (torsades de pointes).

6. **Correct answer - B**

Oliguria and anuria do not occur in hypocalcemia. Bleeding abnormalities occur because calcium helps convert prothrombin to thrombin in the coagulation cascade. The reduced calcium levels cause seizures. Neuromuscular irritability results in bronchospasm and laryngeal stridor.

7. **Correct answer - A**

The patient with hypocalcemia may exhibit labored, shallow breathing and, if respiratory musculature is involved, wheezing and bronchospasm. Neuromuscular irritability can cause airway obstruction and bronchial spasm. The patient may also exhibit muscle tremors, cramps (with minor reductions in calcium level), tetany and generalized tonic clonic seizures (with severe reductions in calcium level), and positive Chvostek's and Trousseau's signs.

8. **Correct answer - C**

Normal saline solution increases the glomerular filtration rate (GFR) and calcium excretion. Consequently, mixing calcium in normal saline solution is inappropriate.

9. **Correct answer - A**

Treatment of hyperkalemia consists of administering calcium, glucose, insulin, and sodium bicarbonate. Glucose and insulin drive potassium into the cells. Sodium bicarbonate corrects the accompanying metabolic acidosis. Calcium stimulates cardiac contractility. Lactulose is used to treat hepatic failure.

10. **Correct answer - B**

Impaired neuromuscular transmission produces intraventricular conduction disturbances. The predominant cardiac abnormalities are repolarization changes, reflected as a peaked T wave, seen in early stages of hyperkalemia. As potassium levels increase, other changes occur, including a prolonged PR interval, an absence of P waves, and widened QRS complex.

11. **Correct answer - B**

Ascending muscle weakness, usually originating in the legs and traveling to the trunk, occurs in hyperkalemia. Because the diaphragm and intercostal muscles are usually spared, respiratory function is not impaired. Cardiac abnormalities include sinus bradycardia, a prolonged PR interval, and a widened QRS complex. Increased peristalsis and oliguria also result. Apathy can occur in hypokalemia or hyperkalemia.

12.   Correct answer - D

Metabolic acidosis is the acid-base imbalance commonly seen with potassium excess. This occurs when potassium, rather than hydrogen, is exchanged for sodium in the kidney. Metabolic acidosis causes a shift of potassium out of the cell into the serum as hydrogen, an acid, enters the cell.

13.   Correct answer - B

Hematuria and flank tenderness indicate renal trauma. Minor contusions are associated with microscopic hematuria, whereas gross blood in the urine is a finding consistent with major damage. Flank tenderness may reflect hemorrhage or extravasation of urine. Colicky pain is associated with obstruction rather than trauma. Bleeding from the urethra indicates urethral trauma; urine output will not initially change as a result of trauma.

14.   Correct answer - C

When trauma ruptures the renal vasculature, bleeding into the retroperitoneal space occurs, as evidenced by ecchymosis around the flank area. The amount of bleeding depends on the degree of injury. This condition may be so severe that the patient succumbs to shock resulting from hemorrhage.

15.   Correct answer - D

A hematoma in the kidney may expand, increasing pain or tenderness. Suspect bleeding if hypotension is present. Although it is appropriate to take a hematocrit sample, the first action should be to assess vital signs, including blood pressure. Drawing a serum electrolyte level yields no valuable information in this situation. Narcotics may be given for pain but their administration is not the primary intervention for bleeding. In some instances, narcotics will be withheld to avoid masking of symptoms, such as increased pain.

16.   Correct answer - C

Renal trauma should be suspected if the patient has a hematoma in the flank area. Other signs and symptoms include flank or microscopic hematuria, flank pain that increases with movement and that radiates to the groin, and abdominal rigidity. Hypotension and hypovolemic shock may result if significant blood loss occurs. Swelling or a mass in the flank area may be present on palpation. Chvostek's sign (facial twitching elicited by tapping the facial nerve) indicates hypocalcemia. Oliguria is seen in prerenal and intrarenal failure. Dysuria (painful urination) is a sign of urinary tract infection and renal calculi.

17.   Correct answer - D

Trauma to the kidneys should be suspected in chest trauma, pelvic fracture, and deceleration injuries. Chest trauma can cause kidney injuries, especially if the lower ribs have been fractured. Deceleration injuries, such as those caused by motor vehicle accidents and contact sports, most commonly cause renal trauma. Most kidney injuries are caused by blunt trauma, but penetrating trauma, such as gunshot or stab wounds, may also cause renal trauma.

18.   Correct answer - C

Renal trauma is best diagnosed by an intravenous pyelogram (IVP). Positive findings include extravasation or delayed excretion of contrast media, distortion of the renal silhouette, and no visualization of the affected kidney. Before this test, the nurse should determine if the patient has a known history of allergy to contrast media or iodine. Methylprednisolone and Benadryl should be available if the allergy history is unknown. A KUB may also help determine renal injury, demonstrating an enlarged kidney shadow on the affected side.

19.   Correct answer - D

Overadministration of phosphate-binding gels causes hypophosphatemia. Acute renal failure, chronic renal failure, and hypoparathyroidism precipitate hyperphosphatemia. In acute and chronic renal failure, the kidneys cannot excrete phosphate. In hypoparathyroidism, parathyroid hormone (PTH) lowers phosphate levels in the kidney.

20.   Correct answer - A

Signs and symptoms of hyperphosphatemia - similar to those of hypocalcemia - include neuromuscular irritability ranging from muscle cramps to tetany. The patient may also develop tetany of the laryngeal or respiratory muscles, producing bronchospasm, and tonic-clonic seizures.

21. **Correct answer - A**

Phosphate reabsorption, an active process that occurs in the proximal tubule, depends on sodium.

22. **Correct answer - C**

Chronic renal failure usually does not result in hypophosphatemia; on the contrary, phosphate levels increase because the kidneys cannot excrete it. Decreased phosphate levels occur in chronic alcoholism (because of inadequate phosphate intake from malnutrition), hyperalimentation (glucose phosphorylation leads to phosphate depletion), and hyperparathyroidism (caused by renal phosphaturia).

23. **Correct answer - D**

Clinical signs of hypophosphatemia, which creates a reciprocal hypercalcemia, include muscle weakness, anorexia, and malaise. Chvostek's and Trousseau's signs and seizures activity are all manifestations of hypocalcemia or hyperphosphatemia.

24. **Correct answer - B**

Nursing interventions for hypophosphatemia include evaluating complete blood count (CBC) and arterial blood gas (ABG) levels because prolonged deficits result in phagocytic activities, platelet dysfunction, hemolysis, hypoxia, and metabolic acidosis. The nurse also must monitor calcium levels closely because hypophosphatemia creates a reciprocal hypercalcemia. Providing frequent rest periods and small, frequent meals helps combat muscle weakness from a lack of intracellular phosphates, which may inhibit the energy-producing metabolic process. Other manifestations of hypophosphatemia are anorexia, malaise, and neuromuscular changes. Administering phosphate-binding medications would cause further hypophosphatemia.

25. **Correct answer - B**

Mannitol exerts an osmotic effect in the tubules, causing diuresis in excess of sodium chloride. Spironolactone (Aldactone) is an aldosterone antagonist, or inhibitor. Aldosterone inhibition promotes sodium secretion into the distal tubule and potassium reabsorption, causing mild diuresis while protecting the body's potassium level.

26. **Correct answer - A**

Nursing interventions for severe hyperkalemia include administration of I.V. glucose, insulin, and sodium bicarbonate to temporarily

249

drive potassium into the cells, I.V. calcium chloride or calcium gluconate to stimulate cardiac contractility (this may be contraindicated in patients on digoxin), and sodium polystyrene sulfonate (Kayexalate) and Sorbitol to reverse hyperkalemia. Because Kayexalate causes exchange of sodium for potassium ions, the nurse must assess sodium gain as well as potassium loss. Plicamycin is indicated for hypercalcemia.

27. **Correct answer - C**

Daily weight is the most reliable indicator of fluid retention in the critically ill patient. A weight gain of 1 kg usually indicates about 1,000 ml of fluid retention.

28. **Correct answer - C**

Adrenal insufficiency, or hypoaldosteronism, causes hyperkalemia. A lack of or decrease in aldosterone alters sodium reabsorption and potassium excretion. In adrenal insufficiency, sodium is not reabsorbed back into the body and potassium cannot be excreted, thus resulting in a low serum sodium level and an elevated serum potassium level. Alkalosis, renal tubular acidosis, and diuretic therapy cause decreased potassium levels. Alkalosis stimulates potassium secretion in the distal tubule and an intracellular shifting of potassium. Renal tubular acidosis and diuretic therapy increase potassium excretion via the kidneys.

29. **Correct answer - D**

Manifestations of hyperkalemia include lethargy, nausea, diarrhea, abdominal cramps, hyperactive bowel sounds, muscle weakness beginning in the legs and ascending toward the trunk and arms, and numbness, tingling, and dysrhythmias from the myocardial depressant effect on conduction and contractility. Paralytic ileus is commonly associated with hypokalemia.

30. **Correct answer - B**

Hyperkalemia produces peaked T waves, a widened QRS complex with associated bradycardia, and disappearance of the P wave, progressing to idioventricular rhythm, asystole, and cardiac arrest. Hypokalemia produces a depressed ST segment, flat or inverted T waves, a U wave, and ventricular dysrhythmias. With hypercalcemia, the ECG reveals shortening of the QT interval and ST segment, whereas hypocalcemia produces a prolonged QT interval and ST segment.

31.   **Correct answer - A**

Factors enhancing potassium excretion include conditions that increase cellular potassium. Elevated cellular potassium levels increase the exchange between sodium and potassium ions. Potassium ions are excreted into urine and sodium ions are reabsorbed. Alkalosis, either metabolic or respiratory, causes movement of potassium ions into cells. Increasing urine flow to the distal portion of the nephron increases the number of available potassium ions and thus the excretion of potassium. Serum potassium levels influence potassium excretion through the aldosterone feedback mechanism. ADH secretion results only in water reabsorption in the distal tubule and collecting ducts.

32.   **Correct answer - A**

Hypercalcemia can result from hyperparathyroidism, metastatic carcinoma, excessive doses of vitamin D, or chronic thiazide therapy. Hyperparathyroidism causes increased tubular reabsorption of calcium. Metastatic carcinoma causes lesions to release calcium into plasma. Excessive doses of vitamin D increase reabsorption of calcium from intestines. Chronic thiazide therapy inhibits calcium excretion. Other causes of hypercalcemia include hypophosphatemia, alkalosis, and immobilization.

33.   **Correct answer - B**

In multiple myeloma, the calcium stores in the bone are released into the extracellular fluid, producing hypercalcemia. In other conditions, hypercalcemia also results from altered renal tubular reabsorption, increased mobilization in primary hyperparathyroidism, and increased intestinal reabsorption secondary to large dietary intake and excessive administration or intake of vitamin D.

34.   **Correct answer - A**

Flank and thigh pain result from renal calculi, which occur in about two-thirds of patients with hypercalcemia. Polyuria results when calcium inhibits ADH secretion in the distal tubules.

35.   **Correct answer - C**

Increased extracellular levels of calcium predispose the patient to repolarization changes (shortening of ST segment) and ultimately, cardiac arrest. If a patient is receiving digitalis therapy, hypercalcemia may enhance the digitalis effect, which can contribute to dysrhythmias or arrest.

36.   Correct answer - D

Increased calcium levels inhibit the action of ADH on the distal and collecting tubules, stimulating gastric acid secretion and the possible development of a peptic ulcer and producing polyuria, nausea, and vomiting. Other manifestations of hypercalcemia include confusion that may progress into coma; hypotonicity, muscle weakness, and pathologic fractures; lethargy; and renal calculi.

37.   Correct answer - A

Normal saline solution is administered to increase the patient's glomerular filtration rate (GFR) and calcium excretion. Loop diuretics are used to prevent tubular reabsorption of calcium. Other therapies for hypercalcemia include corticosteroids to decrease gastrointestinal absorption of calcium, Plicamycin to stimulate bone uptake of calcium, and oral phosphates to bind calcium. Kayexalate, glucose, insulin, and hemodialysis are used to treat hyperkalemia. Thiazide diuretics should be avoided because they decrease calcium excretion.

38.   Correct answer - B

Plicamycin therapy may be used to treat hypercalcemia because the drug stimulates bone uptake of calcium. Other therapies to reduce the serum calcium level include normal saline infusion and diuretics to increase the GFR of calcium excretion, steroids to decrease gastrointestinal absorption of calcium, and oral phosphates to bind calcium.

39.   Correct answer - A

Oliguria is defined as urine output of less than 400 ml/day.

40.   Correct answer - D

Acute renal failure, a syndrome of varying etiologies, comprises prerenal, intrarenal, and postrenal conditions that result in acute deterioration of renal function. Prerenal failure is characterized by diminished kidney perfusion without renal tubular damage. Precipitating factors include hypovolemia, excessive use of diuretics, impaired cardiac function, or bilateral renal vascular obstruction caused by embolism.

41.   Correct answer - C

The patient with a urine output of 200 ml in 24 hours and a urine sodium level of less than 10 mEq/liter is in prerenal failure. Decreased circulating fluid volume and diminished renal perfusion may cause these findings, which suggest that the kidneys are reabsorbing sodium and water - under the influence of aldosterone and ADH, respectively - to increase intravascular volume. In acute tubular necrosis, intrinsic damage prevents the kidneys from reabsorbing sodium; thus, the urine sodium level would be above 40 mEq/liter.

42. Correct answer - A

A urine output of 1,000 ml in 24 hours is normal. A urine sodium level of 26 mEq/liter is on the low side but still within normal range. The findings could indicate that the patient is on a salt-free diet.

43. Correct answer - A

Intrarenal failure, the most common type of acute renal failure, is caused by ischemic or nephrotoxic injury. Ischemic injury occurs if the mean systolic pressure drops below 60 mm Hg for more than 40 minutes. Disorders that cause ischemic injury include massive hemorrhage, transfusion reaction, septic or cardiogenic shock, postsurgical hypotension, and major trauma. Nephrotoxic injury occurs after exposure to nephrotoxic agents, such as antibiotics (aminoglycosides, tetracyclines, and penicillins), carbon tetrachloride, heavy metals, or X-ray contrast media.

44. Correct answer - A

Severe dehydration would lead to prerenal failure, with a urine sodium level of less than 10 mEq/liter. A urine sodium level above 40 mEq/liter in an oliguric patient indicates intrarenal failure with damage to the kidney tissues. Intrarenal failure with cortical involvement includes glomerulonephritis, systemic lupus erythematosus, Goodpasture's syndrome, and malignant hypertension. Intrarenal failure with medullary involvement includes nephrotoxic or ischemic injury.

45. Correct answer - B

A urine of 200 ml in 24 hours indicates oliguria. Although a specific gravity of 1.008 is within the normal range (1.003 to 1.030), the finding is considered low for a patient with oliguria. The kidney's normal response to oliguria is to reabsorb water, thus concentrating the urine to produce a high specific gravity. A specific gravity of 1.008 indicates that the kidney cannot adequately concentrate the urine because of kidney damage from intrarenal failure.

46. **Correct answer - D**

The four most common abnormal laboratory findings in patients with acute renal failure are decreased serum sodium levels and increased serum potassium, blood urea nitrogen (BUN), and creatinine levels. These electrolyte abnormalities occur because of fluid retention and the impaired kidney's inability to conserve sodium and excrete potassium, BUN, and creatinine.

47. **Correct answer - A**

Acute tubular necrosis caused by nephrotoxic drugs affects the epithelial cellular layer. Nephrotoxicity commonly results from antibiotic therapy (gentamicin, amikacin, and cephalosporins). Concomitant use of Lasix may further increase tubular damage and nephrotoxicity as a result of dehydration.

48. **Correct answer - A**

Electrolyte imbalances that result from diuretic therapy include hypokalemia, hyperuricemia, hyponatremia, and hypochloremia. Other complications include volume depletion, azotemia, and metabolic alkalosis.

49. **Correct answer - D**

The loop diuretics (furosemide and ethacrynic acid) are the most potent diuretics available. Their primary site of action is the ascending loop of Henle, resulting in diuresis of isotonic urine. Potassium excretion also occurs. In addition, loop diuretics contribute to increased renal blood flow by exerting a vasodilatory effect on renal vasculature.

50. **Correct answer - B**

Acute tubular necrosis has three phases; oliguric, diuretic, and recovery. The diuretic phase may last for 2 to 3 weeks as renal function begins to return. The glomerular filtration rate increases, but the tubules cannot conserve fluid; this osmotic-diuretic effect is produced by an elevated BUN and impaired ability of the tubules to conserve sodium and water. Severe deficits of potassium (hypokalemia), sodium, and water may lead to electrolyte abnormalities and hypovolemia.

51. **Correct answer - C**

Kidney function gradually returns over 3 to 12 months during the recovery stage, or the third phase, of acute tubular necrosis. At this time, the kidneys ability to concentrate urine improves, resulting in a specific gravity within the normal range of 1.003 to 1.030, a decreased BUN level, and a normal creatinine level.

52. Correct answer - D

Uremic pericarditis caused by accumulation of uremic toxins is a sign of cardiovascular involvement. In uremic pericarditis, a pericardial friction rub can be auscultated, and ST elevations in leads reflecting the involved surface can occur. Tachycardia and heart failure may also occur in the patient with acute renal failure. Elevated potassium levels that occur in the oliguric phase of acute tubular necrosis cause peaked T waves.

53. Correct answer - C

Antacids that do not contain magnesium are used in acute renal failure for bleeding GI ulcers or pain. Maalox and Mylanta, which contain magnesium, may elevate serum magnesium levels to a point requiring dialysis. Amphojel and Basaljel are used in acute renal failure to alleviate GI distress and to lower phosphate levels.

54. Correct answer - C

A protein-restricted diet is essential in patients with renal disease. The metabolite of protein utilization increases the already elevated blood urea nitrogen levels found in patients with renal disease. Nutritional therapy includes maintenance of adequate caloric intake to prevent a negative nitrogen balance and catabolism.

55. Correct answer - D

Phosphate binders, such as Amphojel or Basaljel, are used in chronic renal failure to reduce serum phosphorus levels. Serum calcium levels, meanwhile, increase because the two electrolytes have a reciprocal relationship.

56. Correct answer - B

Patients with renal failure develop a progressive inability to excrete hydrogen because their ability to excrete titratable acid and ammonium ions is diminished; the result is metabolic acidosis.

57. Correct answer - D

Patients with renal failure are susceptible to infection because cellular and hormonal immune responses are decreased secondary to uremic toxins. Anemia and clotting dyscrasias result from decreases in red blood cell production and platelet adhesiveness. Hypertension is common, and metabolic acidosis results from the kidneys' inability to excrete acids. Respiratory acidosis does not result from renal failure, rather, patients hyperventilate to compensate for the metabolic acidosis.

58.   **Correct answer - B**

The glomerulus, located inside Bowman's capsule, is a cluster of tightly coiled capillaries that produces an ultrafiltrate, a portion of which eventually becomes urine.

59.   **Correct answer - B**

The nephron is the kidneys' structural and functional unit. Each kidney has about one million nephrons, so each can compensate for significant nephron destruction by filtering a greater solute load and by hypertrophy of the remaining nephrons. Functional segments of the nephron include the renal corpuscle, which contains the Bowman's capsule and glomerulus, and the renal tubules, segmentally divided into the proximal convoluted tubule, the descending and ascending loops of Henle, the distal convoluted tubule, and the collecting duct.

60.   **Correct answer - D**

The glomerular filtrate flows from the glomerulus to the proximal convoluted tubule, the terminal portion of which descents into the renal medulla. The filtrate then passes into the loop of Henle, a sharp, hairpin loop consisting of a thin descending limb and a thick ascending limb. As the ascending limb enters the renal cortex, the tubule again becomes convoluted. The distal convoluted tubule empties into the collecting ducts, which lead to the ureters and bladder.

61.   **Correct answer - B**

The first step in urine formation is glomerular filtration. The filtrate, a protein-free substance with a specific gravity of 1.010, consists of electrolytes, nonelectrolytes, and water but does not normally contain RBCs. The electrolytes include sodium, potassium, chloride, calcium, magnesium, bicarbonate, and phosphate. Nonelectrolytes are the end products of protein metabolism (urea, uric acid, ammonia, and creatinine), glucose, and amino acids.

62.   **Correct answer - D**

The glomerular filtration rate (GFR), the volume of plasma cleared of a given substance per minute, can be measured clinically by checking creatinine clearance - the amount of plasma cleared of a given amount of creatinine in a given time. In most cases, the creatinine clearance rate is slightly higher in men than in women because men have a larger muscle mass.

63.   Correct answer - D

The normal adult GFR is 125 ml/minute (180 liters/day), while the normal adult urine volume is about 1 liter/day. These figures indicate a greater than 99% reabsorption of the filtrate. Both active and passive transport play a role in the reabsorption and secretion of constituents in the tubules. Active transport occurs when a substance is transported against a concentration gradient and requires energy to exchange ions. Passive transport occurs when a substance is absorbed or secreted without requiring energy.

64.   Correct answer - A

Hypoproteinemia reduces the GFR by lowering the oncotic pressure within the glomerulus. A decreased plasma protein level results in decreased colloid osmotic pressure. A cardiac output of 6 liters/minute and overhydration may increase the GFR. A serum albumin level of 4 is a normal value.

65.   Correct answer - B

The GFR is determined by pressure. Bowman's capsule pressure reflects renal interstitial pressure; urinary tract obstruction, nephron destruction, and interstitial edema of the kidney may alter the pressure within Bowman's capsule. Colloid osmotic pressure results from oncotic pressure of plasma protein in the glomerular blood supply; dehydration, hypoproteinemia, and hyperproteinemia alter oncotic pressure. Changes in glomerular hydrostatic pressure, which reflects cardiac output, also influence the GFR.

66.   Correct answer - C

Sixty to eighty percent of the glomerular filtrate is reabsorbed in the proximal tubule. Most sodium, chloride, calcium, phosphate, magnesium ions, uric acid, glucose, and amino acids are reabsorbed by active transport. The reabsorption rate depends on how long the filtrate is present. In hypovolemia, the GFR decreases, reabsorption increases, and urine output decreases. Conversely, in hypervolemia, the GFR increases and tubular reabsorption decreases, causing increased urine output.

67. Correct answer - A

The loop of Henle is primarily concerned with the concentration or dilution of urine. When the glomerular filtrate reaches the loop of Henle, it is greatly reduced in volume because of the large percentage of water reabsorption in the proximal tubule. The descending segment of the loop of Henle is permeable to water only. As the filtrate passes through the descending limb, water diffuses into the bloodstream and sodium enters the filtrate from the blood, producing a more hypertonic filtrate. The thick limb of the ascending segment actively transports sodium and chloride.

68. Correct answer - C

The distal convoluted tubule receives hypotonic urine from the ascending loop of Henle. Major functions include reabsorption of water, sodium chloride, and sodium bicarbonate and secretion of potassium, ammonia, and hydrogen. Water permeability at this side is controlled by antidiuretic hormone (ADH), and sodium reabsorption is determined by aldosterone.

69. Correct answer - B

Osmolality is the weight of solid particles per kilogram of solvent. The normal value is 285 to 295 mOsm/liter. Serum osmolality is regulated through reabsorption, secretion, and excretion of various particles and substances processed by the glomerulus. The serum osmolality may be calculated from specific laboratory values.

70. Correct answer - A

Sodium, the main extracellular electrolyte, plays an important role in maintaining extracellular fluid volume. An osmotically active solute, sodium is a major determinant of serum osmolality.

71. Correct answer - A

ADH is synthesized in the hypothalamus and stored in and released from the posterior pituitary gland. ADH makes the cells of the distal tubule and collecting ducts permeable to water. Sodium reabsorption increases in the renal tubules during aldosterone secretion and when the GFR decreases secondary of renal hypoperfusion (for example, in shock or congestive heart failure). Aldosterone is a mineralocorticoid secreted from the adrenal cortex. Its major effect is to increase renal tubular reabsorption of sodium and to control selective renal excretion of potassium.

72. **Correct answer - C**

The renin-angiotensin-aldosterone system is a mechanism for controlling blood pressure. Such factors as decreased blood pressure, reduced serum sodium, and increased sympathetic stimulation of the kidneys trigger the juxtaglomerular apparatus to release renin, which acts on angiotensinogen to produce angiotensin I. This is then converted into angiotensin II, which stimulates aldosterone secretion and produces a pronounced vasoconstriction throughout the body.

73. **Correct answer - D**

A lack of ADH, hypercalcemia, or uncontrolled diabetes mellitus with osmotic diuresis can precipitate hypernatremia. Without ADH secretion, water loss exceeds sodium loss. Hypercalcemia causes polyuria and dehydration. Osmotic diuresis secondary to hyperglycemia increases the proportion of water loss to sodium loss, so a relative hypernatremia occurs. Hypoaldosteronism, the lack of aldosterone, results in hyponatremia.

74. **Correct answer - C**

Hypernatremia may result from excessive water loss or sodium retention; nursing implications depend on the etiology. In patients with excessive water loss, the goal is to lower the serum sodium level by water replacement, using a solution of dextrose 5% in water. The nurse must monitor serum sodium levels and serum and urine osmolality. Frequent assessment of hydration status is vital because rapid correction of sodium levels can lead to pulmonary edema. In hypernatremia from sodium retention, the goal is to promote sodium loss by administering diuretics of fluids. Serum sodium levels and urine and serum osmolality should be monitored closely because rapid correction can cause cerebral edema due to fluid shift, demanding frequent neurologic assessments and correlation with serum sodium levels.

75. **Correct answer - A**

If sodium loss occurs with water excess, the patient shows signs of malaise, headache, confusion, and seizures, along with muscular weakness and abdominal cramps. If sodium and water losses coexist, expect lassitude, apathy, tachycardia, orthostatic hypotension progressing to shock, decreased gastric mobility leading to constipation, azotemia, oliguria, and muscle spasms. A severe imbalance, such as a serum sodium level below 120 mEq/liter, is associated with seizures.

76. Correct answer - A

Good skin turgor and weight gain are seen in the patient with dilutional hyponatremia as a result of water intoxication. Dilutional hyponatremia also decreases serum osmolarity, fostering a shift of fluid into the cells. The increased intracellular fluid, especially in the brain, results in central nervous system symptomatology, such as headache, confusion, seizures, and coma. Other physical findings may include hypertension and jugular vein distention.

77. Correct answer - A

Usually, 1.5% glucose dialysate solutions are used during peritoneal dialysis. The higher the percentage of glucose, the larger the amount of fluid that is removed from the body. Dialysis is never carried out exclusively with 4.25% glucose solutions, although these are substituted for the 1.5% solutions at certain intervals during therapy.

78. Correct answer - D

A nursing responsibility during peritoneal dialysis is to observe the characteristic of the dialysate drainage, which is normally clear and straw-colored. Cloudy drainage may indicate contamination; a brownish tinge, bowel perforation; and amber, bladder perforation. Blood-tinged drainage (from insertion of a dialysis catheter) is considered normal from the first to the fourth exchange.

79. Correct answer - D

Inadequate drainage is the most common complication of peritoneal dialysis. Drainage can usually be facilitated by turning the patient from side to side, elevating the head of the bed, or gently massaging the abdomen. Inserting a stylet into the peritoneal catheter, as ordered and using strict sterile technique, can also remedy the problem.

80. Correct answer - D

The principles of peritoneal dialysis and hemodialysis are the same. A semipermeable membrane serves as a filter across which solutes and fluids are exchanged. Water and solutes move across the semipermeable membrane by osmosis, diffusion, and ultrafiltration. Osmosis is the movement of water across a semipermeable membrane from an area of lesser osmolality to one of greater osmolality. Diffusion is the movement of molecules from an area of higher concentration of one of lower concentration. Filtration is the movement of particles through a semipermeable membrane by hydrostatic pressure.

81. **Correct answer - B**

When using 4.25% dialysate solution, monitor closely for hyperglycemia - particularly if the patient is diabetic - because the solution has a high glucose concentration. Also, because this solution may draw off more fluid than a 1.5% glucose dialysate solution, monitor dialysate outflow closely.

82. **Correct answer - D**

Complications of peritoneal dialysis include atelectasis and pneumonia (from decreased mobility and an elevated diaphragm during dialysate dwell), bowel perforation and peritonitis (which may occur before and during dialysis), and hypoproteinemia.

83. **Correct answer - A**

Sulkowitch's test is a laboratory urine test for hypercalcemia. Histocompatibility tests, which determine tissue compatibility between donor and recipient, include ABO blood typing, white cell crossmatching, and human leukocyte antigen (HLA) typing. ABO blood typing is performed to ensure compatibility of red blood cells; without ABO compatibility, immediate rejection of the transplanted organ would occur. White-cell crossmatching identifies preformed, circulating, cytotoxic antibodies in the potential recipient; a negative crossmatch is essential before transplantation HLA typing compares the genetic makeup of donor and recipient to select the most compatible donor.

84. **Correct answer - B**

Acute organ rejection most commonly occurs about 2 weeks after transplantation but can develop from 1 week to 1 year later. T cells responsible for cellular immunity are the primary mechanisms involved. Major signs and symptoms include anuria or oliguria; a fever over 100° F. (37.8° C.); a transplanted kidney that is swollen, soft, and tender on palpation; hypertension and weight gain from fluid retention; malaise; and changes in BUN, serum creatinine, and serum electrolyte levels.

85. **Correct answer - D**

The kidneys regulate bicarbonate concentration through three processes; reabsorption of bicarbonate in the proximal and distal convoluted tubules; formation of titratable acid, such as phosphate; and synthesis formation of ammonium ion, permitting the addition of HCO_3 into the blood. All three processes require the secretion of hydrogen ions into the renal tubules.

86.   Correct answer - A

The kidney regulates sodium and chloride in a parallel fashion. Thus, a patient with hyponatremia will usually have hypochloremia. Sodium and chloride are reabsorbed at the same time, facilitating hydrogen and potassium excretion. A chloride imbalance occurs in metabolic alkalosis; bicarbonate concentration increases at the expense of chloride concentration. Thus, hypochloremia is a common component of metabolic alkalosis. Common causes of metabolic alkalosis include gastrointestinal losses, hyperaldosteronism, massive blood transfusions, diuretic abuse, and hypokalemia. The body's response to metabolic alkalosis causes pulmonary compensation, such as hypoventilation.

87.   Correct answer - C

Intestinal fluids below the stomach, including pancreatic and biliary secretions, are alkaline. Consequently, severe diarrhea or the removal of these fluids, either by tube drainage or fistulas to the skin, can cause HCO_2 loss and metabolic acidosis. Other causes of metabolic acidosis include renal failure, ketoacidosis, shock, and salicylate poisoning. Metabolic disturbances cause pulmonary compensation; respiratory compensation causes hyperventilation to decrease $PaCO_2$.

88.   Correct answer - A

Signs and symptoms of rapidly developing alkalosis are related to increased irritability of the central and peripheral nervous systems. These signs and symptoms include light-headedness, altered consciousness, paresthesias of the extremities and circumoral areas, cramps, muscle tremors, carpopedal spasm, and seizures. When pH increases, more calcium combines with protein, reducing the concentration of ionized calcium; thus, a patient with alkalosis develops the signs and symptoms of hypocalcemia. Obtundation does not occur in developing alkalosis.

89.   Correct answer - D

The body compensates for metabolic alkalosis by hypoventilation. Thus, hypercapnia (increased CO_2) is the compensatory response to metabolic alkalosis. Compensation for metabolic alkalosis is centrally mediated. A decreased hydrogen level in arterial blood reduces stimulation to chemoreceptors, which ultimately decreases the ventilation rate. The resultant hypoventilation increases $PaCO_2$ and carbonic acid formation.

90. Correct answer - A

Metabolic acidosis can produce abnormalities in neurologic and cardiovascular function. Neurologic symptoms range from headache, confusion, and lethargy or coma. Cardiovascular symptoms include potentially fatal ventricular dysrhythmias, reduced myocardial contractility, and hypotension. Metabolic acidosis also causes hyperventilation (Kussmaul's respirations) as a compensatory response.

91. Correct answer -A

Hypoxia (decreased oxygen supply to the tissues) results in anaerobic metabolism, which increases lactic acid levels, thus producing metabolic acidosis. Shock is the most common cause of metabolic acidosis related to increased lactic acid levels and may occur with sepsis, hemorrhage, pulmonary edema, or cardiac failure. The common denominator in these conditions is decreased oxygen supply to the tissues, which favors anaerobic formation of lactic acid. Diuretic abuse, hypokalemia, and vomiting result in metabolic alkalosis.

92. Correct answer - D

Acidosis moves potassium ions out of the cells so that hydrogen ions can move into the cells. This is a compensatory buffer mechanism to reduce the serum hydrogen content, thus reducing acidosis. For every change of 0.1 in the body's pH, the serum potassium changes by 0.6. Acidosis also decreases the amount of binding between calcium and albumin.

93. Correct answer - C

A suprapubic catheter may be inserted by the urologist to divert urine in urethral trauma. The nurse should not insert an indwelling urinary catheter because it may cause further damage. The urologist will decide whether to insert an indwelling urinary or suprapubic catheter. Before the urologist arrives, the nurse should discourage voiding, because extravasation of urine may occur. The patient usually cannot void, although he may have the desire to, because sphincter damage may have occurred.

94. Correct answer - C

Urethral bleeding will occur if the patient's urethra is completely transected. This bleeding must be distinguished from hematuria, which occurs from injury to other parts of the genitourinary system. If the posterior urethra is completely transected, urinary extravasation seldom occurs because the bladder neck remains competent. Hematuria does not occur in a complete transection because urine cannot travel down the transected urethra.

95.   Correct answer - A

Rupture of the bladder is more likely to occur when it is full. Associated with blunt abdominal trauma and pelvic fracture, the condition occurs equally in men and women.

96.   Correct answer - C

In bladder rupture, the patient should also be assessed for rectal injury, which significantly increases morbidity and mortality. Damage to the iliac vessels also may occur.

97.   Correct answer - D

Hematuria, pelvic discomfort, and difficulty in voiding occur when the bladder is ruptured. Hematuria and pelvic discomfort result from trauma to the tissues. Severity of these symptoms depends on the extent of damage and the existence of other injuries. Difficulty in voiding occurs because the muscles responsible for urination cannot function.

98.   Correct answer - A

Immobilization and elevation of the tests help minimize further bleeding from trauma. Ice packs reduce swelling and pain. Trauma to the testes may also cause bleeding into the penis and scrotal sac. This collection of extravasated blood produces pain. Heat packs would contribute to further bleeding.

CHAPTER 5

GASTROINTESTINAL SYSTEM

Case Study

Questions 1-11 refer to the following Case Study:

Mr. K. age 33, is admitted to the intensive care unit (ICU) with suspected gastric perforation and chemical peritonitis. He has a history of duodenal ulcers. The medical plan includes sending the patient for a Billroth II operation as soon as a surgical suite be comes available

1. Clinical manifestations of perforated gastric ulcer include all of the following *except:*

    A. Parlytic ileus
    B. Shock
    C. Anxiety and respiratory difficulty
    D. Severe upper abdominal pain radiating to the jaw

2. Chemical peritonitis associated with a perforated gastric ulcer is caused by:

    A. Overuse of antacids
    B. Salicylate ingestion
    C. Gastric and intestinal content spillage
    D. Sodium and calcium imbalance

3. A primary response of the peritoneum in peritonitis includes:

    A. Hypomotility of the bowel
    B. Outpouring of plasma-like fluid from the interstitial spaces into the intestinal lumen
    C. Inflammation of the visceral surface but not the parietal surface
    D. Edema and vascular congestion in the subperitoneal tissues

4. On admission, the nurse performs a GI assessment of Mr. K. Absent bowel sounds would be expected in all of the following situations *except:*

    A. Peritonitis
    B. Ileus
    C. Borborygmus
    D. Mesenteric infarction

5. The last step in a GI assessment is:

    A. Auscultation
    B. Palpation
    C. Inspection
    D. Percussion

6. Which would be a normal finding in abdominal palpation?

    A. Smooth, nontender spleen
    B. A large, irregular liver
    C. Involuntary spasm during deep palpation
    D. A smooth liver edge palpable only when the patient takes a deep breath

7. Which statement about abdominal percussion is *false?*

    A. Fluid wave maneuver is a method suitable only with accumulation of ascitic fluid
    B. On inspiration, a change in percussion from tympany to dullness over the left subcostal area suggests splenic enlargement
    C. Liver dullness may be decreased or absent when free air is present below the diaphragm
    D. Decreased tympany of the stomach occurs with upper abdominal distention

8. Which statement concerning auscultation of bowel sounds is *true?*

A. Intensity and frequency of bowel sounds do not depend on the prevailing phase of digestion
B. Borborygmi are not present in early intestinal obstruction
C. The stethoscope bell should be placed firmly against the abdominal wall to auscultate bowel sounds
D. Auscultation of bowel sounds should precede percussion and palpation

9. Postoperatively Mr. K. should be assessed for:

A. Hypocalcemia
B. Metabolic acidosis
C. Hypernatremia
D. Hyperkalemia

10. Postoperatively, Mr. K. develops a paralytic ileus. The nurse would anticipate using which therapy?

A. Performing gastrointestinal suction
B. Limiting the diet to full liquids
C. Decreasing I.V. intake
D. Administering bowel-sterilizing agents

11. Because of the paralytic ileus, total parenteral nutrition (TPN) is initiated. A patient receiving TPN may develop all of the following complications *except:*

A. Hyperkalemia and hyperphosphatemia
B. Hypoglycemia and hypomagnesemia
C. Sepsis and pneumothorax
D. Hyperosmolar nonketotic dehydration

Questions 12-29 refer to the following Case Study:

Mr. N., age 35, is admitted to the ICU complaining of a sudden episode of vomiting blood that morning. He does not complain of pain. Past history includes several hospitalizations for alcohol detoxification and rehabilitation.

12. Spontaneous, painless hemorrhage of the GI tract in an alcohol abuser could suggest:

    A. Mallory-Weiss tear
    B. Peptic ulcer
    C. Gastric ulcer perforation
    D. Duodenal ulcer

13. Mr. N. is diagnosed as in the early stage of cirrhosis. During physical assessment, the nurse palpates Mr. N.'s liver, expecting to find a liver that is:

    A. irregular, large, hard and firm
    B. small, nontender and smooth
    C. large, smooth and tender
    D. large, smooth and nontender

14. Endoscopy confirms bleeding esophageal varices. Mr. N. may develop all of the following complications *except:*

    A. Abnormally low blood urea nitrogen (BUN)
    B. Hepatorenal syndrome
    C. Hepatic encephalopathy
    D. Hemorrhagic shock

15. Nursing interventions for the patient with active esophageal bleeding may include:

A. Stopping bleeding through measures that increase portal venous pressure

B. Assessing the patient's level of consciousness for the possibility of alcohol withdrawal syndrome

C. Administering iced saline lavage, infused 50 ml at a time and removed rapidly

D. Administering vasopressin (Pitressin) at 20 units/minute

16. A Sengstaken-Blakemore tube is inserted by the physician. Which nursing intervention would *not* be appropriate for this patient while the tube is in place?

A. Inflating a gastric balloon with 100 cc of air and checking pressure frequently

B. Inflating an esophageal balloon to 20 to 40 mm Hg and releasing pressure periodically to prevent necrosis

C. Keeping scissors at the bedside to release pressure if the esophageal balloon migrates into air passages

D. Decompressing an esophageal balloon and then deflating a gastric balloon to evaluate the status of bleeding varices

17. Vasopressin therapy is initiated for Mr. N. A patient receiving a vasopressin drip should be monitored for:

A. Excessive diuresis

B. Decreases blood pressure

C. Myocardial ischemia

D. Increased portal pressures

18. Mr. N. may develop all of the following complications *except:*

A. Mesenteric infarction

B. Myocardial infarction

C. Myocardial ischemia

D. Hypotension

19. The next day, Mr. N. develops jaundice and ascites. The physician orders serum indirect and direct bilirubin. Indirect bilirubin is:

   A. Fat-soluble and unconjugated
   B. unbound to albumin
   C. found in liver cells
   D. stored in the gallbladder

20. Direct bilirubin is:

   A. Bound with glucuronic acid in the liver
   B. A water-soluble bilirubin
   C. A conjugated bilirubin
   D. All of the above

21. When a patient develops jaundice, the tests to differentiate the pathophysiology are:

   A. Lactate dehydrogenase (LDH) and ammonia level
   B. Serum gluamic-oxaloacetic transaminase (SGOT) and urobilinogen
   C. Serum glutamate pyruvate transaminase (SGPT) and alkaline phosphatase
   D. Indirect and direct bilirubin

22. An elevated *indirect* bilirubin suggests a patient has:

   A. Biliary tract obstruction
   B. Liver dysfunction
   C. Gallbladder disease
   D. Cholelithiasis

23. An elevated *direct* bilirubin suggests a patient has:

   A. Biliary tract obstruction
   B. Hepatitis
   C. Cirrhosis
   D. Hepatic insufficiency

24. Which of the following is *not* usually found during abdominal assessment in ascites?

A. Shifting dullness
B. Fluid wave
C. Tympanic percussion note
D. Taut skin over the abdomen

25. Which of the following factors contributes to ascites formation?

A. Portal hypertension
B. Increased serum colloid osmotic pressure
C. High osmotic pressure within liver tissue
D. Decreased hepatic lymph formation resulting in fluid shift

26. In ascites, all of the following complications may develop *except:*

A. Hydrothorax
B. Reflux esophagitis
C. Inguinal and femoral hernias
D. Tension pneumothorax

27. The most common cause of portal hypertension is:

A. Hepatic cystic disease
B. Hepatitis
C. Cirrhosis
D. Metastatic disease

28. A Denver shunt is inserted in Mr. N. Shunt surgery is primarily performed to:

A. Decompress esophagogastric varices
B. Decrease the incidence of encephalopathy
C. Minimize hepatic perfusion
D. Prevent hemorrhage

29. Which of the following is the *least* desirable treatment for ascites?

A. Paracentesis
B. Sodium restriction
C. Water restriction
D. Aldactone administration

Case Study
Questions 30-40 refer to the following Case Study.

Mrs. O., age 57, is admitted to the ICU with severe abdominal pain and fatty, foul-smelling stools. Serum lipase and amylase levels are elevated. Acute pancreatitis is diagnosed.

30. The exocrine function of the pancreas is controlled by secretory units called the:

A. Islets
B. Alpha cells
C. Beta cells
D. Acinar cells

31. Which of the following medical histories is most likely to contribute to acute pancreatitis?

A. Posttraumatic injury to the pancreas
B. Alcoholism
C. Choletithiasis
D. Biliary tract disease

32. The pathophysiology of acute pancreatitis includes:

A. A severe inflammatory response to endotoxins
B. Overproduction of vasoactive enzymes from acinar cells
C. Overwhelming infection of the pancreatic ducts
D. The autodigestion of the pancreas caused by its enzymes

33. Mrs. O. should be assessed for which complications associated with acute pancreatitis

    A.   Severe, intermittent right upper quadrant pain and vomiting
    B.   Hyperactive bowel sounds and diarrhea
    C.   Lethargy and increased PCO_2
    D.   Hyperventilation and restlessness

34. Which of these physical findings is consistent with the diagnosis of acute pancreatitis?

    A.   Severe epigastric pain
    B.   Rebound tenderness
    C.   Rigidity in the abdominal wall
    D.   All of the above

35. Which clinical sign would *not* be present in acute pancreatitis?

    A.   Chvostek's sign
    B.   Trousseau's sign
    C.   Cullen's sign
    D.   Homans' sign

36. Pulmonary complications of acute pancreatitis may include:

    A.   Atelectasis
    B.   Adult respiratory distress syndrome (ARDS) and pleural effusions
    C.   Elevation of the diaphragm and basilar crackles
    D.   All of the above

37. Mrs. O. may develop which of the following complications?

    A.   Hypovolemic shock and disseminated intravascular coagulation (DIC)
    B.   Respiratory failure
    C.   Renal failure and pancreatic pseudocysts
    D.   All of the above

38. Which of the following analgesics is the drug of choice in managing acute pancreatic pain?

A. Demerol (meperidine)
B. Morphine sulfate
C. Codeine
D. Dilaudid (hydromorphone hydrochloride)

39. Which intervention would be *inappropriate* for Mrs. O?

A. Maintaining her on a low-fat diet for up to 6 weeks after she resumes eating
B. Performing peritoneal lavage
C. Initiating aggressive antibiotic therapy to control inflammation of the pancreas
D. Performing nasogastric suction and prohibiting ice chips

40. On discharge, Mrs. O. should be instructed to follow which diet?

A. Low fat and no alcohol or caffeine
B. Low fat and low cholesterol
C. Low salt, low sugar, and no caffeine
D. No alcohol, caffeine, or sugar

41. A Whipple's operation is scheduled for a patient with chronic pancreatitis. All of the following statements about this procedure are true *except:*

A. It is also known as a pancreatoduodenal resection
B. It involves removal of the gallbladder, the distal portion of the stomach, the duodenum, and the head of the pancreas
C. The remaining parts of the pancreas, stomach, and common bile duct are anastomosed to the jejunum
D. It involves removing the pancreas, the gallbladder, and part of the liver

42. Complications that may develop immediately after pancreatic surgery include all of the following *except:*

A. Pancreatic fistula and anastomotic leak
B. Insulin dependence and steatorrhea
C. Hemorrhage
D. Pancreatic abscess and peritonitis

43. Which of the following statements is *true* about total pancreatectomy for the patient with pancreatic carcinoma?

A. Metabolic derangements are more manageable than in Whipple's procedure
B. Complications are more severe in total pancreatectomy
C. The operative technique is more complicated in total pancreatectomy
D. Surgery time is shortened in total pancreatectomy

Case Study
Questions 44-52 refer to the following case study.

Mr. A. age 68, is admitted to the ICU with a diagnosis of possible bowel obstruction. In the past 5 days, he has experienced abdominal cramping and distention, with nausea, vomiting and constipation.

---

44. The correct sequence for assessing and evaluating Mr. A.'s abdomen is:

A. Auscultation, percussion, inspection and palpation
B. Auscultation, inspection, percussion and palpation
C. Inspection, auscultation, percussion and palpation
D. Inspection, auscultation, palpation, and percussion

45. The primary cause of large-bowel obstruction in adults is:

A. Adhesions
B. Volvulus
C. Carcinoma
D. Diverticulitis

46. The most common findings in large-bowel obstruction are:

    A. Early vomiting and abdominal distention
    B. High-pitched bowel sounds with large third-space fluid loss
    C. Marked abdominal distention and pain of long duration
    D. Early excessive vomiting and no bowel sounds

47. Laboratory findings indicating a bowel obstruction include all of the following *except:*

    A. Increased white blood cell count
    B. Increased hematocrit
    C. Decreased bicarbonate
    D. Decreased blood urea nitrogen

48. An intestinal tube is ordered for decompression. Which of the following tubes is *not* used as an intestinal tube?

    A. Miller-Abbot
    B. Cantor
    C. Salem sump
    D. Metler-Rawson

49. Mr. A.'s bowel obstruction is in the bend in the colon at the right upper quadrant where it joins the transverse colon. This area is called the:

    A. Cecum
    B. Splenic flexure
    C. Hepatic flexure
    D. Ascending flexure

50. Factors that enhance colonic motility include all of the following *except:*

    A. High-residue diets
    B. Bacterial endotoxins
    C. Anticholinergic drugs
    D. Hyperosmolar solution

51. Main functions of the large intestine include all of the following *except:*

A. Absorption of water and electrolytes
B. Synthesis of vitamin K and folic acid
C. Urea breakdown
D. Absorption of waste products

52. Which vessel supplies the large intestine with blood?

A. Celiac artery
B. Inferior mesenteric artery
C. Superior mesenteric artery
D. Intestinal artery

53. A patient with a functional paralytic ileus probably has:

A. Adhesions
B. Hypokalemia
C. High-pitched bowel sounds
D. No abdominal distention

54. Which of the following is *true* regarding a leaking anastomosis in the postoperative esophagogastrectomy patient?

A. The patient may exhibit acute chest pain mimicking pulmonary embolism
B. The patient develops high temperatures with substernal fullness
C. The patient develops inflammation and fluid accumulation in the pericardial space
D. The leakage occurs immediately after the surgical procedure

55. A patient with vitamin D deficiency will develop which condition?

A. Hypolipidemia
B. Hypocalcemia
C. Beriberi
D. Scurvy

Questions 56-68 refer to the following case study.

Mrs. W., age 47, is admitted to the ICU with chronic, persistent hepatitis B and stage II portal-systemic encephalapathy (PSE).

56. The liver receives blood that is rich in amino acids, fats, and sugars because the blood has traversed the walls of the intestinal tract via the:

A. Portal vein
B. Portal artery
C. Hepatic vein
D. Hepatic artery

57. Which statement about the liver is *false?*

A. It forms ammonia to remove urea
B. It stores fat-soluble vitamins
C. It synthesizes globulin and blood factors
D. It provides the phagocytic action of the reticuloendothelial system

58. The liver's contribution to digestion includes:

A. Secretion of proteolytic enzymes
B. Secretion of bile salts
C. Gluconeogenesis
D. All of the above

59. Which liver structure is responsible for destroying old blood corpuscles and detoxifying toxic substances?

A. Liver sinusoids
B. Splenic cells
C. Kupffer's cells
D. Hepatocytes

60. The liver synthesizes all of the following blood-clotting components *except:*

A. Vitamin K
B. Factors II, V and VII
C. Factors VIII, IX, and X
D. Prothrombin and fibrinogen

61. In caring for a patient with hepatitis, the nurse should know that:

A. Isolation precautions with hepatitis A can be discontinued when jaundice begins
B. Isolation and enteric precautions must be maintained for 2 weeks after jaundice subsides
C. Strict isolation is necessary for a patient with non-A, non-B hepatitis
D. Isolation precautions are unnecessary for a patient with any form of hepatitis

62. Mrs. W., who is in stage II of PSE, may exhibit which of the following manifestations?

A. Stuporous, marked confusion
B. Loss of deep tendon reflexes
C. Confusion and asterixis
D. Deep coma

63. The toxic substance that leads to the clinical manifestations of PSE is:

A. Blood urea nitrogen (BUN)
B. Ammonia
C. Bilirubin
D. Uric acid

64. Mrs. W. is assessed as having asterixis, a pathologic sign occurring in patients with:

A. Cirrhosis of the liver
B. Pancreatic pseudocyst
C. Hepatitis
D. Hepatic failure

65. Nursing interventions in PSE include all of the following *except:*

A. Administering neomycin via nasogastric tube
B. Restricting dietary protein
C. Reducing dosage of or avoiding sedatives
D. Administering thiazide diuretics to reduce fluid volume

66. Lactulose can be instrumental in treating PSE because it:

A. Acts as a chelating agent of ammonia
B. Acts as an osmotic agent that induces diarrhea
C. Promotes ammonia excretion by changing intestinal pH
D. All of the above

67. Which of the following findings indicates developing hepatorenal syndrome?

A. Hypokalemic alkalosis
B. Oliguria and azotemia
C. Loss of renal ability to concentrate urine
D. Weight loss or more than 1 kg/day

68. Which dietary elements are most commonly restricted in hepatic dysfunction?

A. Protein and sodium
B. Fluid and starches
C. Sodium and potassium
D. Potassium and protein

Case Study
Questions 69-77 refer to the following case study.

Mr. G. a 52-year-old businessman, is admitted to the ICU with complaints of severe epigastric pain after eating dinner. Past history includes multiple bouts of indigestion and frequent antacid usage. A diagnosis of possible perforated ulcer is made.

---

69. The structure that keeps gastric contents in the stomach is the:

A. Hypopharyngeal sphincter
B. Pyloric sphincter
C. Gastroesophageal sphincter
D. Cardiac sphincter

70. Which statement about gastric gland secretions is *true?*

A. Chief cells secrete pepsinogen and intrinsic factor
B. G cells secrete gastrin in the stomach's antral area
C. Oxyntic cells secrete pepsin and hydrochloric acid (HCL)
D. Parietal cells secrete intrinsic factor only

71. Stimulation of gastric secretion occurs by the interaction of:

A. Gastrin, acetylcholine, and histamine
B. Pepsin, gastrin, and mucus
C. Cholinergic response, pepsin, and histamine
D. HCl, pepsinogen, and intrinsic factor

72. Ranitidine (Zantac) is ordered for Mr. G to:

A. Neutralize gastric pH
B. Decrease HCl production by the parietal cells
C. Prevent histamine interaction in H_2 receptors
D. Block pancreatic enzyme stimulation

73. A function of the stomach's distal portion is to:

A. Mix food
B. Secrete HCl
C. Secrete pepsinogen
D. Act as a reservoir for chyme

74. Which factor is a potent inhibitor of gastric emptying?

A. Chyme with a high lipid content
B. Hypo-osmolar chyme
C. Anger
D. All of the above

75. Which factor would increase the rate of gastric emptying?

A. Pain and anxiety
B. Duodenal hormones
C. Gastrin
D. High fat content

76. Perforated ulcers are most commonly located in the:

A. Stomach
B. Jejunum
C. Duodenum
D. Ileum

77. Pancreatitis occurs as a complication of perforated duodenal ulcer when:

A. Serum amylase is elevated to dangerous levels
B. The perforation erodes into the pancreas
C. The patient has a high alcohol intake
D. The pancreatic duct is obstructed

Case Study

Questions 78-84 refer to the following case study.

Mr. Z. age 49, is driving while intoxicated and becomes involved in a motor vehicle accident with severe front-end damage. Three left ribs are fractured. He is hypotensive on admission to the ICU, and blunt abdominal trauma is suspected.

---

78. Which of Mr. Z.'s organs has probably sustained trauma?

    A.   Liver
    B.   Small intestine
    C.   Spleen
    D.   Colon

79. Which type of solution should be administered to restore circulatory volume for Mr. Z?

    A.   Hypertonic
    B.   Hypotonic
    C.   Isotonic
    D.   Hypo-osmolar

80. Two diagnostic tools used for detecting intra-abdominal injury are paracentesis and peritoneal lavage. Peritoneal lavage is contraindicated in the patient who:

    A.   Has a colostomy
    B.   Is unconscious
    C.   Has multiple abdominal scars
    D.   Is between ages 2 and 10

81. A diagnostic peritoneal lavage may yield a false-negative result in:

    A.   Splenic bleeding
    B.   Diaphragmatic rupture
    C.   Bladder tear
    D.   Retroperitoneal hematoma

82. Six hours after admission Mr. Z.'s blood test results reveal suddenly elevated alkaline phosphatase and lactic dehydrogenase levels. Which situation is suspected?

    A.   Liver injury
    B.   Alcoholism
    C.   Hepatitis
    D.   Pancreatitis

83. Patients with blunt abdominal trauma commonly suffer injuries to the:

    A. Liver and spleen
    B. Kidneys and spleen
    C. Pancreas and spleen
    D. Pancreas and liver

84. Which statement about splenic injury is *false?*

    A. The normal spleen is palpable below the lower left costal margin
    B. The spleen is injured more often than any other abdominal organ
    C. The high incidence of splenic injury is directly related to the organ's high vascularity
    D. A positive Kehr's sign is evident in about 50% of patients with splenic injury

85. The mucoprotein necessary for intestinal absorption of vitamin B_{12} is:

    A. Intrinsic factor
    B. Cholecystokinin
    C. Secretin
    D. Lipase

86. Which structures in the small intestine are responsible for nutrient absorption?

    A. Crypts of Lieberkuhn
    B. Brunner's glands
    C. Peyer's patches
    D. Villi

87. Basic mechanisms for nutrient absorption include:

    A. Active transport
    B. Passive transport
    C. Facilitated diffusion
    D. All of the above

88. Which of the following absorbs 90% of nutrients and 50% of water and electrolytes?

A. Stomach
B. Duodenum
C. Jejunum
D. Ileum

89. Bile salts must be present for the small intestine to absorb:

A. Vitamin C
B. Vitamin B₁
C. Calcium
D. Vitamin D

90. The prime function of bile salts in digestion is to:

A. Emulsify fats
B. Break down complex carbohydrates
C. Neutralize gastric juices
D. Activate proteases

Mental Humor Break

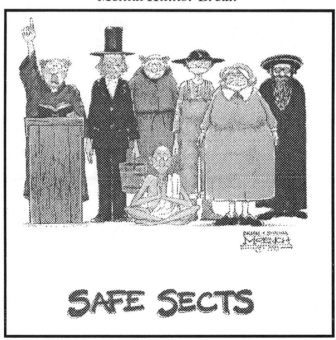

SAFE SECTS

In Your Face
800-658-8508

1.   **Correct answer - D**

Paralytic ileus, shock, anxiety, respiratory difficulty, and severe upper abdominal pain radiating to the shoulders are clinical signs of perforated gastric ulcer. The radiating pain is caused by irritation of the diaphragm and phrenic nerves.

2.   **Correct answer - C**

Chemical peritonitis is caused by a rapid escape of gastric and intestinal contents after perforation. Spillage of these irritating digestive juices stimulates a severe inflammatory response.

3.   **Correct answer - D**

Peritonitis is an inflammation of a portion or all of the abdominal cavity's parietal and visceral surfaces. Primary responses of the peritoneum to injury include edema and vascular congestion in the subperitoneal tissues, hypermotility of the bowel, and an outpouring of plasma-like fluid from the extracellular, vascular, and interstitial compartments into the peritoneal space. Secondary responses from this fluid shift include decreases in venous return and urine output, producing hypovolemia and progressive systemic acidosis. Progressive abdominal distention leads to respiratory compromise.

4.   **Correct answer - C**

Normal bowel sounds occur when air and water move through the intestine. These sounds range from faint, low reverberations to loud, high-pitched noises. Abnormal or absent bowel sounds can air diagnosis of various conditions. For example, borborygmus (an intense, loud, rushing sound heard early in peristalsis) may indicate an intestinal obstruction; absent bowel sounds may be noted late in intestinal obstruction, peritonitis, ileus, and mesenteric infarction.

5.   **Correct answer - B**

Inspection, auscultation, percussion, and palpation are used when assessing the abdomen. Palpation, the last step, can help detect and characterize masses, define the normal abdominal organs, verify organomegaly, and differentiate pain. Because the organs have minimal pain receptors, visceral pain is generalized and dull. When the peritoneum is inflamed, the associated pain is localized and sharp. Rebound tenderness - the excruciating pain provoked when the palpating hand is suddenly lifted off the abdomen - indicates peritoneal inflammation.

6. Correct answer - D

The edge of the liver, palpable as the patient takes a deep breath, normally presents as a sharp, firm object with a smooth surface. If the liver is enlarged, hard, firm, and irregular, cancer is suspected. In cirrhotic patients, the liver is usually enlarged, smooth, and nontender. If the edge is tender, hepatitis should be suspected. The spleen must increase its surface area about 3 times before it is palpable.

7. Correct answer - D

Percussion is used to establish distention, tumors, fluids, or enlargements of viscera. The normal liver and the normal spleen are dull when percussed; the normal stomach is tympanic when empty. Increased tympany of the stomach occurs in upper abdominal distention.

8. Correct answer - D

Auscultation should precede percussion and palpation because the latter procedures may alter the frequency of bowel sounds. In auscultation, the diaphragm of the stethoscope is placed lightly against the abdominal wall to avoid distracting sounds resulting from friction and compression of vessels. If the nurse listens in all four quadrants for 2 to 5 minutes, normal sounds occur intermittently at 5 to 34/minute. Intensity and frequency depend on the phase of digestion; bowel sounds are loudest when a meal is overdue. Early intestinal obstruction produces loud, rushing, high-pitched sounds (borborygmi). Absent bowel sounds may signal paralytic ileus, peritonitis, mesenteric infarction, and advanced intestinal obstruction.

9. Correct answer - A

Hypocalcemia may result after a Billroth II operation (gastrojejunostomy) because of reduced absorption of calcium and vitamin D resulting from rapid transit through the bowel. Postoperatively, nasogastric suction is performed until peristalsis returns. Hyponatremia, hypochloremia, hypokalemia, and metabolic alkalosis may result from prolonged nasogastric suction.

10.   Correct answer - A

A paralytic ileus can result from such factors as abdominal surgery, hypokalemia, trauma, and spinal fractures. This functional intestinal obstruction presents with abdominal pain, nausea, vomiting, and distention. Therapy includes gastrointestinal suction, maintenance of fluid and electrolyte balance, and measures to alleviate pain.

11.   Correct answer - A

Complications of total parenteral nutrition (TPN) are caused by catheter, sepsis, or metabolic disorders. Numerous problems may arise with insertion of the subclavian catheter, including hemothorax, pneumothorax, and air embolism. Sepsis may occur from lack of asepsis during catheter insertion, infection around the catheter, or solution contamination. Hyperglycemia and increased temperature are often initial signs of sepsis. Either hyperglycemia or hypoglycemia may develop as a complication of TPN, with hypoglycemia usually resulting from abrupt cessation of the TPN infusion. Infusion of dextrose 10% in water will prevent symptomatic hypoglycemia. Serum levels of phosphate and magnesium must be monitored closely because patients receiving TPN may develop deficiencies in these electrolytes. Hypokalemia may develop as cellular rebuilding uses large amounts of potassium. Because TPN is a hypertonic solution, the patient is at risk for developing hyperosmolar nonketotic dehydration.

12.   Correct answer - A

Spontaneous, painless hemorrhage of the GI tract in an alcohol abuser suggests esophageal varices or a Mallory-Weiss tear. Alcoholism precipitates reflux esophagitis, which erodes and weakens the esophagus; retching or coughing produces an esophageal, or Mallory-Weiss, tear. Hemorrhage from peptic ulceration, gastric perforation, or a duodenal tear usually is associated with pain.

13. **Correct answer - D**

An enlarged liver with a smooth, nontender edge suggests early cirrhosis. As cirrhosis progresses, the liver becomes smaller from malnutrition. An enlarged, smooth, tender liver indicates hepatitis or passive congestion from right ventricular failure. Suspect cancer if the liver is enlarged, hard, firm, and irregular.

14. **Correct answer - A**

Portal hypertension from cirrhosis precipitates esophageal varices, complications of which include hepatic encephalopathy, hepatorenal syndrome, and hemorrhagic shock. Esophageal varices result in plasma protein in the GI tract; the protein is degraded by bacteria into ammonia, thus precipitating hepatic encephalopathy. Hepatorenal syndrome, a condition of decreased renal perfusion and performance from liver dysfunction, may also develop. A decrease in circulating blood volume from esophageal bleeding stimulates renin release, which causes vasoconstriction, thereby reducing urine output. Blood in the GI tract breaks down into nitrogen, which increases the blood urea nitrogen (BUN) level.

15. **Correct answer - B**

An important nursing intervention in active esophageal bleeding is to reduce portal venous pressure. This can be done by giving I.V. vasopressin (Pitressin) at 0.2 units/minute. If pharmacologic therapy fails to reduce portal hypertension and control esophageal bleeding, a Sengstaken-Blakemore tube can be used. This stops acute variceal hemorrhage in 90% of patients. Lastly, the nurse should assess the patient's level of consciousness and be alert for the possibility of alcohol withdrawal syndrome, since varices occur in patients with alcohol-induced cirrhosis. Ice lavage does not stop esophageal bleeding because saline is instilled into the stomach.

16. **Correct answer - A**

Balloon tamponade may be used to control esophageal bleeding from varices. The Sengstaken-Blakemore tube exerts direct pressure on bleeding varices in the esophagus and upper stomach. The gastric balloon is usually inflated with 200 to 400 cc of air and traction is applied to exert firm pressure against the esophagogastric junction. The esophageal balloon is then inflated to 20 - 40 mm Hg and clamped. About every 24 hours, the esophageal balloon is decompressed and the gastric balloon is deflated to evaluate the status of the bleeding varices. Balloon tamponade carries several risks. If either balloon is inflated for too long or with excessive pressure, ulceration and necrosis in the stomach or esophagus can develop. Airway obstruction may also result from migration of the esophageal balloon into air passages. Scissors must be kept at the bedside to release the air in the balloon to prevent respiratory distress.

17.   **Correct answer - C**

Vasopressin (Pitressin), a synthetic antidiuretic hormone (ADH), lowers portal pressure, thus lessening esophageal bleeding. The usual dose is 0.2 units/minute. Administration requires constant monitoring for myocardial ischemia because the drug causes vasoconstriction. Vasopressin is contraindicated in patients with angina. Side effects include abdominal cramping, pallor, decreased urine output, and water retention.

18.   **Correct answer - D**

Intravenous vasopressin (Pitressin) is given to patients with bleeding esophageal varices because it causes vasoconstriction. Infusion may cause myocardial ischemia and infarction. The drug can also be administered via the superior mesenteric artery. Severe abdominal cramping may develop during infusion; if infiltration occurs, a mesenteric infarction may ensue because of lack of blood flow from the vasoconstriction.

19.   **Correct answer - A**

Once a red blood cell's membrane becomes fragile, it ruptures, causing a release of hemoglobin, which splits into globin and heme. The reticuloendothelial cells convert the heme into bilirubin and release it into the bloodstream to be transported to the liver. This unconjugated, or indirect, bilirubin is fat-soluble and bound to albumin. The bilirubin is soluble enough for transport but not for excretion. The next processing step occurs in the liver.

20.   **Correct answer - D**

Albumin-associated bilirubin travels in the bloodstream to the liver, where the bilirubin is removed from the albumin. It then is bound with glucuronic acid in a new, water-soluble formation. This conjugated, or direct, bilirubin, can now be excreted into the bile.

21.   Correct answer - D

Measuring conjugated and unconjugated bilirubin blood levels can help determine the pathophysiology of jaundice. Lactate dehydrogenase (LDH), serum glutamic-oxaloacetic transaminase (SGOT), and serum glutamate pyruvate transaminase (SGPT) levels are elevated in liver dysfunction but are not useful in diagnosing jaundice.

22.   Correct answer - B

A healthy liver converts indirect (unconjugated) bilirubin into direct (conjugated) bilirubin. A diseased liver cannot make this conversion. Thus, an elevated indirect bilirubin level indicates liver dysfunction.

23.   Correct answer - A

After a healthy liver converts indirect bilirubin into direct bilirubin, the latter is excreted into hepatic ducts and stored as bile. Thus, an elevated direct bilirubin level suggests biliary tract obstruction. Hepatitis, cirrhosis, and hepatic insufficiency result in elevated levels of indirect bilirubin because the damaged liver cannot convert it.

24.   Correct answer - C

When a patient with ascites accumulates 1,000 ml or more of peritoneal fluid, shifting dullness is audible on abdominal percussion. The patient's abdomen is taut and his umbilicus is flat or protruding. Palpation initiates a fluid wave. Tympanic percussion note usually does not occur; fluid accumulation produces a dull percussion sound.

25.   Correct answer - A

Portal hypertension plays a significant role in formation of ascites, the accumulation of fluid within the peritoneal cavity. Increased pressure within the portal system elevates hydrostatic pressure inside the vessel, favoring movement of fluid into the peritoneal cavity. Other factors that contribute to ascites formation include decreased albumin production by the liver, causing a decreased serum colloid osmotic pressure, and increased hepatic lymph formation, which exceeds the capacity of the lymphatic ducts to remove it, causing transudation of fluid from the liver surface into the peritoneal cavity.

26.   Correct answer - D

When ascites is evidenced by a distended abdomen, severe complications may develop. The intra-abdominal pressure elevates the diaphragm, interfering with lung expansion; if ascitic fluid moves through the diaphragm into the pleural cavity, a hydrothorax may develop. This increased intra-abdominal pressure predisposes the patient to inguinal and femoral hernias. The lower esophageal sphincter can become incompetent from the elevated pressure in the peritoneal cavity, leading to a reflux esophagitis and irritation of esophageal varices. Tension pneumothorax does not occur.

27.   Correct answer - C

Portal pressure is elevated by an obstruction of blood flow through the liver. More than 90% of portal hypertension cases stem from cirrhosis secondary to chronic alcoholism. Cirrhosis results in fibrous tissue and regenerating nodules, which compress the sinusoids and outflow vessels and interrupt blood flow through the liver.

28.   Correct answer - A

Hepatic cirrhosis and its sequela, portal hypertension, are among the leading causes of death in American men. More than one-third of these deaths follow esophageal or gastric variceal hemorrhage; thus, shunt surgery for portal hypertension is performed to decompress esophagogastric varices and maintain optimal portal perfusion. Shunt surgery also lessens the incidence of variceal rebleeding.

29.   Correct answer - A

Controlling dietary sodium is the cornerstone of therapy for ascites. Restricting sodium to 200 to 500 mg/day limits the amount of fluid formed. Fluid restriction and diuretic therapy are also important. A l d a c t o n e (spironolactone) is administered to inhibit aldosterone secretion, thereby reducing sodium reabsorption. Thiazide diuretics are avoided in patients with ascites. Paracentesis, a last resort in managing ascites, is used primarily to relieve respiratory distress and to provide comfort to the terminally ill patient. Only a small amount of ascitic fluid is withdrawn from the abdomen during paracentesis. Excessive fluid removal can cause fluid shifts, resulting in hypovolemia and protein loss and can contribute to development of hepatorenal syndrome or portal-systemic encephalopathy. Paracentesis is a temporary, palliative measure, as new ascitic fluid rapidly accumulates because of the persistent, primary pathophysiologic derangements.

30. **Correct answer - D**

The exocrine function of the pancreas is controlled by the acinar cells, which secrete a high concentration of sodium bicarbonate, water, sodium, potassium, and digestive enzymes constituting about 1,500 ml of the total daily secretion of intestinal juices. The enzymes lipase, amylase, and trypsin break down fats, carbohydrates, and proteins, respectively. The endocrine function of the pancreas is performed by the beta cells from the islets of Langerhans, which secrete insulin, and by the alpha cells, which secrete glucagon.

31. **Correct answer - B**

Alcoholism triggers about 60% of acute pancreatitis cases. Studies indicate that chronic alcohol ingestion leads to changes in pancreoltic exocrine secretion with the development of protein precipitates within the pancreatic ducts. These precipitates cause ductal obstruction and subsequent inflammation. Biliary tract disease is the second most common cause of pancreatitis, accounting for about 20% of such cases. Passage of gallstones (in choleithiasis) through the distal common bile duct and possibly into the ampulla of Vater can also lead to pancreatitis. Other precipitating factors include trauma, drugs, such as steroids and thiazide diuretics, and infections, such as the mumps and coxsackie virus.

32. **Correct answer - D**

Acute pancreatitis is an autodigestive disease believed to be caused by the escape of activated enzymes from the acinar cells. Activated enzymes most commonly found to cause injury are trypsin, phospholipase A, and elastase.

Trypsin enters pancreatic ducts, causes edema and necrosis, and activates other enzymes. Elastase produces necrosis of vessel walls and leads to hemorrhage. Phospholipase A damages acinar cell membranes; the inflammatory process ensues, causing necrosis of fat in the pancreas.

33. Correct answer - D

The patient with acute pancreatitis presents with severe, constant epigastric pain radiating to the back and associated with nausea, vomiting, and fever. Other signs include abdominal distention and absent bowel sounds caused by paralytic ileus. Restlessness and hyperventilation may occur in severe cases, as a result of adult respiratory distress syndrome (ARDS) and hypoxia. Hypotension results from hemorrhage and loss of plasma into pancreatic tissue.

34. Correct answer - D

Clinical presentation in acute pancreatitis includes severe, constant epigastric pain that often radiates to the back. Pain eases when the patient leans forward. Abdominal distention follows the pain, and paralytic ileus ensues as intestinal motility ceases. Rigidity may be evident on abdominal palpation and rebound tenderness.

35. Correct answer - D

A patient with acute pancreatitis may develop Chvostek's sign or Trousseau's sign, indicating hypocalcemia, an electrolyte abnormality caused by precipitation and use of calcium from fat necrosis during pancreatic autodigestion. Chvostek's sign (facial twitching) is elicited by tapping the facial nerve. Trousseau's sign (carpal spasm contracture) is elicited by applying pressure to the brachial nerve. Hemorrhagic pancreatitis causes blood to pool retroperitoneally, producing a bluish discoloration of the flank (Grey-Turner's sign) and umbilicus (Cullen's sign). Homans's sign indicates deep-vein thrombosis; when the toe is passively dorsiflexed, calf pain develops.

36. Correct answer - D

Patients with acute pancreatitis develop various pulmonary complications. The inflamed pancreas results in an elevated diaphragm with bilateral basilar crackles. Pleural effusion occurs in 5% to 17% of patients, usually on the left side. Diffuse alveolar consolidation and pulmonary atelectasis may occur in severe cases. Pancreatitis releases vasoactive enzymes, which may decrease surfactant levels in the lungs, precipitating ARDS.

37. Correct answer - D

Complications of acute pancreatitis include hypovolemic shock, which results from the vast amount of plasma released into the peritoneum or from blood loss caused by hemorrhage. Other complications associated with shock from acute pancreatitis include disseminated intravascular coagulopathy (DIC) and acute renal failure. Respiratory failure may ensue from the resulting diffuse alveolar consolidation and ARDS. Pseudocyst formation in the pancreas also is common.

38. Correct answer - A

The analgesic drug of choice in acute pancreatitis is Demerol (meperidine), given 50 to 100 mg every 4 hours as needed. Other analgesics, such as morphine, hydromorphone (Dilaudid), and codeine, should be avoided because they cause spasm of the sphincter of Oddi.

39. Correct answer - C

Nursing interventions in pancreatitis include nasogastric suctioning to decrease gastric and intestinal distention and the flow of acid into the duodenum, thus reducing pancreatic stimulation. The patient should be cautiously started on clear liquids when symptoms improve and advanced to low-fat, full liquids. A low-fat diet can then be initiated, as tolerated, and should be maintained for up to 6 weeks. Peritoneal lavage typically is used in acute pancreatitis; the intraperitoneal space is rinsed with fluid to remove toxic substances released from the pancreas. Antibiotics are contraindicated because they may mask the causative organism of pancreatic sepsis.

40. Correct answer - A

A low-fat, no-alcohol diet minimizes pancreatic stimulation. Prohibiting caffeine limits stimulation of gastric acid secretion, which initiates pancreatic activity.

41.   Correct answer - D

A pancreaticoduodenal resection, or Whipple's procedure, involves the removal of the gallbladder, the distal portion of stomach, the duodenum, and the head of the pancreas. The remaining pancreas, stomach, and common bile duct are anastomosed to the jejunum.

42.   Correct answer - B

Complications that may develop immediately after pancreatic surgery include pancreatic fistula, anastomotic leaks, hemorrhage, and the development of a pancreatic abscess with possible peritonitis. Long-term postoperative complications include insulin dependence and steatorrhea.

43.   Correct answer - A

Pancreatic carcinoma is often multifocal. A total pancreatectomy is less complicated than Whipple's procedure, and the severity and frequency of complications are decreased. Many patients who undergo Whipple's procedure eventually develop pancreatic insufficiency and diabetes; with a total pancreatectomy, metabolic derangements are more manageable.

44.   Correct answer - C

After inspection of the abdomen, auscultation precedes percussion and palpation to prevent distortion of auscultatory findings related to pressure on the abdominal wall. Percussion precedes palpation to screen for an enlarged spleen before deep palpation.

45.   Correct answer - C

The primary cause of large-bowel obstruction in adults is carcinoma. Diverticulitis is the second most common cause, and volvulus the third.

46.   Correct answer - C

Intestinal obstruction is marked by an accumulation of intestinal secretions, fluids, and gas. Distention increases intraluminal pressure, compromising circulation to the bowel layers. Intestinal obstruction has mechanical causes (such as physical blockage by adhesions, tumors, or hernias) and functional causes (such as paralytic ileus from abdominal surgery, hypokalemia, and trauma). Clinical presentation depends on whether the obstruction occurs in the small or large bowel. Small-bowel obstruction produces great fluid loss from third-space fluid shifting, little distention, early vomiting, and short, sharp pain. Large-bowel obstruction presents with marked distention, pain of long duration, and late vomiting. Obstruction to either the small or the large bowel precipitates nausea, vomiting, rebound tenderness, and rigidity. Bowel sounds may be absent or high-pitched with a partial obstruction.

47. Correct answer - D

Laboratory findings in bowel obstruction include leukocytosis (increased white blood cell count), a result of the toxic proliferation of bacteria across the damaged membrane; increased hematocrit and other blood chemistry values, usually reflecting hemoconcentration from hypovolemia and dehydration; and a decreased bicarbonate level caused by systemic acidosis.

48. Correct answer - C

Gastrointestinal tubes are of two types: nasogastric and intestinal. Nasogastric tubes include the Salem sump (a double-lumen tube) and the Levin (a single-lumen tube). One advantage of the Salem sump is that its narrow lumen prevents development of excessive negative pressure by breaking the vacuum when the stomach mucosa is aspirated into the other lumen. Low, constant suction should be used, with the narrow lumen positioned above the patient's midline. Intestinal tubes include the Miller-Abbott, Cantor, and Metler-Rawson; gravity and peristalsis facilitate their passage into the small intestine.

49. Correct answer - C

The large intestine, which is 5 to 6 feet long, extends from the ileum to the anus. Its anatomic divisions are the cecum; the ascending, transverse, descending, and sigmoid colons; and the rectum. The large intestine has two flexures: the hepatic flexure in the right upper quadrant and the splenic flexure in the left upper quadrant.

50.   Correct answer - C

Factors that enhance colonic motility include high-residue diets, morphine, and parasympathomimetic drugs (such as bethanechol and neostigmine). Coloni irritation from increased bile salts, bacterial endotoxins, hyperosmolar fluids, or such diseases as ulcerative colitis also stimulate colonic motility. Factors that inhibit colonic motility include low-residue diets and anticholinergic drugs, such as atropine.

51.   Correct answer - D

The large intestine performs several functions. It absorbs water and electrolytes, with the ascending and transverse colons absorbing about 1 liter of water per day. Sodium and chloride also are absorbed, and potassium and bicarbonate are secreted into the lumen for excretion. The main anaerobic bacteria, *Bacteroides fragilis,* and the aerobic bacteria, *Escherichia coli*, partially synthesize folic acid, riboflavin, vitamin K, and nicotinic acid. Mucosal cells of the colon break down blood urea, a metabolic waste product, into ammonia. Lastly, the large intestine eliminates fecal material.

52.   Correct answer - B

The arterial supply of the GI tract stems from the aorta. The branching of the celiac artery supplies the upper GI tract. The gastric, hepatic, and gastroduodenal arteries supply the stomach; the cystic artery supplies the gallbladder; and the splenic artery supplies the pancreas and spleen. The superior mesenteric artery supplies the middle GI tract. Its branch stems from the abdominal aorta and supplies the jejunum, ileum, cecum, ascending colon, and part of the transverse colon. Thus, the major blood supply to the small intestine is via the superior mesenteric artery. The inferior mesenteric artery supplies the lower GI tract. Also from the abdominal aorta, this branch provides the   rectum and the transverse, descending, and sigmoid colons with arterial flow. Thus, the major blood supply to the large intestine is via the inferior mesenteric artery.

53.   Correct answer - B

In a functional paralytic ileus, decreased mobility is caused by a physiologic dysfunction rather than an anatomic obstruction. Hypokalemia decreases motor activity of the GI tract. A patient with paralytic ileus presents with marked abdominal distention, moderately severe abdominal pain, nausea, vomiting, and no bowel sounds.

54. Correct answer - A

A leaking anastomosis is usually apparent 1 week to 10 days after surgery. Signs include a low-grade fever, inflammation, and fluid accumulation in the pleural space; the patient may exhibit acute chest pain mimicking pulmonary embolism. If the leakage persists, an intercostal catheter is inserted to drain the pleural space. A nasogastric tube commonly is left in place 1 to 2 days after the patient starts oral feedings.

55. Correct answer - B

Calcium absorption from the small intestine depends on activated vitamin D (1,25-dihydroxycholecalciferol). Thus, a patient with a vitamin D deficiency secondary to chronic renal failure, hepatic failure, or rickets develops hypocalcemia. Beriberi results from a B_1 deficiency, and scurvy develops from a vitamin C deficiency.

56. Correct answer - A

Both the portal vein and the hepatic artery bring blood to the liver. The hepatic artery delivers oxygenated blood and the portal vein brings venous blood, which has traversed the walls of the intestinal tract and is rich in amino acids, fats, and sugars. Blood leaves the liver via the hepatic veins, which empty into the inferior vena cava.

57. Correct answer - A

The liver, the largest internal organ, has several important functions. It controls synthesis of amino acids, albumin, globulin, prothrombin, fibrinogen, and other blood factors; stores fat-soluble vitamins; synthesizes ketone bodies, acetate, and cholesterol; and forms urea to remove ammonia from blood. Phagocytic action of the reticuloendothelial system by Kupffer's cells destroys old red blood cells and detoxifies toxic substances.

58.   Correct answer - B

The liver does not secrete digestive hormones or enzymes. Its only contribution to digestion is the secretion of bile salts, which play an important role in digestion; they emulsify fats and assist in fatty acid absorption. Gluconeogenesis - the formation of glucose from noncarbohydrate sources, such as amino acids and fats is a liver function but does not contribute to digestion.

59.   Correct answer - C

Kupffer's cells - the phagocytes of the reticuloendothelial system - destroy old blood corpuscles and detoxify toxic substances.

60.   Correct answer - A

The liver synthesizes the following blood-clotting components: Factors II, V, VII, VIII, IX, and X, prothrombin and fibrinogen. Vitamin K, essential for blood clotting, is stored in the liver but is synthesized in the large intestine.

61.   Correct answer - A

All patients with suspected hepatitis should be isolated from other patients and enteric and blood precautions must be observed. In hepatitis A cases, enteric precautions are recommended; with the arrival of jaundice, the patient is no longer infectious. With acute hepatitis B patients, isolation and enteric precautions can be discontinued when jaundice subsides. In cases of acute non-A, non-B hepatitis, isolation is controversial, but blood precautions are probably advisable throughout the incubation period (7 to 50 days).

62.   Correct answer - C

The initial mental slowness in stage I of portal-systemic encephalopathy (PSE) progresses to disorientation to time, place, or person. Stage II presents with more prominent clinical manifestations, such as mental confusion and asterixis. Stage III is characterized by progressive, marked confusion and stupor. The patient can be aroused - but usually to a violent or agitated state. During stage IV, the patient becomes unresponsive and progresses into a deep coma; deep tendon reflexes are absent. The patient with PSE fluctuates among the four stages. Particularly in the early stages, the nurse must frequently assess neurologic status.

63. Correct answer - B

Abnormal ammonia metabolism contributes to the clinical manifestations of PSE. Elevated ammonia levels interfere with normal cerebral metabolism by decreasing the amount of energy produced by brain cells. The diseased liver cannot detoxify ammonia into urea, so the serum ammonia level rises.

64. Correct answer - D

Asterixis, or "liver flap," occurs in patients with hepatic failure who have progressed into PSE. A flapping tremor of the hands, asterixis can be elicited by having the patient raise both arms with the forearms fixed and hands dorsiflexed. Asterixis can also be noted when the patient rests his arms on a flat surface and extends his hands upward. These positions allow detection of rapid flexion and extension movements of the writs. The clinical manifestation probably indicates impaired cerebral metabolism and may also occur in other end-stage metabolic diseases, such as respiratory failure and uremia.

65. Correct answer - D

Ammonia contributes to development of PSE, so measures must be instituted to lower serum ammonia levels. Such drugs as neomycin and lactulose can be administered to reduce bacterial breakdown of protein substances in the bowel. Restriction or elimination of dietary protein is necessary because intestinal bacteria break down protein in the GI tract to produce ammonia. Therapy also involves restricting potentially hepatotoxic drugs, especially sedatives, narcotics, and barbiturates. Thiazide therapy is avoided because it may induce hepatic coma.

66. Correct answer - D

In the bowel, bacteria convert lactulose, a disaccharide, to lactate and other organic acids. This creates an acidic environment in the bowel, causing ammonia to leave the blood and move into the colon, where the ammonia is trapped and cannot be absorbed. As a result, serum ammonia levels fall. A high-molecular-weight sugar, lactulose also creates an osmotic gradient; water is drawn into the bowel by the osmotically active lactulose molecules. The increased water content exerts a laxative effect and facilitates ammonia elimination. The desired effects of lactulose are an acidic fecal pH and two to three soft stools daily. Side effects include abdominal cramping, bloating, diarrhea, nausea, and vomiting.

67.   Correct answer - B

Hepatorenal syndrome is sudden renal failure associated with progressive liver disease in a patient with previously normal renal function. It commonly occurs in end-stage cirrhosis associated with ascites, hypoalbuminemia, splenomegaly, and portal hypertension. Hepatorenal syndrome does not produce anatomic or histologic changes in the kidneys; rather, the syndrome appears to be a functional disorder. Initial manifestations include the abrupt development of oliguria and azotemia; blood urea nitrogen (BUN) and serum creatinine levels rise progressively.

68.   Correct answer - A

In hepatic dysfunction, protein intake may be cut to 40 g/day or stopped completely. Restriction or elimination is necessary because protein in the GI tract is broken down into ammonia, which may contribute to development of hepatic encephalopathy. Sodium intake is restricted to decrease ascites.

69.   Correct answer - C

The esophagus and the stomach each contain two sphincters. In the esophagus, the hypopharyngeal sphincter (at the top of the esophagus) is closed at rest and opens when the sphincter contracts during swallowing or vomiting. At rest, the gastroesophageal sphincter (at the junction of the stomach and esophagus) is tonically closed to keep gastric contents in the stomach. Inappropriate relaxation of the gastroesophageal sphincter, called reflux, can be caused by hiatal hernia, increased abdominal pressure, or pregnancy. The two stomach sphincters, the cardiac and the pyloric, control the rate of foot passage. The cardiac sphincter is at the opening from the esophagus, and the pyloric sphincter is at the opening into the duodenum.

302

70. **Correct answer - B**

The gastric glands are located in the stomach's fundic and antral areas. The fundic area contains the chief cells, which secrete pepsinogen and mucus; the oxyntic, or parietal cells, which secrete HCl and the intrinsic factor; and the mucous neck cells, which secrete mucus. In the antral area, G cells are responsible for secreting gastrin.

71. **Correct answer - A**

Gastric secretion is stimulated by the interaction of three main classes of compounds; the hormone gastrin, acetylcholine, and histamine. Gastrin is released by the G cells of the antral area. Acetylcholine promotes acid release and increases gastric motility; gastric distention and vagal stimulation. Histamine is also a potent stimulator of acid secretion; the gastric mucosa can manufacture and store large quantities of histamine.

72. **Correct answer - C**

HCL secretion occurs when histamine combines with H_2 receptors on the parietal (oxyntic) cells. Ranitidine and cimetdine are H_2 receptor-antagonists, which block the action of histamine on the parietal H_2 receptor site, preventing HCL secretion. Ranitidine and cimetidine may not be given together with antacids, such as Mylanta and Maalox, because antacids would decrease their efficacy.

73. **Correct answer - A**

Digestive juices, such as HCL and pepsinogen, begin to break down food as it enters the stomach. This secretory function occurs in the top, or fundic, portion of the stomach. The mixing of food occurs in the stomach's distal portion.

74. **Correct answer - A**

Factors that inhibit gastric emptying include chyme with a high lipid content, high acidity in the antrum of the stomach, pain, anxiety, and sadness, as well as intestinal hormones such as secretin and cholecystokinin. Factors accelerating gastric emptying include ingestion of liquids, increase in stomach volume contents, anger, and aggression.

75.   Correct answer - C

Sympathetic and parasympathetic pathways and gastric hormones influence emptying of the stomach, or gastric motility; release of the hormone gastrin augments that rate. Gastrin release promotes HCL and pepsin production by stimulating the parietal (oxyntic) and chief cells. Gastrin affects gastric emptying primarily by increasing antral motility, which enhances the rate of gastric emptying; stimuli from the duodenum, on the other hand, decrease that rate. The duodenum inhibits gastric peristalsis and constricts the pyloric sphincter in response to fat, high osmolarity, and acidity. Emotional factors also affect the rate of gastric emptying, with pain and anxiety slowing it.

76.   Correct answer - C

About 80% of ulcers are duodenal and 20% are gastric. Duodenal ulcers usually occur in patients aged 30 to 50; gastric ulcers are typically seen in later years.

77.   Correct answer - B

Perforation of a duodenal ulcer with ensuing peritonitis erodes the wall of the pancreas, causing pancreatitis.

78.   Correct answer - C

The spleen, located in the left upper abdominal quadrant, is the organ most commonly injured in abdominal trauma. It is a highly vascular organ, and trauma may result in intrasplenic bleeding; thus, a large mass may be palpated in the left upper abdominal quadrant. A normal spleen cannot be palpated. The liver is located in the right upper abdominal quadrant. Damage to the small intestine or colon usually is associated with lower quadrant injuries.

79.   Correct answer - C

To restore circulatory volume, fluid replacement is essential in blunt injury with suspected trauma to internal organs. An isotonic solution, such as lactated Ringer's or normal saline solution, is given intravenously. This solution maintains the same osmotic pressure as blood serum, so cellular.

constituents remain unchanged. Isotonic solutions are administered until blood products are available, maintaining blood volume until surgery can be performed.

80.   **Correct answer - C**

Peritoneal lavage is contraindicated in a patient with a history of many abdominal operations. Adhesions increase the likelihood that the bowel will be penetrated and the lavage will be trapped, making its return difficult. Peritoneal lavage also is contraindicated in pregnant patients because of possible fetal damage.

81.   **Correct answer - D**

Hemorrhage from retroperitoneal structures does not cause bleeding into the abdominal compartment; hence, a false-negative lavage may result.

82.   **Correct answer - A**

Acute liver injury may cause a sudden rise in the liver enzymes alkaline phosphatase and lactic dehydrogenase. Levels would have been elevated on admission in alcoholism or hepatitis. Pancreatitis causes a rise in serum amylase or lipase.

83.   **Correct answer - B**

Some abdominal organs are more likely to be injured than others, depending on the injury's location and how it occurred. Abdominal trauma occurs most commonly in the spleen, followed by the kidneys, intestines, liver, and pancreas.

84.   **Correct answer - A**

The spleen, injured more often than any other abdominal organ, is located in the left upper abdominal quadrant, under the diaphragm and near the abdominal wall. Partly protected by the left lower ribs, it cannot be palpated until triple its normal size. Kehr's sign (referred pain to the left shoulder from blood irritating the diaphragm) is evident in about 50% of splenic injuries. Incidence of splenic injury is so high because the spleen is the most vascular organ in the body. Splenic lacerations and ruptured

hematomas are notorious sources of persistent bleeding into the peritoneal cavity.

85.   Correct answer - A

Intrinsic factor is secreted by the parietal (oxyntic) cells in the fundus of the
stomach. This mucoprotein is necessary for intestinal absorption of vitamin
B_{12} by the ileum. Cholecystokinin and secretin, released from the cells of
the duodenum, control contraction of the gallbladder and secretion of
pancreatic fluid. Lipase, a digestive enzyme in pancreatic fluid, breaks
down triglycerides to fatty acids and glycerol.

86.   Correct answer - D

Villi are fingerlike projections of the mucosa and submucosa prominent
in the duodenum and jejunum. Each villus contains a lacteal and a capillary
bed to aid in absorption of fats, carbohydrates and protein. Individual cells
of the villi contain small projections called microvilli, which increase the
absorption area. Lieberkuhn's crypts are found between the villi; epithelial
cells of these crypts produce intestinal secretions that are reabsorbed into
the villi. Peyer's patches, cells in the mucosa and submucosa of the small
intestine, control antibody synthesis. Brunner's glands, located in the
duodenum, are cells that secrete alkaline mucus, which protects the
duodenal lining from the acidic gastric juices.

87.   Correct answer - D

The small intestine's most important functions are to digest and absorb
food. Active transport, one of the three basic absorption mechanisms, is
movement of a substance against a concentration gradient. Energy is
required to move the substance into or out of a cell. Amino acids, sodium,
potassium, sugars, calcium, and chloride require active transport. Passive
diffusion is movement of a substance along a concentration gradient. No
energy is required to move the substance from an area of high concentration
to one of low concentration. Examples of passive diffusion include fatty
acids and water. Facilitated diffusion is movement of a substance by a
carrier from an area of high concentration to one of low concentration; the
substance can cross the membranes only by binding with the carrier. An
example of facilitated diffusion is glucose. Entry of glucose into the cell is
facilitated through binding with a carrier substance.

88. **Correct answer - C**

Most digestion and absorption take place in the small intestine, primarily in the jejunum. Electrolytes, water, carbohydrates, protein, fats, fat-soluble vitamins (A,D,E, and K), and iron are absorbed there

89. **Correct answer - D**

The fat-soluble vitamins (A,D,E, and K) require bile salts for absorption in the jejunum. Water-soluble vitamins (vitamin C and B complex) are absorbed in all parts of the small intestine by passive diffusion. Vitamin B12 requires the intrinsic factor from the parietal cells and is absorbed in the ileum. Calcium requires vitamin D for absorption, which occurs primarily in the duodenum.

90. **Correct answer - A**

The prime digestive function of bile salts is fat emulsification. Initially, dietary fat is in the form of a triglyceride. Digestion of fats begins in the duodenum, where the pancreatic enzyme lipase splits the triglyceride into fatty acids and glycerol. With the completion of lipolysis, bile salts are necessary for absorption of fats by the jejunum. The breakdown of complex carbohydrates is completed in the duodenum by the pancreatic enzyme amylase. The digestion of protein begins in the stomach and continues in the duodenum. The pancreas secretes protein-splitting enzymes known as proteases.

CHAPTER 6

ENDOCRINE SYSTEM

---

1. Pituitary gland hormone secretion is controlled by:

    A.   The thalamus
    B.   The hypothalamus
    C.   The neurohypophysis
    D.   Hormonal secretions of the thyroid

---

2. Which of the following is *not* secreted by the posterior pituitary gland?

    A.   Adrenocorticotropic hormone
    B.   Antidiuretic hormone
    C.   Oxytocic hormone
    D.   Vasopressin

---

3. Hormonal activity of the thyroid, adrenal, cortex, and gonads is controlled by:

    A.   Adrenocorticotropic hormone
    B.   Neurohypophysis
    C.   Adenohypophysis
    D.   Posterior pituitary gland

Case Study
Questions 4-14 refer to the following case study:

Mr. L. age 47, is comatose when brought to the emergency room. The family reports that he had become confused over the last 72 hours. He had a seizure in the car on the way to the hospital. On arrival, the patient was minimally responsive. His respiratory rate was 32 breaths/minute; his pulse, 110 beats/minute; his blood pressure, 120/90 mm Hg. Initial laboratory work includes complete blood count, serum electrolytes, and urine and serum osmolalities. Chest X-ray reveals a mass in the right upper-lung field.

4. The underlying factor responsible for Mr. L.'s change in mental status is related to:

    A.   Cerebral metastasis from lung cancer
    B.   Syndrome of inappropriate antidiuretic hormone (SIADH)
    C.   Seizure activity from meningitis
    D.   Possible subarachnoid hemorrhage

5. Which of the following would be *inappropriate* treatment for Mr. L.?

    A.   Administration of furosemide (Lasix)
    B.   Administration of 200 to 300 ml of 3% normal saline solution
    C.   Fluid restriction
    D.   Administration of demeclocycline (Ledermycin) 300mg P.O.

6. Which patient is *not* at risk for SIADH?

    A.   A 20-year-old transferred from a skilled nursing facility where he received prolonged positive-pressure ventilation
    B.   A 36-year-old receiving phenytoin (Dilantin)
    C.   A 64-year-old with chronic obstructive pulmonary disease (COPD) complicated by pneumonia
    D.   A 70-year-old with carcinoma of the lung

7. An increase in antidiuretic hormone (ADH) secretion in Mr. L. may be caused by:

    A.   Chlorpropamide therapy
    B.   Head trauma
    C.   Viral respiratory infections
    D.   All of the above

8.   ADH stimulates the kidneys to:

A.   Reabsorb sodium and excrete potassium
B.   Reabsorb water and concentrate urine
C.   Reabsorb water and dilute urine
D.   Reabsorb sodium and retain potassium

9.   A normal releasing stimulus for ADH is:

A.   Decreased aldosterone levels
B.   Decreased serum osmolality
C.   Increased serum osmolality
D.   Increased potassium levels

10.   All of the following factors inhibit ADH release *except:*

A.   Increased serum osmolality
B.   Inflammatory conditions in the pituitary gland
C.   Surgery of the pituitary gland
D.   Decreased serum osmolality

11.   The symptoms of SIADH result from:

A.   Elevated potassium levels
B.   Water intoxication
C.   Increased serum osmolality
D.   Precipitating factors of SIADH

12.   The patient with SIADH would most likely present with which complication?

A.   Tetany
B.   Seizures
C.   Hypotension
D.   Poor skin turgor

13. Which laboratory finding would be present in Mr. L.?

    A. Low serum sodium level
    B. Serum osmolality of 350 mOsm/liter
    C. Urine specific gravity of 1.001
    D. Elevated potassium level

14. An *inappropriate* therapy for the patient with SIADH would be:

    A. Fluid restriction
    B. Eradication of the underlying cause
    C. Administration of hypertonic saline solution
    D. Administration of vasopressin (Pitressin) drip

Case Study
Questions 15-18 refer to the following case study:

Mr. D., a patient recently admitted to the intensive care unit (ICU), has diabetes insipidus. His blood pressure is 100/60, with rapid pulse of 134.

15. Which of the following patients would be *most* likely to develop diabetes insipidus?

    A. An elderly patient receiving thiazides and clofibrate
    B. A young woman with severe pneumonia
    C. A 50-year-old man with esophageal varices who is receiving vasopressin therapy
    D. A young man with head trauma resulting in skull fracture

16. During assessment, which finding would be expected in Mr. D?

    A. Serum osmolality of 250 mOsm/liter
    B. Serum sodium level of 165 mEq/liter
    C. Urine output of less than 600 ml in 24 hours
    D. Urine specific gravity of 1.025

17. A major complication of diabetes insipidus is:

A. Hypovolemic shock
B. Seizures
C. Congestive heart failure
D. Cardiac dysrhythmias from hypokalemia

18. Evaluation of laboratory findings for Mr. D. would show:

A. Increased urine osmolality
B. Urine specific gravity between 1.001 and 1.005
C. Decreased serum sodium level
D. Decreased serum osmolality

19. Resistance to vasopressin therapy may be caused by:

A. Administration of vasopressin with calcium blockers
B. Inadequate warming or agitation of the medication vial
C. Mixing vasopressin with normal saline solution
D. Failure to keep medication refrigerated

20. Vasopressin must be used cautiously in a patient with:

A. Liver dysfunction
B. Brain tumor
C. Angina pectoris
D. Kidney transplant

Case Study
Questions 21-26 refer to the following case study:

Mrs. V., a 60-year-old woman with postoperative small-bowel re-section, is admitted to the surgical intensive care unit (SICU). She has a history of hypothyroidism. She appears extremely lethargic, her temperature is 94.6°F. (34.8° C.) Myxedema coma is diagnosed.

21. Which factor would *not* precipitate Mrs. V.'s myxedema coma?

   A. Thyroidectomy
   B. Pituitary tumor
   C. Hypophysectomy
   D. Discontinuation of antithyroid medication

22. The nurse would suspect myxedema coma in a patient with:

   A. Hypothermia and tachycardia
   B. Hypoventilation and hypertension
   C. Seizure activity and hypothermia
   D. Hypotension and hyperpnea

23. Intolerance to cold, periorbital edema, gland hypertrophy, and dry skin are effects of:

   A. Increased levels of triodothyronine (T_3)
   B. Increased levels of thyrocalcitonin
   C. Decreased levels of thyroxine (T_4)
   D. Decreased levels of thyrocalcitonin

24. Further assessment of Mrs. V. may reveal all of the following *except:*

   A. Audible bruit over the thyroid gland
   B. Pleural effusion
   C. Pericardial effusion
   D. Paralytic ileus

25. Evaluation of Mrs. V.'s diagnostic studies would demonstrate:

   A. Increased serum sodium
   B. Decreased O_2
   C. Decreased CO_2
   D. Increased serum osmolarity

26. An appropriate intervention while caring for Mrs. V. would be to:

A. Administer fluid challenges of normal saline solution to raise the blood pressure
B. Give 3% sodium chloride at 100 ml/hour to correct hyponatremia
C. Administer thyroxin intravenously
D. Place the patient on a hyperthermia blanket set at 110° F.

Case Study
Questions 27-34 refer to the following case study:

Mrs. M. has just been transferred to SICU from a surgical floor. She underwent thyroid surgery the day before. A diagnosis of hypoparathyroidism is made.

27. Precipitating factors of hypoparathyroidism include:

A. Surgery of the thyroid gland
B. Radiation injury secondary to thyroid therapy
C. Acute pancreatitis
D. All of the above

28. Parathyroid hormone (parathormone, or PTH) affects serum calcium level by:

A. Increasing bone resorption of calcium
B. Increasing GI absorption of calcium
C. Increasing absorption of calcium and decreasing reabsorption of phosphate by the kidney
D. All of the above

29. Which condition must be present for parathyroid hormone to exert its effects at GI and bone sites?

A. Increased calcium level
B. Decreased phosphate level
C. Adequate vitamin D level
D. A normally functioning thyroid gland

315

30. In assessing Mrs. M.'s hypoparathyroidism, the nurse may observe which of the following:

    A. Numbness and tingling of fingers and toes
    B. Laryngeal stridor, dyspnea, and cyanosis
    C. Confusion, lethargy, and emotional lability
    D. All of the above

31. A carpopedal spasm produced in the hypocalcemic patient is known as:

    A. Positive Trousseau's sign
    B. Positive Chvostek's sign
    C. Carpal tetany
    D. Cullen's sign

32. Which statement regarding hypocalcemia is *false?*

    A. Resulting low calcium levels may cause the patient to exhibit Chvostek's sign
    B. A prolonged QT interval appears on the ECG
    C. I.V. calcium should not be mixed with saline for infusion
    D. Decreased secretion of calcitonin by the parathyroid gland results in hypocalcemia

33. Appropriate care for a patient with hypoparathyroidism includes all of the following *except:*

    A. Administration of oral calcium supplements with caution if the patient is on digitalis
    B. Administration of phosphates to maintain adequate phosphorus levels
    C. Administration of vitamin D to increase calcium absorption
    D. Administration of oral calcium supplements with meals but not dairy products - if the patient develops GI upset

34. Which condition would be expected to precipitate tetany in the hypocalcemic patient?

    A. Hypoventilation
    B. Decreased calcitonin levels
    C. Increased parathormone stimulation
    D. Alkalosis

Case Study
Questions 35-47 refer to the following case study:

Mrs. T. is transferred to the ICU from a medical unit. She was admitted with pneumonia and has a history of hyperthyroidism. Her temperature is 103° F. (39.4° C.); blood pressure, 170/80; and pulse, 120 beats/minute. She is anxious and irritable. Thyroid storm is diagnosed.

35. The thyroid gland produces which of the following?

    A. Thyroxine
    B. Tri-iodothyronine
    C. Calcitonin
    D. All of the above

36. Which hormone would lower Mrs. T.'s serum calcium level?

    A. PTH
    B. Parathyroid hormone
    C. Calcitonin
    D. Glucocorticoid

37. The normal effects of calcitonin secretion include:

    A. Reduction of plasma calcium by inhibiting bone resorption
    B. Increase in urine sodium, chloride, magnesium, and calcium excretion
    C. Lysis and assimilation of bone
    D. All of the above

38. Secretion of thyroid hormone is regulated by hormones from which glands?

    A. Anterior pituitary and the hypothalamus
    B. Anterior pituitary and the thalamus
    C. Posterior pituitary and the parathyroid
    D. Posterior pituitary and the adrenal cortex

39. The biochemical and physiologic response of thyrotoxic crisis in Mrs. T. results from:

    A. An increase in systemic adrenergic activity
    B. A defect in thyroid hormone synthesis
    C. An increase in iodine uptake by thyroid cells
    D. An overstimulation of the thyroid gland by thyrotropin-releasing hormone (TRH) from the pituitary

40. Which of the following would *not* be caused by increased levels of T_4 in Mrs. T.?

    A. Diarrhea
    B. Decreased tolerance to heat
    C. Weight loss
    D. Cardiomegaly and heart failure

41. Which factor would *not* precipitate a thyroid storm in a patient with hyperthyroidism?

    A. Overdose of antithyroid medication
    B. Trauma, infection, and stress
    C. Ketoacidosis
    D. Vigorous palpation of thyroid gland in a hyperthyroid patient

42. Mrs. T. would exhibit which of the following symptoms?

    A. Hypothermia and flushing
    B. Hypotension and tachycardia
    C. Emotional lability and psychosis
    D. Bradycardia and hypoventilation

43. Which finding in Mrs. T. would *not* be a result of thyrotoxic crisis?

A. Widening pulse pressure and systolic murmurs
B. Decreased pulse pressure and diastolic murmurs
C. S$_3$ heart sounds
D. Increased pulse pressure and hypertension

44. All of the following decrease thyroid hormone synthesis and release *except:*

A. Guanethidine (Ismelin)
B. Propylthiouracil (Propyl-Thyracil)
C. Lithium carbonate (Eskalith)
D. Sodium iodide (Iodotope Therapeutic)

45. Specific care to decrease a hypermetabolic state of thyrotoxic crisis includes all of the following actions *except:*

A. Instituting hypothermic measures
B. Modifying environmental stimuli
C. Administering corticosteroids and sedatives
D. Administering aspirin for hyperthermia

46. Which medication is administered to support myocardial function in the patient with thyroid storm?

A. Epinephrine (Adrenalin)
B. Isoproterenol (Isuprel)
C. Propranolol (Inderal)
D. Dopamine (Intropin)

47. The nurse would suspect common complications caused by thyrotoxic crisis to include:

A. Tetany and seizures
B. Dehydration and congestive heart failure
C. Hypertensive crisis and cerebrovascular accident
D. Respiratory distress and respiratory arrest

Questions 48-61 refer to the following case study:

B.J., a 17-year-old male, is admitted to the critical care unit in a comatose state. He has poor skin turgor, scant urine output, a blood pressure of 86/50, and a pulse of 130 beats/minute. Diabetic ketoacidosis (DKA) is diagnosed.

48. Precipitating factors in the development of DKA include:

    A. Failure to take or resistance to insulin
    B. Pancreatitis
    C. Surgery or trauma in a patient with diabetes mellitus
    D. All of the above

49. The patient with DKA typically presents with all of the following *except:*

    A. Acetone breath odor and slow respirations
    B. Polyuria and signs of dehydration
    C. Altered level of consciousness and Kussmaul's respirations
    D. Tachycardia and possible hypotension

50. The most obvious sign or symptom of DKA observed in B.J. is:

    A. Elevated serum potassium
    B. Elevated blood pH
    C. Increased rate and depth of breathing
    D. Oliguria

51. The primary cause of intracellular dehydration in DKA is:

    A. Elevated temperature from cellular depletion
    B. Kidney excretion of water and excess glucose
    C. Elevated blood glucose level
    D. Shifting of potassium into the intravascular space

52. B.J. is at risk for which complication?

    A. Septic shock
    B. Oliguria
    C. Hypercalcemia
    D. Hypokalemia

53. Which electrolyte abnormality may develop in B.J.?

    A. Hypomagnesemia
    B. Hypophosphatemia
    C. Hyperchloremia
    D. Hypercalcemia

54. Which of the following patients with insulin-dependent diabetes mellitus is most at risk for DKA?

    A. The child with otitis media
    B. The child who participates in a gym class
    C. The child who requires insulin twice a day
    D. The child who self-administers insulin

55. Which of the following initial diagnostic studies would *not* reflect DKA?

    A. Decreased arterial pCO_2, decreased arterial pH, and decreased HCO_3^-
    B. Elevated serum potassium and decreased bicarbonate levels
    C. Elevated urine specific gravity and elevated blood urea nitrogen level
    D. Decreased serum potassium and decreased hematrocrit levels

56. Which of the following would be an *inappropriate* intervention for B.J.?

   A.   Administration of isophane insulin suspension (NPH) by continuous infusion of 4 to 8 units/hour
   B.   Rapid administration of fluids, initially at 1,000ml/hour
   C.   Infusion of dextrose 5% in 0.45% saline solution
   D.   Infusion of potassium replacement as ketosis decreases and insulin therapy is started

57. Initially, for the acutely ill DKA patient, the preferred method of insulin administration is:

   A.   Continuous I.V. infusion of 4 to 8 units/hour
   B.   Loading doses, given I.M. or I.V., of about 20 units
   C.   I.V. bolus of 10 to 25 units/hour
   D.   I.M. dose of 5 to 10 units/hour or subcutaneous (S.C.) dose of 10 to 100 units/hour

58. A common and serious complication of DKA for the diabetic patient is:

   A.   Respiratory acidosis
   B.   Shock from dehydration
   C.   Hyperkalemia
   D.   Metabolic alkalosis

59. B.J.'s hemodynamic status is stabilizing: his blood pressure is 110/70, and his pulse is 96 beats/minute. Which I.V. solution would the nurse anticipate infusing at this time?

   A.   Dextrose 5% in 0.45% saline solution
   B.   0.9% normal saline solution
   C.   Dextrose 5% in normal saline solution
   D.   0.45% normal saline solution

60. Complications from DKA and its treatment include:

A. Shock and cardiac dysrhythmias
B. Pulmonary and cerebral edema
C. Hypoglycemia and hypokalemia
D. All of the above

61. The Somogyi phenomenon is:

A. Hyperglycemia in response to low-dose insulin therapy
B. Rebound hypoglycemia in response to release of stress hormones
C. A neurogenic response to sustained hyperglycemia
D. Rebound hyperglycemia caused by release of stress hormones in response to insulin-induced hypoglycemia

Case Study
Questions 62-75 refer to the following case study:

Mrs. J., age 62, is brought to the hospital by ambulance. She is severely dehydrated, does not respond to verbal stimuli, and withdraws from painful stimuli. Her blood pressure is 90/60, and her pulse is 120 beats/minute. She has a blood glucose level of 1,000 mg/dl. Hyperglycemic hyperosmolar nonketotic coma (HHNK) is diagnosed.

62. Which statement about HHNK is *false?*

A. Hyperglycemia occurs because of a total insulin deficiency
B. Cerebral impairment is a major factor
C. Ketogenesis does not occur
D. Severe dehydration results from an osmotic diuresis

63. Which condition would *not* have predisposed Mrs. J. to develop HHNK?

    A.   Pancreatitis
    B.   Thiazide or steroid therapy
    C.   Total parenteral nutrition (TPN) therapy
    D.   Cerebrovascular accident (CVA)

64. HHNK is frequently misdiagnosed. Which of the following statements is *false?*

    A.   Misdiagnosis delays initiation of aggressive therapy and contributes to high mortality
    B.   HHNK occurs in association with many other conditions, such as pancreatitis, burns, and severe infection
    C.   A patient with HHNK has the same laboratory findings as a patient with DKA
    D.   Signs and symptoms of HHNK are similar to those of other diseases, such as CVA and diabetic coma

65. Which is *not* a precipitating factor in the development of HHNK?

    A.   Undiagnosed mild diabetes in the middle-aged patient
    B.   Use of diuretics, steroids, or hypertonic solutions
    C.   Acute illness, trauma, or stress in a patient over age 50
    D.   Omission of insulin in the diabetic patient

66. The classic signs of HHNK are primarily caused by:

    A.   Rapid decrease in plasma osmolarity
    B.   Markedly elevated serum glucose
    C.   Intravascular dehydration
    D.   Serum electrolyte abnormality

67. The altered mental status in Mrs. J. results from:

    A.   Hyperosmolality of plasma
    B.   Intracerebral dehydration
    C.   Severe osmotic diuresis from hyperglycemia
    D.   Intravascular dehydration

68. Which finding would *not* be present in HHNK?

A. Kussmaul's respirations at 28 breaths/minute
B. Serum glucose level above 650 mg/dl and often greater than 1,000 mg/dl
C. Serum osmolarity above 350 mOsm/liter
D. Severe dehydration and the absence of ketoacidosis

69. Mrs. J.'s laboratory values would include which finding?

A. A serum sodium level of 120 mEq/liter
B. A serum osmolarity of 380 mOsm/liter
C. A urine sodium level of 50 mEq/24 hours
D. A bicarbonate level of 15 mEq/liter

70. With HHNK, Mrs. J. will probably exhibit which signs and symptoms?

A. Shallow respirations, hypertension, and flushed skin
B. Change in level of consciousness, decreased respiratory rate, and hypotension
C. Diaphoretic skin, decreased skin turgor, and tachycardia
D. Weakness, tachypnea, and hypotension

71. The fluid volume deficit characteristic of HHNK results from:

A. Osmotic diuresis
B. Hyperglycemia
C. Hyperosmolarity
D. All of the above

72. Assessment of Mrs. J.'s diagnostic data would reflect:

A. A pH of 7.10
B. 4+ ketone bodies in the urine
C. Azotemia
D. Hematocrit level of 29%

73. Once Mrs. J.'s hemodynamic status is stable, which parenteral solution would correct the intracellular dehydration?

  A. 0.45% saline
  B. 0.9% saline
  C. 5% dextrose and 0.5% saline
  D. 5% dextrose and normal saline

74. Overzealous fluid replacement in the patient with HHNK may cause:

  A. Cardiac failure
  B. Cerebral edema
  C. Seizures
  D. All of the above

75. Which of the following comparative statements about DKA and HHNK is *true?*

  A. HHNK requires less fluid replacement
  B. DKA requires less insulin
  C. HHNK requires more bicarbonate replacement
  D. DKA requires more potassium replacement

Case Study
Questions 76-79 refer to the following case study:

While in the intensive care unit (ICU), Mr. Y., a patient with diabetes, exhibits a decreased level of consciousness. A hypoglycemic reaction is suspected.

---

76. Emergency management of a hypoglycemic comatose patient includes:

A. Drawing a fasting blood glucose specimen and giving sweetened orange juice via a nasogastric tube
B. Drawing a fasting blood glucose specimen and giving 50 ml of dextrose 50% in water I.V.
C. Administering 50 ml of a 50% glucose I.V. push followed by a glucagon injection
D. Infusing 1 liter of dextrose 10% in water and drawing a blood glucose specimen

77. Which of the following would *not* precipitate Mr. Y.'s hypoglycemia?

A. Gastrectomy
B. Pancreatic disease
C. Severe stress
D. Hepatic disease

78. Mr. Y. may exhibit which of these signs and symptoms?

A. Nervousness and tremors
B. Palpitations and tachycardia
C. Confusion, depression and coma
D. All of the above

79. The signs and symptoms identified in Mr. Y. are caused by:

A. Neuroglycopenia
B. Decreased response of the sympathetic nervous system
C. Decreased liver glycogenolysis
D. Glycopenia

Case Study
Questions 80-83 refer to the following case study:

Mrs. W., age 65, is admitted to the ICU after fainting. Physical examination reveals obesity; buffalo hump; hirsutism; thin, fragile extremities with areas of ecchymosis; hypertension; and mild conges-

tive heart failure. She has experienced weakness, fatigue, and altered sleep patterns in the past month.

---

80.   Mrs. W.'s signs and symptoms are characteristic of:

    A.   Conn's syndrome
    B.   Cushing's syndrome
    C.   Diabetes insipidus
    D.   Myxedema coma

---

81.   Weakness, irritability, fat deposition in the face and trunk and wasting of extremities would be detected in a patient with:

    A.   Increased cortisol levels
    B.   Increased aldosterone secretion
    C.   Decreased mineralocorticoid levels
    D.   Decreased glucocorticoid levels

---

82.   Mrs. W. should be monitored for:

    A.   Hyperglycemia
    B.   Hypokalemia
    C.   Hypernatremia
    D.   All of the above

---

83.   A patient with increased levels of mineralocorticoids and glucocorticoids exhibits which of the following?

    A.   Increased heart rate with atrial premature complexes
    B.   Decreased serum osmolarity
    C.   Elevated calcitonin level
    D.   Chvostek's sign

Case Study
Questions 84-100 refer to the following case study:

Mr. G., an obese patient, is transferred to the ICU after surgery. He is ambulatory but exhibits fever, pallor, signs of dehydration, headache, confusion, restlessness, and a rapid, weak pulse. His blood pressure is 90/50. He has an 8-year history of Addison's disease. Laboratory data reveals a serum potassium level of 6.5 mEq/liter, a white blood cell count of 15,000/mm³, a serum glucose level of 55 mg/dl, and a serum sodium level of 124 mEq/liter. Adrenal crisis is diagnosed.

84. The most probable cause of Mr. G.'s adrenal crisis is:

    A. Obesity
    B. Decreased exercise
    C. Increased appetite
    D. Nothing by mouth (NPO) status before surgery

85. The adrenal cortex produces:

    A. Glucocorticoids and androgens
    B. Catecholamines and epinephrine
    C. Norepinephrine and epinephrine
    D. Mineralocorticoids and catecholamines

86. Normal effects of cortisol within the body include all of the following *except:*

    A. Stimulation of gluconeogenesis in the liver
    B. Reduction of blood glucose concentration
    C. Inhibition of glucose utilization in cells
    D. Inhibition of the inflammatory process

87. Factors that may stimulate release of the glucocorticoid cortisol in Mr. G. include:

    A. Adrenocorticotropic hormone (ACTH)
    B. Trauma
    C. Infection and stress
    D. All of the above

88. Which of the following is *not* an effect of aldosterone release?

    A. Increase in sodium reabsorption by the distal and collecting tubules of the kidney
    B. Potassium excretion in exchange for sodium reabsorption by the kidney
    C. Increase in extracellular fluid volume
    D. Decrease in serum sodium levels

89. Which factor would *not* precipitate adrenal insufficiency?

    A.   Excessive steroid therapy
    B.   Waterhouse-Friderichsen syndrome
    C.   Stress after trauma, infection, or surgery
    D.   Adrenalectomy

90. Acute adrenal insufficiency causes:

    A.   Fluid and electrolyte imbalances
    B.   Protein, fat, and carbohydrate metabolism
         disturbances
    C.   Circulatory collapse
    D.   All of the above

91. The *most* life-threatening aspect of adrenal crisis is:

    A.   Hypokalemia
    B.   Hypoglycemia
    C.   Vascular collapse
    D.   Hypernatremia

92. Which diagnostic test is the *most* reliable indicator of Mr. G.'s
    condition?

    A.   Plasma carcinoembryonic antigen (CEA)
    B.   24-hour urine 17-hydroxycorticosteroid
    C.   Plasma cortisol
    D.   ACTH infusion

93. Decreased levels of aldosterone would result in which laboratory
    finding?

    A.   Decreased serum sodium level
    B.   Decreased serum potassium level
    C.   Increased serum osmolarity
    D.   Increased urine potassium level

94. The patient in adrenal crisis would present with:

A. Polyuria, dehydration, and lethargy
B. Hypertension, bradycardia, and restlessness
C. Increased reflexes and decreased level of consciousness
D. Hypotension, mild acidosis, and confusion

95. Which of the following findings is *not* typical of acute adrenal insufficiency?

A. Elevated serum potassium level
B. Decreased serum sodium level
C. Elevated serum glucose level
D. Elevated blood urea nitrogen level

96. Hyperkalemia can cause which of the following ECG changes?

A. T wave depression with prolonged QT interval
B. Tall, tented T waves, wide QRS complexes, and prolonged PR interval
C. Q wave inversion and shortened PR interval
D. Bradycardia and bundle branch block

97. One difference between epinephrine and norepinephrine is that:

A. Epinephrine constricts pupils
B. Epinephrine has a greater vasoconstrictor activity in muscles
C. Epinephrine dilates blood vessels in the heart and in smooth muscles
D. Norepinephrine has a greater effect on cardiac and metabolic activities

98. Which is the *most* appropriate fluid replacement for Mr. G.?

A. Dextrose 5% in lactated Ringer's solution at 100 ml/hour
B. Dextrose 5% with normal saline solution at 1 liter in 2 hours
C. Dextrose 5% in water at 200 ml/hour
D. 0.45% saline solution at 1 liter in 6 hours

99. Which medication should be ordered immediately to treat adrenal insufficiency?

    A.   Levothyroxine sodium (Synthroid) 0.1 mg
    B.   Dexamethasone (Decadron) 200 mg
    C.   Hydrocortisone (Cortef) 200 mg
    D.   Fludrocortisone (Florinef) 0.1 mg

100. Which action would be *inappropriate* in treating Mr. G.?

    A.   Administering hydrocortisone as a bolus
    B.   Administering potassium chloride to maintain normal serum levels
    C.   Checking urine specific gravity to evaluate hydration status and renal function
    D.   Reducing physical and psychological stress

Case Study
Questions 101-103 refer to the following case study:

Mr. K., age 43, is admitted to the intensive care unit (ICU) with uncontrolled hypertension. He has experienced sweating, palpitations, and anxiety for 2 weeks. After an abdominal computed tomography (CT) scan, pheochromocytoma is diagnosed.

101. The signs and symptoms produced by Mr. K.'s pheochromocytoma are caused by:

    A.   Increased renin secretion
    B.   Increased catecholamine secretion
    C.   Excessive cholesterol deposit
    D.   Advanced arteriosclerosis

102. For which abnormality should Mr. K. be assessed?

   A.   Hyperglycemia
   B.   Hyperkalemia
   C.   Hypercalcemia
   D.   Hypocalcemia

103. Mr. K. undergoes surgery to remove the tumor. Which common complication should the nurse watch for immediately after surgery?

   A.   Hypertension
   B.   Pulmonary embolus
   C.   Ketoacidosis
   D.   Hypotension

1.   **Correct answer - B**

The pituitary gland (hypophysis) is located at the brain's base in the sella turcica of the sphenoid bone. The hypothalamus controls the pituitary via a portal vascular system; hormones produced and released by the hypothalamus in response to negative feedback mechanisms control secretory activities. The posterior lobe (neurophypophysis) is connected to the hypothalamus by neural tissue; nerve impulses originating in the hypothalamus in response to stimuli from other body parts regulate secretion.

2.   **Correct answer - A**

The posterior pituitary gland, or neurohypophysis, secretes antidiuretic hormone (ADH), also known as vasopressin, and oxytocic hormone, also known as oxytocin. ADH is produced in the hypothalamus. Adrenocorticotropic hormone (ACTH) is one of the seven hormones produced by the anterior pituitary gland (adenohypophysis); the other six are growth hormone (GH), thyroid-stimulating hormone (TSH), melanocyte-stimulating hormone (MSH), follicle-stimulating hormone (FSH), prolactin (PRL), and luteinizing hormone (LH).

3.   **Correct answer - C**

The adenohypophysis (anterior pituitary gland) releases TSH, which influences the thyroid gland's hormonal activity; ACTH, which affects the adrenal gland's hormonal activity; and LH and ICSH (interstitial cell-stimulating hormone), which influence the gonads.

4.   **Correct answer - B**

Oat cell carcinoma, tumor in the apical lung field, may cause syndrome of inappropriate antidiuretic hormone (SIADH), whose symptoms include hyponatremia and an altered mental status. Subarachnoid hemorrhage, characterized by acute headache with the change in mental status, may be associated with hyponatremia from SIADH. Cerebral metastasis usually produces neurologic dysfunction of one area or side of the body. Acute purulent meningitis could cause an altered mental status without such dysfunction, but the lack of fever or elevated white blood cell count makes meningitis a less likely diagnosis.

5.   **Correct answer - D**

The dilutional hyponatremia and resultant decreased osmolarity can cause seizures. The goal is to raise the serum sodium level to at least 125 mEq/liter to improve the patient's mental status. Administering furosemide will produce diuresis, thus decreasing fluid volume; hypertonic saline solution, such as 3% NaCl, also is administered and fluids are restricted. Use of demeclocycline or other drugs that block the ADH's effect on the renal tubules may be appropriate treatment for chronic - but not acute - SIADH.

6.   **Correct answer - B**

Phenytoin (Dilantin), which decreases ADH production, is not associated with SIADH (unlike other drugs, such as chlorpropamide, vincristine, vinblastine, cyclophosphamide, and tricyclic antidepressants). Lung carcinoma is the most common cause of SIADH; oat-cell carcinoma accounts for 80% of all SIADH cases. The tumor tissue synthesizes, stores, and releases ADH. Positive-pressure ventilation has been associated with SIADH, probably because it reduces left atrial filling and stimulates central ADH release. Pneumonia, tuberculosis, lung abscesses, and empyema also have been associated with SIADH; the probable mechanism is ADH release from the inflamed pulmonary tissue.

7.   **Correct answer - D**

Increased ADH secretion by the posterior pituitary causes SIADH. Precipitating factors include tubercular meningitis; extracranial malignant tumors, especially bronchogenic and pancreatic tumors; skull fractures; medications, such as chlorpropamide, thiazides, and clofibrate; and viral respiratory infection.

8.   **Correct answer - B**

ADH stimulates renal tubules to reabsorb water, thereby concentrating urine. Aldosterone is responsible for sodium reabsorption and potassium excretion via the kidney.

9. **Correct answer - C**

ADH is released from the posterior pituitary gland when serum osmolality increases. This release causes the renal tubules to reabsorb water into the circulation in an attempt to dilute the serum concentration, thereby reducing serum osmolality.

10. **Correct answer - A**

ADH, one of the hormones secreted by the neurohypophysis, promotes constriction of arterioles and causes increased water reabsorption by the renal tubules. Factors that inhibit ADH release include surgery, inflammation of the pituitary gland, and decreased serum osmolality. Increased serum osmolality stimulates ADH release.

11. **Correct answer - B**

Nursing care of the patient with SIADH includes interventions to prevent or treat symptoms caused by water intoxication. Edema may not always occur with water intoxication; symptoms include weakness, confusion, hostility, increased blood pressure, vomiting, abdominal cramps, and seizures. If symptoms persist after treatment, coma and death may result.

12. **Correct answer - B**

Water intoxication dilutes serum sodium levels, producing hyponatremia and neurologic changes. As hyponatremia and water intoxication progress, manifestations vary from a mild headache to seizures. If symptoms persist after treatment, coma and death may result.

13. **Correct answer - A**

Increased ADH secretion promotes excessive water retention by the kidneys, producing marked decreases in the serum sodium level and serum osmolality. Hypokalemia also results. Urine output decreases because of the increased water reabsorption, producing concentrated urine with a high specific gravity and osmolality.

14. **Correct answer - D**

Treatment for SIADH includes fluid restriction (elevated ADH levels cause fluid retention), eradicating of the syndrome's underlying cause, and administration of a hypertonic saline solution, such as 3% sodium chloride, to counter hyponatremia and prevent cerebral edema and seizures.

15. **Correct answer - D**

Diabetes insipidus develops most commonly in neurosurgical patients. The second major cause is head trauma, especially basilar skull fractures. Other precipitating factors include inflammatory or degenerative conditions, such as tubercular meningitis, syphilis, sarcoidosis, Hodgkins's disease, and tumors. Thiazide and clofibrate therapy, severe pneumonia, and excessive amounts of vasopressin can predispose the patient to develop SIADH.

16. **Correct answer - B**

Diabetes insipidus is characterized by excessive urine output. Without ADH, the renal tubules cannot reabsorb water, producing polyuria of 6 to 24 liters/day. The urine remains diluted, with a specific gravity below 1.005. As the body loses water, the serum sodium level increases, causing an increased serum osmolality greater than the normal range of 275 to 295 mOsm/liter.

17. **Correct answer - A**

Diabetes insipidus can be complicated by severe volume depletion and dehydration, leading to hypovolemic shock. The nurse must meticulously record the patient's intake and output, monitor his vital signs, and weigh him daily.

18. **Correct answer - B**

Diabetes insipidus results from a defect in release or synthesis of ADH within the pituitary gland or a defect in renal tubular response to ADH. Because the kidneys fail to conserve water, the serum sodium level rises, increasing serum osmolality. The urine remains diluted, resulting in a decreased urine osmolality and a specific gravity between 1.001 and 1.005.

19.   **Correct answer - B**

The drug of choice in managing diabetes insipidus is vasopressin (Pitressin). If Pitressin Tannate 2.5 to 5 units I.M. is prescribed, the vial must be warmed under hot water for several minutes and then shaken vigorously. Brown specks may appear in the vial, which is normal. Other forms of vasopressin include Aqueous Pitressin, a shorter-acting preparation lasting about 4 hours, and lysine vasopressin, a nasal spray providing an alternative mode of administration.

20.   **Correct answer - C**

Vasopressin increases water reabsorption by the kidneys and constricts smooth muscle of arterioles. Because its vasoconstrictive properties can precipitate myocardial ischemia, vasopressin must be used cautiously in a patient with heart disease.

21.   **Correct answer - D**

Discontinuing antithyroid medication would precipitate thyroid crisis, not myxedema coma. Factors contributing to myxedema coma include thyroidectomy and any dysfunction of the hypothalamic-pituitary axis, such as pituitary tumor, pituitary infarction, and hypophysectomy (removal of the pituitary gland).

22.   **Correct answer - C**

The nurse would suspect myxedema coma in a patient with seizure activity and hypothermia. Seizure activity may occur as hyponatremia develops, fostering fluid shifting into the intracellular compartment, and as cerebral edema ensues. Clinical presentation also includes hypothermia, hypoventilation, hypotension, bradycardia, and coma.

23.   **Correct answer - C**

Decreased levels of thyroxine (T4) result in hypothyroidism. This disease produces hypertrophy of the gland and decreases metabolic activity, causing lethargy, fatigue, weight gain, and constipation. A decreased T4 level also produces dry skin and hair, intolerance to cold, cardiomegaly, heart failure, and periorbital edema.

24.   Correct answer - A

Assessment of a patient in myxedema coma would reveal pericardial effusion, pleural effusion, and paralytic ileus. Myxedema results in interstitial accumulation of a mucopolysaccharide substance that attracts water, causing nonpitting edema and fluid accumulation around organs, thus leading to pericardial and pleural effusions. An audible bruit over the thyroid gland is found in hyperthyroidism.

25.   Correct answer - B

Diagnostic studies of a patient in myxedema coma would reveal a decreased O2 and an increased CO2 level from hypoventilation. Hyponatremia and a decrease in serum osmolarity may occur from water retention.

26.   Correct answer - C

Appropriate nursing interventions in myxedema coma include administering thyroxin intravenously. Fluid restriction is indicated to correct the resulting hyponatremia. If the serum sodium level is lower than 120 mEq/liter, a 3% sodium chloride solution is given no faster than 50 ml/hour. Rewarming should be done gradually, using only blankets. A hyperthermia blanket is strongly contraindicated because rapid rewarming can precipitate vasodilation, which can cause cardiac dysrhythmias or cardiovascular collapse.

27.   Correct answer - D

Precipitating factors of hypoparathyroidism include thyroid gland surgery, radiation injury from thyroid therapy, and acute pancreatitis.

28.   Correct answer - D

Parathyroid hormone (PTH), also known as parathormone, maintains normal calcium levels or increases low calcium levels. PTH increases bone resorption of calcium, increases renal and GI absorption of calcium, and decreases phosphate reabsorption in the renal tubules.

29.   Correct answer - C

Adequate vitamin D must be present for parathyroid hormone to exert in its hormonal effects at GI and bone sites.

30.   Correct answer - D

Hypocalcemia causes symptoms of hypoparathyroidism, including numbness and tingling of fingers and toes, laryngeal stridor, dyspnea, cyanosis, confusion, lethargy, and emotional lability. Seizures and tetany may also occur.

31.   Correct answer - A

A carpopedal spasm (hand folding in) occurs in a patient with hypocalcemia when the circulation is interrupted with a blood pressure cuff. This diagnostic finding is known as a positive Trousseau's sign. A positive Chvostek's sign (twitching of muscles along the facial nerve when the side of the face is tapped) may also be elicited. Cullen's sign is an ecchymosis around the umbilicus during acute hemorrhagic pancreatitis.

32.   Correct answer - D

Decreased parathormone secretion by the parathyroid gland causes hypocalcemia. Calcitonin is secreted from the thyroid gland. A positive Chvostek's sign indicates a calcium deficit. Hypocalcemia also produces a prolonged QT interval on ECG because of the increase in ventricular refractory period. Parenteral calcium must not be mixed with saline for infusion, because this increases calcium excretion by the kidneys.

33.   Correct answer - B

The patient with hypocalcemia has elevated phosphorus levels, so phosphate administration is contraindicated. The first priority is to reestablish normal serum calcium levels by administering calcium supplements. These supplements should be given with caution to a patient on digitalis because the medications have similar effects on the myocardium. If GI upset develops, the supplements can be given with meals, but not with dairy products, because phosphorus may lessen calcium absorption. Vitamin D is administered to increase calcium absorption. When giving calcium intravenously, the nurse should avoid infiltration to prevent tissue irritation, necrosis, sloughing and should not mix calcium in saline solution for infusion because this increases calcium excretion by the kidneys. The nurse must also monitor the patient closely for changes in cardiac rhythm, rate, and blood pressure.

34.   Correct answer - D

When treating hypocalcemia, the nurse should prevent conditions that can precipitate tetany by modifying the patient's environmental stimuli and limiting visitors to decrease stress. Stress-related hyperventilation causes alkalosis from a decrease in CO_2 levels; alkalosis decreases serum calcium levels, thus precipitating tetany in the already hypocalcemic patient.

35.   Correct answer - D

The thyroid gland consists of two lobes connected by a strip of tissue called the isthmus. Located across the second and third tracheal rings in the neck's anterior middle portion, distinct cells of the thyroid produce three hormones: thyroxine (T_4), tri-iodothyronine (T_3), and calcitonin (also called thyrocalcitonin). T_3 and T_4 are produced by the follicular cells, and calcitonin is produced by the parafollicular cells. T_4 constitutes 90% of the secreted thyroid hormones. T_3 binds with plasma protein for transport, constitutes 10% of the secreted thyroid hormones, and is four times more potent than T_4. Calcitonin reduces the plasma calcium level and increases urine phosphate, sodium, magnesium, and calcium excretion. T_4 and 3% increase protein synthesis, bone growth, carbohydrate and fat metabolism, and cyclic AMP (adenosine monophosphate) in muscle cells.

36.   Correct answer - C

Calcitonin, produced and released by the thyroid gland, reduces serum calcium levels. Factors that cause calcitonin's release include an increase in serum calcium and administration of magnesium and glucagon.

37.   Correct answer - D

Calcitonin reduces serum calcium levels by inhibiting bone resorption - lysis and assimilation of bone - and by increasing urine calcium excretion.

38.   Correct answer - A

Thyroid hormone secretion is regulated by thyroid-stimulating hormone from the anterior pituitary gland, which in turn is regulated by thyrotropin-releasing hormone from the hypothalamus.

39.   Correct answer - A

The biochemical and physiologic response in thyrotoxic crisis occurs from a marked increase in systemic adrenergic activity caused by excessive quantities of thyroid hormones. The effects of hypersecretion of thyroid hormone are caused by a heightened sensitivity of effector organs to adrenergic stimuli.

40.   Correct answer - D

Cardiomegaly and heart failure are found in hypothyroidism (decrease in T_4 levels). Increased levels of T_4 may produce an increase in gland size, weight loss, and a decreased tolerance to heat. Other effects include tachycardia, tremors, muscle weakness, and diarrhea. Cardiomegaly and heart failure are found in hypothyroidism.

41.   Correct answer - A

Precipitating factors of thyrotoxic crisis include trauma; infection, stress, or vigorous palpation of the thyroid gland in a hyperthyroid patient; subtotal thyroidectomy, ketoacidosis; and abrupt withdrawal of antithyroid drugs. Overdose of antithyroid drugs precipitates hypothyroidism or myxedema coma.

42.   Correct answer - C

Clinical presentation in thyrotoxic crisis includes hyperthermia, flushing, hypertension, tachycardia, psychosis, and emotional lability. Stupor and coma may ensue. GI symptoms include nausea, vomiting, and diarrhea. Bradycardia and hypoventilation occur in severe hypothyroidism or myxedema coma.

43.   Correct answer - B

In assessing the thyrotoxic patient's cardiovascular status, the nurse would note a widened pulse pressure, hypertension, systolic murmurs, and an S_3 heart sound caused by a hyperdynamic heart. Other findings include a bruit heard over the enlarged thyroid, hyperactivity, and a flushed and diaphoretic appearance.

44.   Correct answer - A

Propylthiouracil blocks thyroid hormone synthesis and is given by mouth; its abrupt withdrawal may precipitate thyroid crisis. Sodium iodide, given by mouth or intravenously, and lithium carbonate block thyroid hormone release. Guanethidine is an anthypertensive drug.

45.   Correct answer - D

Aspirin therapy must be avoided in thyrotoxic crisis. Salicylates interfere with the binding of T_3, T_4, and the circulating thyroid-binding protein. Increases in T_3 and T_4 exacerbate hypermetabolism.

46.   Correct answer - C

Propranolol, a beta-adrenergic blocker, deters the effects of epinephrine and norepinephrine on the endocrine glands, including sympathetic stimulation. Propranolol decreases heart rate, helps control dysrhythmias, and reduces the force of myocardial contractions, which lowers blood pressure and oxygen consumption. Epinephrine, isoproterenol, and dopamine are adrenergic stimulators that potentiate sympathetic stimulation and thyrotoxic crisis.

47.   Correct answer - B

Complications from thyrotoxic crisis include dehydration and congestive heart failure. Dehydration results from hyperthermia, a temperature of 104°F. (40°C.) and a persistent respiratory rate above 30 breaths/minute may cause insensible fluid loss of more than 2,500 ml. Congestive heart failure results from cardiac dysrhythmias. Excessive thyroid hormone increases the metabolic rate, accelerating the heart's myocardial oxygen consumption; this causes cardiac dysrhythmias, such as tachycardia and premature ventricular contractions. Other complications include seizures, hyperglycemia, hypercalcemia, and psychological disturbances.

48.   Correct answer - D

Precipitating factors of diabetic ketoacidosis include failure to take or resistance to insulin, pancreatitis (because it interferes with insulin production and release), and surgery or trauma in a patient with diabetes mellitus. These conditions produce stress, thereby increasing glucocorticoid release and blood glucose levels.

49.   Correct answer - A

Clinical presentation in DKA includes an altered level of consciousness, poor skin turgor, and hypotension and tachycardia, all from dehydration. Hyperglycemia promotes osmotic diuresis, producing polyuria, polydipsia, and cellular and intravascular fluid depletion. The breakdown of body fats releases excessive ketones, producing metabolic acidosis. The patient develops an acetone breath odor and compensates for the acidosis by increasing rate and depth to blow off carbon dioxide, a response known as Kussmaul's respirations.

50.   Correct answer - C

Metabolic acidosis decreases blood pH, and the patient compensates with Kussmaul's respirations, with an increased rate of breaths and depth in order to blow off carbon dioxide, an acid. Initially the osmotic diuretic effect of hyperglycemia causes polyuria. Although the serum potassium level does increase because of ketone induced metabolic acidosis, this symptom is not an obvious sign or symptom.

51.   Correct answer - C

The primary cause of intracellular dehydration in DKA is an elevated blood glucose level. Hyperglycemia increases the serum osmolarity or concentration, causing a shift of intracellular water into the intravascular space.

52. Correct answer - D

After therapy begins, hypokalemia usually occurs from acidosis correction or insulin therapy. Once intravascular fluid depletion has been reversed, 20 to 40 mEq of potassium should be added to each liter of I.V. fluid.

53. Correct answer - B

Hypophosphatemia, manifested by muscle weakness, may occur in DKA if diuresis and acidosis totally deplete phosphate levels. Initial phosphate and potassium measurements may be normal or high but typically drop after therapy. Phosphate and potassium can be replaced by administering I.V. potassium phosphate.

54. Correct answer - A

Infection (such as otitis media), emotional stress, and noncompliance with therapy predispose the child with insulin-dependent diabetes mellitus to DKA. Younger children tend to develop more infections, whereas adolescents are more likely to experience emotional stress and exhibit noncompliance. Increased activity may precipitate hypoglycemia by lowering insulin requirements.

55. Correct answer - D

Initial diagnostic studies of the DKA patient reveal decreased arterial pH, HCO_3 and CO_2 levels because of metabolic acidosis and respiratory compensation. Blood urea nitrogen and hematocrit levels increase from dehydration. Acidosis also results in a shift of potassium from the cells into the intravascular fluid in exchange for a hydrogen shift into the cells. This compensatory mechanism attempts to buffer the acidosis, producing an elevated serum potassium level.

56. Correct answer - A

Nursing interventions for the patient with DKA aim to restore fluid balance; re-establish normal carbohydrate, fat, and protein metabolism; and maintain electrolyte balance and function of related systems. Rapid-acting (regular) insulin - not NPH - is administered to re-establish normal carbohydrate, fat, and protein metabolism. Rapid administration of up to

1,000 ml/hour may be ordered initially to restore fluid balance. When the patient's plasma glucose level falls to 250 mg/dl, initial solutions of 0.45% or 0.9% normal saline should be changed to dextrose 5% in 0.45% saline solution to prevent hypoglycemia, hypokalemia, and cerebral edema. Administration methods include continuous I.V. infusion at 4 to 8 units/hour (the preferred method), I.M. or I.V. loading doses, or an I.V. bolus at 10 to 25 units/hour. During patient treatment, the nurse should monitor electrolyte levels, especially potassium, for hypokalemia.

57. Correct answer - A

The preferred insulin administration method in DKA is continuous intravenous infusion at 4 to 8 units/hour. During therapy, blood and urine glucose levels must be monitored hourly.

58. Correct answer - B

A common and serious complication of DKA for the diabetic patient is shock from dehydration. Sustained hyperglycemia not only leads to intracellular dehydration but also results in intravascular fluid loss after excessive polyuria from osmotic diuresis.

59. Correct answer - D

Administration of a hypotonic solution, such as 0.45% normal saline, promotes intracellular hydration. An isotonic solution of 0.9% normal saline or hypertonic solutions of dextrose 5% in 0.45% saline and dextrose 5% in normal saline would promote intravascular hydration, which is not required by a patient whose hemodynamic status is stabilizing.

60. Correct answer - D

Complications can arise from DKA or its treatment. Severe dehydration may lead to shock. Electrolyte imbalances, especially hyperkalemia or hypokalemia, can trigger cardiac dysrhythmias. Hyperkalemia usually occurs in DKA from acidosis; hypokalemia can result from correction of acidosis and insulin therapy. Pulmonary and cerebral edema may develop from excessive fluid replacement; hypoglycemia, from excessive insulin therapy.

61.   Correct answer - D

The Somogyi phenomenon (also called the Somogyi effect) is a paradox - insulin causing a high blood glucose level. The effect is a rebound hyperglycemia caused by the release of stress hormones (adrenaline, ACTH) in response to insulin-induced hypoglycemia.

62.   Correct answer - A

In hyperglycemic hyperosmolar nonketotic coma (HHNK), hyperglycemia occurs because of decreased peripheral glucose uptake related to a relative (although not total) insulin deficiency. Because lipolysis from adipose tissue is inhibited, ketogenesis (ketone production) does not occur. Osmotic diuresis caused by an elevated glucose level leads to severe dehydration. Intracellular dehydration ensues, causing cerebral cellular dehydration and neurologic impairment.

63.   Correct answer - D

A cerebrovascular accident (CVA) would not predispose a patient to develop HHNK. Risk factors include pancreatitis; Thiacide or steroid therapy; total parenteral nutrition or high-caloric feedings; diet-controlled diabetes; and old age.

64.   Correct answer - C

A patient in HHNK does not have the same laboratory findings as one with DKA. HHNK produces a higher serum glucose level and shows no evidence of acidosis from ketone excess. HHNK is commonly misdiagnosed, however, because its symptoms mimic those of other diseases. For instance, cerebral dehydration in HHNK can produce neurologic symptoms found in CVA. HHNK also occurs in association with many other conditions, such as pancreatitis, burns, and severe infection. Misdiagnosis typically delays initiation of aggressive therapy and contributes to HHNK's high mortality.

65.   Correct answer - D

HHNK produces a relative insulin deficiency in which the patient has enough insulin to prevent ketone body formation but not enough to maintain

347

normal serum glucose levels. Hyperglycemia becomes marked, and hyperosmolarity of the extracellular fluid develops, causing cellular dehydration. Cerebral dehydration leads to central nervous system (CNS) dysfunction. Precipitating factors include undiagnosed or recent-onset mild diabetes; acute illness, trauma, or stress; and administration of diuretics, steroids, or hypertonic solutions. Insulin omission in the diabetic patient precipitates DKA.

66.   Correct answer - B

The classic signs of HHNK result from a markedly elevated serum glucose level. Hyperglycemia produces osmotic diuresis, causing severe intracellular and intracerebral dehydration. Clinical signs in HHNK include poor skin turgor, dry mucous membranes, hypotension, tachycardia and weight loss. Cerebral dehydration causes neurologic dysfunction: lethargy, disorientation, seizures, stupor, and coma.

67.   Correct answer - B

The patient in HHNK presents with CNS dysfunction from severe intracerebral dehydration. Symptoms include an altered mental state, such as dull sensorium, hallucinatory behavior, disorientation, stupor, and coma. Vestibular dysfunction, focal neurologic disturbances, and seizures may also develop.

68.   Correct answer - A

The patient in HHNK presents with a serum glucose level above 650 mg/dl and commonly greater than 1,000 mg/dl. Such severe hyperglycemia raises the serum osmolarity above 350 mOsm/liter, causing osmotic diuresis and severe dehydration. In HHNK, the patient does not have Kussmaul's respirations; ketoacidosis does not occur, so increasing the respiratory rate and depth to blow off CO_2 is unnecessary.

69.   Correct answer - B

Normal serum osmolarity is between 275 and 295 mOsm/liter. In HHNK, serum osmolarity usually is higher than 350 mOsm/liter because of the osmotic diuresis. The resulting dehydration elevates the serum sodium level and decreases the urine sodium level (to retain water, the kidneys attempt to hold onto sodium). The bicarbonate level is normal (between 23 and 27 mEq/liter) because ketosis does not occur.

70.   Correct answer - B

Clinical presentation in HHNK includes weakness, polyuria, decreased skin turgor, and flushed, dry skin from the osmotic effects of hyperglycemia; hypotension and tachycardia from intravascular depletion; and shallow breathing, altered level of consciousness, seizures, and nystagmus from severe intracerebral dehydration.

71.   Correct answer - D

Several factors cause the fluid volume deficit that characterizes HHNK. Hyperglycemia produces a hyperosmolar state that leads to osmotic diuresis, resulting in intracellular and intravascular dehydration.

72.   Correct answer - C

Diagnostic studies would reflect azotemia (elevated BUN) hemoconcentration, an elevated serum creatinine level, an elevated plasma glucose level (often over 1,000 mg/dl), no significant ketosis, and a relatively normal pH.

73.   Correct answer - A

A hypotonic solution (one with an osmolarity less than 275 mOsm/liter) would hydrate the intracellular compartment. Thus, .45% saline (155 osmolarity) would be administered after stabilizing hemodynamic status. Normal saline is an isotonic solution, whereas 5% dextrose and 0.5% saline and 5% dextrose and normal saline are hypertonic solutions.

74.   Correct answer - D

Cardiac failure, cerebral edema, and seizures may occur during overzealous fluid replacement in the patient in HHNK. I.V. fluid administration initially lowers serum osmolarity, while intracellular (especially intracerebral) osmolarity is high. Fluid then shifts to an area of higher concentration of osmolarity. Overzealous fluid therapy causes a rapid shift of water into the intracerebral cells, cerebral edema, and seizures. Cardiac failure may occur if the patient receives fluid volume that his heart cannot effectively pump. Because HHNK usually is found in patients age 50 or older, cardiac failure may be a common complication of fluid therapy.

75.   Correct answer - D

A patient with DKA requires more potassium replacement than one in HHNK because DKA requires much more insulin therapy, which lowers potassium levels. During therapy for DKA, sodium bicarbonate is given to correct ketoacidosis. Acidosis does not occur in HHNK. Because a patient in HHNK has a higher serum glucose level than one with DKA, the resulting dehydration from the osmotic diuresis warrants more fluid replacement.

76.   Correct answer - C

Emergency management of a hypoglycemic comatose patient includes administering 50 ml of a 50% glucose I.V. push followed by a glucagon injection. If in doubt about whether a comatose patient has hypoglycemia or hyperglycemia, the nurse should first draw a blood glucose specimen, not a fasting blood glucose specimen.

77.   Correct answer - C

Gastrectomy, pancreatic disease, and hepatic disease may precipitate hypoglycemia. The decrease in blood glucose results from a defect in the process by which blood glucose normally increases, such as inadequate carbohydrate absorption, excessive insulin release, or an inability to form glucose from nonglucose sources (gluconeogenesis) or to mobilize glucose from glycogen (glycogenolysis).

78.   Correct answer - D

Two neurologic responses cause hypoglycemia's signs and symptoms. As hypoglycemia progresses, norepinephrine and epinephrine are released from the adrenal medulla, producing tachycardia, palpitations, sweating, and tremors. This adrenergic discharge causes the release of glucocorticoids and glucagon, which attempt to raise the blood glucose by stimulating hepatic glycogen breakdown. As the blood glucose level falls below normal, progressive cerebral function impairment ensues, causing nervousness, confusion, depression, blurred vision, seizures, and possibly coma. These changes occur when the cerebral cortex is deprived of its main energy supply.

79.   Correct answer - A

The identifiable signs and symptoms of hypoglycemia are caused by neurologic responses, also known as neuroglycopenia.

80.   Correct answer - B

These clinical manifestations are a classic presentation of Cushing's syndrome with associated protein catabolic, gluconeogenic, mineralocorticoid, androgenic, and behavioral effects.

81.   Correct answer - A

With an increased cortisol level, the patient exhibits wasting of extremities, thinning of skin, and fat deposition in the face and trunk. Weakness, fatigue, irritability, depression, hypertension, and hyperglycemia also develop.

82.   Correct answer - D

A patient with Cushing's syndrome should be monitored for mineralocorticoid effects, including increased serum sodium, decreased serum potassium, hypertension, and edema. The increased blood glucose level is a gluconeogenic effect manifested by glucose intolerance.

83.   Correct answer - A

In a patient with Cushing's syndrome, hypokalemia produces an increased heart rate, often with atrial premature complexes. An elevated serum aldosterone level increases serum osmolarity and produces hypernatremia. Chvostek's sign occurs with hypocalcemia.

84.   Correct answer - D

Although Addison's disease can be controlled with corticosteroids, the patient could not take his medication before surgery, so the blood level of corticosteroids decreased. Abrupt discontinuation of steroid therapy precipitated the adrenal crisis.

85.   Correct answer - A

The adrenal glands lie retroperitoneally at the apex of each kidney and have two divisions, the cortex and the medulla. The cortex produces three types of hormones - glucocorticoids, mineralocorticoids, and androgens. The medulla produces the catecholamines epinephrine and norepinephrine.

86.   Correct answer - B

Cortisol stimulates gluconeogenesis in the liver, inhibits glucose utilization in cells, slows the rate of protein synthesis, and promotes fatty acid mobilization from adipose tissue, increasing blood glucose concentrations. Cortisol also helps inhibit inflammation.

87.   Correct answer - D

The most important glucocorticoid released by the adrenal cortex is cortisol. Release-stimulating factors include adrenocorticotropic hormone (ACTH), stress, trauma, and infection.

88.   Correct answer - D

Aldosterone is a mineralocorticoid produced and released by the adrenal cortex. Aldosterone increases sodium reabsorption and potassium excretion by the kidneys. The extracellular fluid volume also increases because the kidneys retain water when they reabsorb sodium.

89.   Correct answer - A

Precipitating factors of adrenal insufficiency include abrupt cessation of steroid therapy; stress after trauma, infection, or surgery; Water-house-Friederichsen syndrome (adrenal hemorrhage from meningococcal meningitis); and adrenalectomy.

90.   Correct answer - D

Acute adrenal insufficiency is a rapid, overwhelming exacerbation of chronic, primary adrenal insufficiency (Addison's disease). It may also follow trauma, overwhelming infection, or pituitary infarction. The condition is characterized by a deficiency in cortisol and aldosterone that leads to protein, fat, and carbohydrate metabolism disturbances, fluid and electrolyte imbalances, and circulatory collapse.

91.   Correct answer - C

The most serious threat in adrenal crisis is peripheral vascular collapse; as much as 20% of extracellular fluid volume may be lost. Thus, the first goal of emergency treatment is fluid replacement.

92.   Correct answer - C

The most reliable diagnostic test for adrenal crisis is measurement of plasma cortisol levels; abnormally low levels indicate adrenocortical insufficiency. Although ACTH and 24-hour urine 17-hydroxycorticosteroid measurements are used in diagnosing adrenal disorders, they are contraindicated in adrenal crisis because of the potentially life-threatening delay associated with the tests. Plasma carcinoembryonic antigen (CEA) levels are used in diagnosing cancer or abnormal cells in the body.

93.   Correct answer - A

Aldosterone causes sodium reabsorption and potassium excretion by the renal tubules. A decreased aldosterone level would lower the serum sodium level - and serum osmolarity - and increase the serum potassium level. If sodium is not reabsorbed by the renal tubules, urine sodium increases and urine potassium decreases.

94.   Correct answer - D

Clinical signs and symptoms of adrenal crisis include confusion, restlessness, and a decreased level of consciousness. The patient is usually hypotensive and has a rapid, thready pulse and oliguria. He may also have abdominal pain, weight loss, and flaccid extremities. Decreased renal function and hypotension may cause mild metabolic acidosis.

95.   Correct answer - C

The patient with acute adrenal insufficiency has decreased sodium and glucose and increased potassium because of a deficiency in aldosterone and cortisol. Blood urea nitrogen and creatinine increase when the extracellular fluid volume decreases, a result of aldosterone deficiency. Aldosterone regulates sodium reabsorption and water retention by the renal tubules.

96.   **Correct answer - B**

When adrenal crisis is complicated by hyperkalemia, the ECG shows a prolonged PR interval, a wide QRS complex, and a tall, tented T wave. Hyperkalemia may cause bradycardia but is not associated with a bundle branch block or T wave depression.

97.   **Correct answer - C**

Epinephrine and norepinephrine are hormones of the adrenal medulla. Although each catecholamine influences both alpha and beta receptors, epinephrine has a stronger beta effect, which mediates adrenergic influences for vasodilation, cardioacceleration, and bronchial relaxation. Norepinephrine has a greater alpha effect on the adrenergic receptors, producing mydriasis (pupil dilation), widespread vasoconstrictive properties, and increased blood pressure with reflex bradycardia.

98.   **Correct answer - B**

To combat fluid deficit, an I.V. of 5% dextrose in normal saline should be infused at an extremely rapid rate - usually within 1 to 2 hours - barring complications, such as cardiac or renal disease. Fluid replacement raises blood pressure by volume expansion and contributes needed glucose and sodium. After the first liter, the patient may require additional fluids at a rate of 1 liter every 3 to 4 hours. A .45% saline solution and dextrose 5% in lactated Ringer's solution are inappropriate because they do not contain enough sodium to correct the hyponatremia that occurs in adrenal crisis.

99.   **Correct answer - C**

Hydrocortisone, a soluble cortisol replacement, is used to replace the glucocorticoids lost in adrenal crisis. The usual dose is 100 to 200 mg I.V. immediately, then every 6 hours. Levothyroxine sodium is used for thyroid disease. Dexamethasone and fludrocortisone, mineralocorticoid replacements, may be used to treat adrenal crisis but are not urgently required because saline solution and hydrocortisone adequately compensate for lost mineralocorticoids.

100.   Correct answer - B

Specific care in adrenal insufficiency focuses on restoring adequate blood volume, monitoring vital functions, initiating nursing interventions for hyperpyrexia, reducing physical and psychological stress, and implementing nursing interventions related to the underlying cause of crisis. To restore adequate blood volume, hydrocortisone is administered as a bolus dose or given as an intravenous infusion. Plasma and vasopressors also may be used. The nurse should frequently assess central venous pressure readings, urine output, and urine specific gravity to evaluate hydration status and renal function and should monitor ECG readings and cardiac function for complications from hyperkalemia. Other appropriate interventions include maintaining the patient on strict bed rest and providing reassurance and a quiet environment to reduce stress.

101.   Correct answer - B

Signs and symptoms of pheochromocytoma are produced by increased secretion of the catecholamines norepinephrine and epinephrine. Uncontrolled hypertension and the symptoms of the "flight or fight" response are the major signs of pheochromocytoma, a usually benign tumor of the adrenal medulla.

102.   Correct answer - A

Hyperglycemia occurs in response to increased epinephrine secretion. Epinephrine stimulates the conversion of glycogen to glucose in the liver, preparing the body for "flight or fight."

103.   Correct answer - D

Postoperatively, hypotension is a major problem because circulating catecholamines are depleted 24 to 48 hours after surgery until the body adapts to the tumor's absence. Hemorrhage is also a major problem because the adrenal gland is vascular. Adrenal insufficiency can occur if a large portion of the gland is removed.

CHAPTER 7

HEMATOLOGIC AND IMMUNOLOGIC SYSTEM

Case Study
Questions 1-12 refer to the following case study:

Mr. H., age 31, is admitted to the intensive care unit (ICU) with a diagnosis of acquired immunodeficiency syndrome (AIDS) with possible Pneumocystic carinii pneumonia. He is confused, emaciated, and dyspneic with purplish lesions over his body. For the last 2 months at home, he has been taking zidovudine (Retrovir). He is unmarried and lives with a male companion. Mr. H.'s mother, who lives in another city, is presently visiting.

---

1. Mr. H. should be placed in which type of precaution?

    A. Blood and body fluid precautions and protective care
    B. Blood and body fluid precautions, protective care, and respiratory isolation
    C. Blood and body fluid precautions
    D. Protective care

---

2. Zidovudine is prescribed as an:

    A. Antibiotic against *Pneumocystic carinii* pneumonia
    B. Antiviral agent to decrease replication of HIV (human immunodeficiency virus)
    C. Antituberculosis drug
    D. Antifungal for thrush

---

3. Mr. H. would have which of the following laboratory test results?

    A. Lymphocyte count of 3,000
    B. A white blood cell count of 6,000
    C. PH 7.49, HCO_3 32 meq/l
    D. CD_4 count of 50

4. Erythropoetin (Epogen, Epoetin) injections are begun on Mr. H. Which statement by his significant other demonstrates correct understanding for this therapy?

A. "It is given because the other medications cause anemia"
B. "His kidneys are failing, which is causing the anemia"
C. "The medications are causing bleeding. This medication will stop it"
D. "This medication will stop his spleen from destroying the red blood cells"

5. Mr. H.'s dementia is most likely caused by:

A. An adverse reaction to medication
B. Human immunodeficiency virus (HIV) infection of the brain
C. Kaposi's sarcoma
D. I.V. drug abuse

6. Which of the following is indicated to treat *Pneumocystic carinii* pneumonia?

A. Zidovudine (Retrovir)
B. Fluconazole (Diflucan)
C. Pentamidine (Pentam 300)
D. No treatment is available

7. Which nursing diagnoses should be observed to document the development of complications of the above therapy?

A. Potential for injury related to nausea and vomiting
B. Fluid volume deficit related to nausea and vomiting
C. Nutrition alteration related to impaired glucose metabolism
D. Fluid volume deficit related to diarrhea

8. Which of the following has the *least* amount of HIV concentration?

A. Blood
B. Saliva
C. Vaginal secretions
D. Semen

9. Mr. H. is now started on dideoxyinosine (DDI, Videx). In assessing for one of the most common side effects of this therapy, the nurse should monitor the serum:

   A. Creatinine
   B. Amylase
   C. Calcium
   D. Potassium

10. A physician wants to perform an open lung biopsy on Mr. H. Who should sign the consent form?

    A. The patient
    B. The male companion
    C. The mother
    D. Two physicians

11. Mr. H.'s condition progressively deteriorates. His male companion and mother begin to ask about a DNR (do not resuscitate) order. The most appropriate method for changing the patient to DNR status is:

    A. Writing "DNR" on the Kardex
    B. Having the physician write a DNR order after talking with the mother and male companion
    C. Waiting for the patient to become more oriented to talk with him about it
    D. Telling the family it is best to obtain a court order

12. While on duty in the intensive care unit, the nurse receives a telephone call from a person claiming to be Mr. H.'s employer. The person requests information about Mr. H.'s status. The appropriate response is to:

    A. Give him the information
    B. Give him the information after asking the patient
    C. Refer him to the physician
    D. Tell him it is confidential information and refuse to give it

Questions 13-18 refer to the following case study:

Mr. T., age 36, is admitted to the ICU and scheduled for a renal transplant. He has been on hemodialysis for five years and has a history of diabetes.

13. Preoperative evaluation of Mr. T. is necessary to detect which of the following contraindications for transplantation?

    A. Hypertension
    B. Hyperglycemia
    C. Congestive heart failure
    D. Infection

14. Preoperative immunologic testing of donor and transplant recipient include:

    A. ABO compatibility only
    B. HLA compatibility only
    C. ABO and HLA compatibility
    D. ABO, Rh, and HLA compatibility

15. The day before surgery, Mr. T. should receive:

    A. Dialysis
    B. Renal angiogram
    C. An intravenous pyelogram
    D. A renal biopsy

16. In the immediate postoperative period, which of the following urine outputs best indicates a well-functioning renal transplant?

    A. 200-300 ml/hr
    B. 50/100 ml/hr
    C. 30-50 ml/hr
    D. 15-30 ml/hr

17. In a well-functioning renal transplant, the nurse should anticipate which electrolyte abnormality?

   A. Serum potassium - 6.0 mEq/L
   B. Serum sodium - 150 mEq/L
   C. Serum calcium - 7.0 mEq/L
   D. Serum bicarbonate - 15 mEq/L

18. Which of the following findings is most critical to report in the postoperative renal transplant patient?

   A. Temperature - 100.6° F
   B. Hemoglobin - 9.6 g/dl
   C. A decrease in creatinine
   D. A blood glucose of 260 mg/dl

Case Study
Questions 19-30 refer to the following case study:

Mr. C., age 52, is admitted to the coronary care unit with a diagnosis of acute myocardial infarction. He meets the criteria as a candidate for thrombolytic therapy. During infusion of strep-tokinase, he develops an anaphylactic reaction.

19. The type of immunity that secretes antibodies specific to an antigen is provided by:

   A. Interferon
   B. T lymphocytes
   C. B lymphocytes
   D. Neutrophils

20. Which statement accurately describes the mechanism of anaphylactic reactions?

   A. They are triggered by the sensitization of T lymphocytes
   B. Large amounts of IgG antibodies are produced
   C. Antibodies bind with mast cells and basophils to become sensitized to the antigen
   D. Antibody-antigen reactions trigger mediators, such as histamine, that cause systemic reactions hours after exposure to the antigen

361

21. Which type of antibodies react in anaphylaxis?

    A. IgE
    B. IgD
    C. IgG
    D. IgM

22. Which leukocytes function during an allergic response?

    A. Basophils
    B. Neutrophils
    C. Monocytes
    D. Myeloblasts

23. Hemodynamically, anaphylactic shock is accompanied by:

    A. A rise in systemic vascular resistance
    B. A low cardiac output
    C. An elevated pulmonary capillary wedge pressure
    D. Decreased pulmonary capillary permeability

24. In most patients, anaphylaxis is precipitated by:

    A. Insect venom
    B. Food allergies
    C. Antibiotic use
    D. Blood transfusions

25. After exposure to an allergen, a patient typically develops the symptoms of anaphylaxis within:

    A. 2 to 20 minutes
    B. 20 to 60 minutes
    C. 48 hours
    D. 3 days

26. Which clinical manifestation has the *lowest* priority for intervention?

   A. Inspiratory wheezing
   B. Stridor
   C. Hoarseness
   D. Angioneurotic edema

27. Which of the following is *not* a classic manifestation of anaphylaxis?

   A. Inspiratory wheezing
   B. Laryngeal edema with bronchospasm
   C. Hypotension
   D. Paresthesias

28. All of the following treatments are used in initial emergency management of anaphylaxis *except:*

   A. Methylprednisolone (Meprolone)
   B. I. V. fluids
   C. Epinephrine (Adrenalin)
   D. Diphenhydramine (Benadryl)

29. The drug *least* likely to be used during treatment of the patient with anaphylaxis is:

   A. Hydrocortisone (Hydrocortone)
   B. Dobutamine (Dobutrex)
   C. Aminophyline (Aminophylin)
   D. Diphenhydramine (Benadryl)

30. Which nursing action should receive the *highest* priority when caring for a patient with a history of allergies?

    A. Avoiding known allergens and unnecessary patient exposure by administering drugs only when indicated

    B. Observing any patient given penicillin closely for at least 30 minutes

    C. Initiating current skin-testing procedures to identify allergens

    D. Obtaining an accurate, thorough drug history that identifies and describes previous drug reactions

Case Study
Questions 31-33 refer to the following case study:

Mrs. A., age 51, is admitted to the intensive care unit (ICU) with a diagnosis of pneumonia. She has no known allergies. One hour after an intravenous infusion of penicillin, she complains of difficulty breathing, she wheezes audibly. An erythematous rash, not seen on admission, has appeared over her entire body.

31. Signs and symptoms of anaphylaxis for which Mrs. A. should be assessed include:

    A. Bradydysrhythmias

    B. Cheyne-Stokes respirations

    C. Acute pulmonary hyperinflation

    D. Hypertension

32. Which statement about anaphylactic drug reactions is *true?*

    A. The eruption begins as macules spread in a symmetrical pattern, first on the head and arms

    B. First episodes of exanthematous reactions always occur 1 week after the drug is started

    C. When a patient has received a drug many times without a reaction, a reaction will not develop

    D. The eruption's morphology provides clues to its cause

33. Immediate treatment of a severe drug reaction includes:

A. Oxygen therapy
B. Norepinephrine (Levophed)
C. Furosemide (Lasix)
D. Prednisone (Deltasone)

Case Study
Questions 34-43 refer to the following case study:

Mr. Q., age 71, is admitted to the ICU with upper GI bleeding. He was taking warfarin (Coumadin) at home for deep vein thrombosis. His blood pressure is 86/54, his pulse is 112 beats/minute, and his respiratory rate is 26 breaths/minute. Hemoglobin is 7.0 g/dl, hematocrit is 24%, and reticulocyte count is 3%.

---

34. Warfarin (Coumadin) interferes with the coagulation process by:

A. Inhibiting plasmin
B. Promoting fibrinolysis
C. Inducing thrombocytopenia
D. Blocking the action of vitamin K

---

35. Mr. Q.'s reticulocyte count indicates:

A. Hemorrhage
B. Renal disease
C. Infection
D. Leukemia

---

36. On first assessing Mr. Q., the nurse should be particularly alert for:

A. Facial flushing
B.. Petechiae
C. Pruritus
D. Hypertension

37. During long-term anticoagulant therapy, serious hemorrhagic complications occur most commonly in the:

A. Gastrointestinal tract
B. Genitourinary tract
C. Respiratory system
D. Capillary vasculature

38. Which therapy should *not* be implemented for the patient with hemorrhagic complications from oral anticoagulants?

A. Volume replacement
B. Whole blood
C. Fresh frozen plasma
D. Protamine sulfate

39. The nurse should teach the patient receiving anticoagulant therapy to:

A. Avoid excessive alcohol intake
B. Avoid electric razors
C. Avoid soft-bristle toothbrushes
D. Trim corns and calluses weekly

40. Packed red blood cells (RBCs) are ordered for transfusion. The patient is typed and crossmatched. His blood type is AB. Which statement is *true* of this blood group?

A. The antibodies in the plasma are A and B
B. The antigens in the plasma are A and B
C. The antigens on the red cell membrane are A and B
D. This blood group possesses neither A nor B antigens

41. Which statement about packed RBCs and whole blood is *true?*

A. Both RBCs and whole blood cause hemoglobin and hematocrit levels to increase at the same rate
B. Fresh packed RBCs provide the necessary blood components, including platelets and coagulation factors
C. RBCs decrease the risk of hepatitis transmission
D. RBCs are indicated for massive hemorrhage and hypovolemia

366

42. Which of the following statements about transfusing RBCs is *true?*

A. Lactated Ringer's and normal saline are the solutions that may be used when administering blood products
B. The patient's vital signs must be assessed once before and once after the transfusion
C. The temperature of a blood warmer should not exceed 101°F. (38.3°C.)
D. 18G or 20G catheters may be used during a blood transfusion

43. One hour after the transfusion begins, Mr. Q. complains of chills. His temperature is 103.1°F. (38.5°C.). He is probably experiencing a:

A. Febrile, nonhemolytic transfusion reaction
B. Hemolytic transfusion reaction
C. Delayed hemolytic transfusion reaction
D. Bacterial transfusion reaction

Case Study
Questions 44-45 refer to the following case study:

Mr. F., age 67, is admitted to the ICU with thrombocytopenia. He has been taking quinidine gluconate for 2 months for a cardiac dysrhythmia. His platelet count is 50,000/ml.

44. Mr. F. should *not* be given:

A. Acetaminophen (Tylenol)
B. Iron Replacements
C. Antibiotics
D. Aspirin (Bayer Aspirin)

45. After quinidine therapy in a thrombocytopenic patient is discontinued, the platelet count should return to normal in:

A. 24 hours
B. 72 hours
C. 1 week
D. 2 weeks

Case Study
Questions 46-56 refer to the following case study:

Mr. V., age 68, is admitted to the intensive care unit (ICU) after a motor vehicle accident. He has a fractured pelvis and has just returned from surgery for an open reduction of a fractured left femur. His blood has been typed and crossmatched for 4 units of packed RBCs, and the doctor has ordered transfusion of 2 units. The laboratory indicates that his blood has tested positive for cold agglutinins.

---

46. Which occurs *first* in hemostasis caused by a traumatized vessel?

    A.   Formation of the platelet plug
    B.   Vascular spasm
    C.   Activation of the intrinsic pathway
    D.   Activation of the extrinsic pathway

---

47. Which ion is necessary for blood clotting?

    A.   Bicarbonate
    B.   Potassium
    C.   Iron
    D.   Calcium

---

48. Which statement about cold agglutinins is accurate?

    A.   They result from a congenital, sex-linked trait
    B.   They form after exposure to multiple bouts of influenza
    C.   They are a concern only during blood transfusions
    D.   They are part of an autoimmune process

---

49. The test for agglutination of two blood specimens is called:

    A.   Coombs' test
    B.   Typing
    C.   Crossmatching
    D.   Complement fixation

50. Which blood component does *not* require typing and crossmatching before administration?

    A. Fresh frozen plasma
    B. Platelets
    C. Cryoprecipitate
    D. Albumin

51. Which blood type contains no red cell antigens but has anti-A and anti-B antibodies?

    A. Type A
    B. Type B
    C. Type O
    D. Type AB

52. Which statement about the differences between packed RBCs and whole blood is *correct*?

    A. RBCs increase the incidence of heart failure
    B. RBCs increase the hemoglobin and hematocrit levels more quickly
    C. RBC transfusion increases the risk of plasma protein reactions
    D. Whole blood must be transfused at a slower rate than RBCs

53. Transfusion of stored blood may lead to which condition?

    A. Hypokalemia
    B. Hypercalemia
    C. Clotting factor deficiency
    D. Acidosis

54. Ten minutes after the transfusion is begun, Mr. V.'s temperature is 102°F. (38.9°C.), and he complains of chills, headache, and chest and back pain. His blood pressure is 70/52, and he is having difficulty breathing. The physician diagnoses an acute hemolytic transfusion reaction, which is typically caused by incompatibility of:

A. Plasma proteins
B. Major blood group
C. Leukocytes
D. Platelets

55. Treatment of hemolytic blood transfusion reaction may include administration of:

A. Sodium bicarbonate
B. Epinephrine (Adrenalin)
C. Aspirin (Bayer Aspirin)
D. Diphenhydramine (Benadryl)

56. Which laboratory finding will be seen in Mr. V., after an acute hemolytic blood transfusion reaction?

A. Myoglobinuria
B. Positive cold agglutinins
C. Leukocytosis
D. Hemoglobinemia

Case Study
Questions 57-64 refer to the following case study:

Mrs. B., age 32, is transferred to the ICU from the maternity unit after giving birth to a healthy baby girl. She had a large amount of lochia after delivery, losing about 500 ml of blood. Disseminated intravascular coagulation (DIC) is diagnosed.

57. Obstetric incidents leading to DIC are caused by:

A. Thromboembolism from bed rest and microemboli formation
B. Placental and fetal tissue activating the clotting mechanism
C. Fetal enzyme release that results in hemolysis of RBCs
D. The normal thrombocytopenic state accompanying pregnancy

58. The extrinsic clotting mechanism is activated by:

A. Vascular injury
B. Tissue injury
C. Platelet aggregation
D. Vitamin K

59. Which test studies the functioning of the intrinsic clotting mechanism?

A. Platelet count
B. Ivy bleeding time
C. Partial thromboplastin time
D. Prothrombin time

60. The nurse should assess Mrs. B. for dysfunction of which of the following organs which may result in blood clotting factor abnormalities?

A. Liver
B. Spleen
C. Bone marrow
D. Thymus gland

61. The nurse evaluates Mrs. B.'s laboratory results, expecting to find an increase in:

A. Platelet count
B. Fibrin split products
C. Erythrocyte sedimentation rate
D. Fibrinogen level

62. Cyoprecipitate is ordered for Mrs. B. This transfusion replenishes which portion of blood?

A. Red blood cells
B. White blood Cells
C. Platelets
D. Clotting factors

63. The physician then orders a continuous heparin infusion for Mrs. B. Heparin is used in DIC because it:

A. Contains clotting factors
B. Increases circulating platelets
C. Reverses the effects of aminocaproic acid (Amicar)
D. Neutralizes thrombin

64. Heparin interferes with coagulation by:

A. Inhibiting plasmin
B. Inactivating thrombin
C. Promoting fibrinolysis
D. Inactivating vitamin K

65. Anemia associated with prosthetic heart valves results from:

A. Rupture of RBCs from hitting the valves
B. Blood loss from anticoagulant administration
C. Accumulation of RBCs along the prosthesis
D. Vitamin B_{12} deficiency from anorexia

66. Erythropoietin release into the blood is stimulated by:

A. Hypoxia
B. Erythropoietic-stimulating factor
C. Bone marrow activity
D. Immature RBCs

67. Development of antibodies after a hepatitis vaccine is called:

A. Natural immunity
B. Active acquired immunity
C. Autoimmunity
D. Passive acquired immunity

68. Which statement about Hodgkin's disease is *true*?

A. Radiation is usually ineffective as a treatment
B. The immune system becomes hypersensitive
C. Disease typically arises in multiple sites
D. Proliferation of many blood cells can occur

69. Which electrolyte abnormality may occur with lymphoma?

A. Hypocalcemia
B. Hypercalcemia
C. Hypokalemia
D. Hyperkalemia

70. Which body element is responsible for lysing clots?

A. Antithrombin factor
B. Streptokinase
C. Plasmin
D. Christmas factor

71. A Coombs' test may be performed to:

A. Crossmatch blood
B. Diagnose sickle cell anemia
C. Identify chronic inflammation
D. Detect syphilis

72. Patient care in multiple myeloma includes preventing:

A. Hepatic failure
B. Hypocalcemia
C. Gastrointestinal bleeding
D. Bone fractures

73. Anemia is associated with which condition?

    A.   Chronic obstructive pulmonary disease
    B.   Congestive heart failure
    C.   Dehydration
    D.   Malignancy

74. The spleen performs the hematologic function of:

    A.   Stimulating erythropoiesis
    B.   Forming clotting factors
    C.   Synthesizing vitamin K
    D.   Producing antibodies

75. Aplastic anemia is associated with:

    A.   Chronic blood loss
    B.   Agranulocytosis and thrombocytopenia
    C.   Deficiency of clotting factors and vitamin K
    D.   Vitamin B_{12} and folic acid deficiency

1. Correct answer - C

Acquired immunodeficiency syndrome (AIDS) is transmitted via blood and other body fluids, so the patient should be placed on blood and body fluid precautions. Protective care does not alter the risk of nosocomial infection, although meticulous hand washing - as with all patients - should be used. Because *Pneumocystic carinii* is a common parasitic protozoa that rarely infects a person with a normal immune response, respiratory isolation is unnecessary.

2. Correct answer - B

Zidovudine (Retrovir), an antiviral agent that decreases replication of human immunodeficiency virus (HIV), is used to treat patients with AIDS or AIDS-related complex (ARC). A patient taking zidovudine has higher CD_4 lymphocyte counts, is less likely to develop severe opportunistic infections, and typically lives longer than one not taking the drug. Zidovudine was formerly called azidothymidine (AZT).

3. Correct answer - D

A patient with AIDS has lymphocytopenia, thrombocytopenia, and a low CD_4 count. HIV attacks CD_4 lymphocytes, copying its own genetic material into the DNA of the CD_4 cell, which then replicates as HIV. CD_4 cells include helper and inducer cells. Helper cells activate cytotoxic (killer) T cells and stimulate B cells to produce antibodies. Inducer cells initiate T cell development. T_8 cells, which are not directly attacked by HIV, include cytotoxic T cells and suppressor cells (which suppress the action of the other cells). Allowed to proliferate, suppressor cells further impair CD_4 cells.

4. Correct answer - A

Side effects of medications such as Zidovudine and pentamidine cause anemia through bone marrow suppression. Erythropoietin hormone injections have been found to be effective in raising the hemoglobin and hematocrit in this population, thus decreasing the need for blood transfusions.

5.   Correct answer - B

The patient's dementia is most likely due to HIV brain infection. This type of dementia is progressive and affects 30% to 40% of AIDS patients.

6.   Correct answer - C

Treatment of *Pneumocystic carinii* pneumonia includes pentamidine, an antiprotozoal agent, and trimethoprim - sulfamethoxazole (Bactrim, Septra), an antibiotic. Initially, these medications are administered intravenously. Pentamidine can be administered as long-term therapy in aerosol form to prevent further infection. Zidovudine decreases replication of human immunodeficiency virus and is used to treat patients with AIDS or ARC. Fluconazole is an antifungal agent commonly used to treat fungal diseases associated with HIV.

7.   Correct answer - C

A common side effect of pentamidine, especially when parenterally administered, is impaired glucose metabolism. Initially hypoglycemia may occur with the later development of diabetes mellitus. Patients taking pentamidine should have their blood glucoses closely monitored.

8.   Correct answer - B

Saliva has the least concentration of HIV; no documented case of AIDS has been spread through saliva. Blood, semen, and vaginal secretions - three major sources of transmission in adults - have high HIV concentrations.

9.   Correct answer - B

Monitoring the serum amylase will assess for the common side effect of pancreatitis in the patient taking dideoxyinosine.

10.   Correct answer - C

The mother should sign the consent form because she is the closest living relative. The patient cannot sign it because of his dementia, and the male companion is not a blood relative. The male companion could sign the consent if he was designated the durable power of attorney for healthcare decisions. Two physicians need not sign an emergency consent when a relative is available.

11.   **Correct answer - B**

A DNR (do not resuscitate) order should be written by the physician after he talks with the mother and male companion. This is the most ethically and legally sound procedure because relatives may bring legal suit if they question the care given the patient. Having the physician talk with the mother and male companion allows them to become fully informed of the situation and to ask questions about what will happen to the patient. Writing an order also clarifies the situation with the health team to prevent uncertainty about what to do when the patient dies.

12.   **Correct answer - D**

Information about the patient's health status and diagnosis is confidential; discussing it on the telephone- especially with an employer who may be concerned about the person's ability to return to his job - is an invasion of privacy.

13.   **Correct answer - D**

The presence of an active infection is a contraindication for transplantation since immunotherapy is begun in the immediate postoperative period. Since Mr. T is in end-stage renal disease and is a diabetic, it is anticipated that he probably would be hypertensive, hyperglycemic and have some signs and symptoms of congestive heart failure.

14.   **Correct answer - C**

It is imperative that donor and recipient have ABO compatibility and a close match on HLA (Human Leukocyte Antigen) testing. RH compatibility has not been found to be a factor in the development of rejection.

15. **Correct answer - A**

Dialysis should be performed the day prior to surgery in order to have the transplant recipient in an optimal state of fluid and electrolyte balance.

16. **Correct answer - A**

In the immediate postoperative period, massive diuresis indicates a well-functioning transplanted kidney. Urine outputs from 100 - 1000 ml/hr may be observed.

17. **Correct answer - D**

Electrolyte deficits of bicarbonate, potassium, and sodium may accompany the massive diuresis seen in postoperative renal transplant patients with well-functioning kidneys.

18. **Correct answer - A**

Even a slight rise in temperature may indicate infection in the transplant patient and should be reported promptly. Slight rises in temperature from an infectious process occur because of immunosuppression. A low hemoglobin and high blood glucose may be anticipated since this patient was in end-stage renal disease and is a diabetic. A decrease in creatinine is beneficial, indicating good kidney function.

19. **Correct answer - C**

B lymphocytes provide humoral immunity. When they recognize an antigen, they divide into plasma cells, secreting one type of antibody specific to that antigen. The antigen is neutralized and lysed. T lymphocytes, which provide cell-mediated immunity, directly attack the antigen after becoming sensitized to it, bind to it, and kill it with the assistance of macrophages. T cells are responsible for rejection of organ transplants. The phagocytic activity of neutrophils is nonspecific, occurring through the localization and destruction of antigens or with specific immunologic mechanisms. Interferon is an immunologic agent that attacks and inactivates specific viral antigens, inhibiting viral replication.

20. **Correct answer - C**

Anaphylaxis stimulates B lymphocytes to secrete specific IgE antibodies. After binding with the mast cells and basophils, IgE antibodies react with the antigen to stimulate production of mediators, such as histamine, slow-reacting substance of anaphylaxis, platelet-activating factor, and eosinophil chemotactic factor of anaphylaxis. These mediators cause the immediate, systemic reaction of anaphylaxis - wheezing, vasodilation, and shock.

21. **Correct answer - A**

IgE antibodies react in anaphylaxis. IgE is an immunoglobulin called a reagin; it responds to allergens that enter the body, causing an allergic reaction. When this reaction is severe, the IgE antibodies attach to other cells - such as mast cells, eosinophils, and basophils - causing them to rupture, inducing anaphylaxis.

22. **Correct answer - A**

Basophils function during an allergic response, stress, or chronic inflammation and serve as an anticoagulant. These polymorphonucleated granulocytes constitute 0.5% of the white blood cell count. Basophils contain and can liberate heparin and histamine and are physiologically similar to mast cells in the connective tissue near capillaries. Eosinophils also seem to increase during an allergic response and migrate to the site of the antibody-antigen reaction. The reaction causes the basophils and eosinophils to rupture, releasing histamine from the basophils, and the eosinophils may attempt to destroy the toxic proteins.

23. **Correct answer - B**

Hemodynamically, anaphylactic shock is accompanied by a low cardiac output. Anaphylaxis is a hypersensitive reaction to an antigen that causes increased secretion of histamine, which produces vasodilation and increases capillary permeability. Large fluid losses occur from the intravascular to the extravascular space; hypovolemia and hypotension result; and all hemodynamic parameters are depressed.

Hemodynamic treatment includes fluid and vasopressor therapy.

24.   Correct answer - C

Anaphylaxis most commonly is precipitated by antibiotic use, although any compound capable of acting as an allergen may cause an anaphylactic reaction. Common allergens include antibiotics, especially penicillin, medicines derived from animal sources, insect bites and stings, and iodinated radioactive contrast media.

25.   Correct answer - A

After exposure to an allergen, the patient develops life-threatening symptoms of anaphylaxis within 2 to 20 minutes. A reaction that occurs 20 minutes to 48 hours after exposure is called an accelerated reaction and is rarely life-threatening, manifesting itself principally as urticaria and occasionally as laryngeal edema. A delayed reaction may develop 3 days or more after drug administration starts and usually consists of a rash.

26.   Correct answer - D

Angioneurotic edema is a cutaneous manifestation seen initially in anaphylaxis. Stridor, hoarseness, and inspiratory wheezing indicate respiratory compromise. Airway obstruction and severe respiratory distress may follow quickly; therefore, these have the highest priority for intervention.

27.   Correct answer - D

Classic manifestations of anaphylaxis include the triad of urticaria, laryngeal edema and bronchospasm, and hypotension. The initial signs usually are cutaneous; diffuse erythema, pruritus, urticaria, or angioneurotic edema. These are commonly followed by bronchospasm, laryngeal edema, These are commonly followed by bronchospasm, laryngeal edema, or both. The patient typically has stridor and wheezing. Airway obstruction may progress rapidly and lead to severe respiratory distress. Cardiovascular collapse may occur before or after the cutaneous and pulmonary manifestations.

28. **Correct answer - A**

Although methylprednisolone is used in long-term management of anaphylaxis, epinephrine is the initial drug of choice because it can reverse bronchospasm and hypotension. Diphenhydramine can also assist in causing bronchodilation by decreasing the action of histamine. I.V. fluids are indicated to restore the circulating volume depleted by hypotension.

29. **Correct answer - B**

Vasodilation - not loss of myocardial contractility - causes hypotension in anaphylaxis. Thus, a drug with vasoconstrictive effects, such as dopamine, would be desirable. Dobutamine has little vasoconstrictive effect. Aminophylline is used if bronchospasm occurs. Antihistamines, such as diphenhydramine, are useful in relieving urticaria, and hydrocortisone decreases inflammation.

30. **Correct answer - D**

The most important intervention in caring for a patient with a history of allergies is to obtain an accurate and thorough drug history, identifying and describing previous drug reactions. Other actions are necessary, but the drug history has the highest priority.

31. **Correct answer - C**

Signs and symptoms of anaphylaxis include acute pulmonary hyperinflation caused by airway obstruction or by laryngeal edema, urticaria, or vascular collapse.

32. **Correct answer - A**

An anaphylactic drug reaction typically begins as a macular eruption on the head and arms before spreading in a symmetrical pattern. First episodes of exanthematous reactions usually occur within 1 week after the patient starts taking the drug, although the rash can appear as long as 14 days after the drug has been discontinued. A patient may be treated with a drug many times before developing a reaction. Because the eruption's morphology gives no clue to the cause, a proper diagnosis cannot be made without a careful history of all medications and other substances that have entered the body.

33.   Correct answer - A

Immediate treatment includes oxygen therapy if the patient has signs of systemic anaphylaxis. Treatment is aimed at impairing absorption of the antigen, enhancing oxygenation and treating or preventing hypotension. Emergency treatment also includes epinephrine, aminophylline, and hydrocortisone. Neither norepinephrine nor furosemide reverse bronchospasm. Prednisone, an oral steroid, is not indicated in the emergency treatment of anaphylaxis.

34.   Correct answer - D

Warfarin interferes with the coagulation process by blocking vitamin K's action in the liver. Vitamin K synthesizes prothrombin and Factors VII, IX, and X. The half-lives of prothrombin and Factors IX and X are longer than 24 hours. Thus, it takes 2 to 3 days before warfarin can effectively block these components. The prothrombin test measures the effectiveness of prothrombin, Factor IX, and Factor X - all part of the extrinsic mechanism of coagulation. The goal of warfarin therapy is to prolong the prothrombin time by 50% to 100%.

35.   Correct answer - A

An elevated reticulocyte count occurs in hemorrhage. A reticulocyte, an immature red blood cell (RBC), is normally present in the blood as 1% of the RBC count. A reticulocyte matures into an erythrocyte 2 days after being expelled from the bone marrow. An elevated reticulocyte count in anemia caused by hemorrhage indicates the bone marrow is responding to the anemia. The reticulocyte count drops in leukemia (because the bone marrow is depressed) and renal disease (because erythropoietin is not produced). Infection should not alter the reticulocyte count.

36.   Correct answer - B

Signs and symptoms of anticoagulant overdose include petechiae, tachycardia, hypotension, hematuria, epistaxis, bleeding gums, ecchymoses, tarry stools, and coffee-ground vomitus.

37. **Correct answer - A**

In long-term anticoagulant therapy, serious hemorrhagic complications occur intracranially and in the GI tract. GI hemorrhage is commonly associated with underlying lesions, such as ulcers. Minor bleeding is caused by capillary rupture and may include epistaxis and hematuria. Genitourinary and pulmonary bleeding are rare but may occur after instrumentation.

38. **Correct answer - D**

Protamine sulfate neutralizes the effects of the parenteral anticoagulant heparin and is used to treat heparin overdose. Therapy for hemorrhagic complications from oral anticoagulants includes volume replacement, vitamin K administration, and transfusions of clotting factors, fresh frozen plasma, and whole blood. Vitamin K acts as a pharmacologic antagonist to oral anticoagulants and may be given orally or parenterally.

39. **Correct answer - A**

Excessive alcohol should be avoided by a patient on anticoagulant therapy. He should also wear gloves while gardening, use an electric razor rather than straight-edge blades, and use a soft-bristled toothbrush. The patient should be encouraged to wear a medical identification bracelet and cautioned not to trim corns or calluses himself.

40. **Correct answer - C**

In a patient with type AB blood, the antigens on the red cell membrane are A and B. The four main blood groups of the ABO system are A, B, AB, and O. The antigens for this system are on the RBC membrane and are the same as the blood group. The antibodies of the ABO system are in the serum. These antibodies do not correspond to the antigens on the RBC membrane, because antibodies cannot be produced against present antigens.

41. **Correct answer - C**

Packed RBCs decrease the risk of hepatitis transmission. A unit of whole blood, which contains the necessary blood components, including platelets and coagulation factors, is centrifuged to separate the RBCs from the plasma. The packed cells consist of the same RBC mass as whole blood with only small amounts of plasma, leukocytes, and platelets. The small amount of plasma decreases the risk of hepatitis and plasma protein reaction. A transfusion of packed RBCs causes the hemoglobin and hematocrit levels to rise faster than a whole blood transfusion does. In the average patient, hemoglobin rises 1 gm/dl and hematocrit rises 2% to 3% for each unit of packed cells transfused. In whole blood transfusion, a similar rise takes about 24 hours. Packed RBCs restore or maintain oxygen-carrying capacity and are indicated in anemia or surgical blood loss or to increase RBC mass. Whole blood is indicated with massive hemorrhage.

42.   Correct answer - D

For blood transfusions, 18G or 20G catheters may be used. To prevent hemolysis, 18G catheters are usually recommended, although 20G catheters are acceptable for average transfusion rates. Only normal saline solution may be used when administering blood products. Lactated Ringer's solution causes agglutination, and dextrose solutions cause hemolysis. The patient's vital signs should be assessed before initiation of the transfusion, every 15 minutes for the first hour, and after completion of the transfusion. The temperature of a blood warmer should not exceed 98.6° F. (37° C.); RBCs heated above that point may hemolyze.

43.   Correct answer - A

A febrile, nonhemolytic transfusion reaction is the most common of the immediate reactions. Signs and symptoms include fever, chills, headache, hypotension, lumbar pain, palpitations, and malaise. The fever typically occurs 1 to 6 hours after the transfusion starts. This reaction typically occurs in a patient with multiple transfusions. A hemolytic reaction occurs immediately because of ABO blood group incompatibility; clinical findings include fever that may exceed 104.9° F. (40.5° C.), facial flushing, chills, lumbar pain, hypotension, headache, chest pain, dyspnea, oliguria, and shock. A bacterial reaction, caused by bacterial contamination of the blood product, is rare; signs and symptoms include high fever, severe hypotension, pain in the abdomen and extremities, vomiting, bloody diarrhea, and dry, flushed skin. A delayed hemolytic reaction, which occurs 2 or more days after a transfusion, typically develops in a patient who has received previous transfusions; signs and symptoms include continued anemia, hemoglobinuria, and bilirubinemia.

44.   Correct answer - D

In normal doses, aspirin can prolong clotting time by impairing platelet aggregation. This can occur after one dose and persist for several days, even in a healthy person; thus, aspirin is contraindicated in a patient with thrombocytopenia or bleeding disorders, such as hemophilia. Other medications with the same reaction include dipyridamole and low-molecular-weight dextran.

45.   Correct answer - C

After quinidine therapy is stopped, thrombocytopenia begins to recede within 24 hours and a normal platelet count returns within 1 week. About one in 100,000 persons taking quinidine develops this idiosyncratic reaction of platelet antibody formation with resultant thrombocytopenia, which can develop 12 hours after initiation of therapy.

46.   Correct answer - B

In normal hemostasis, the first response to a traumatized vessel is vascular spasm - an attempt to control bleeding. The more a vessel is traumatized, the more spasm occurs (thus, crushing injuries produce more vasoconstriction than sharp wounds do). The spasm lasts 20 to 30 minutes, until the clot forms and retracts. Next, the platelet plug forms over the hole while activators, such as platelet factor 3 and thromboplastin, are released from platelets and the injured blood vessel to activate the intrinsic and extrinsic pathways . These pathways convert prothrombin to thrombin, which activates fibrinogen to form the fibrin threads of a clot. The clotting mechanism begins 15 seconds to 2 minutes after the trauma, and a clot is formed in 3 to 6 minutes. After 30 minutes, the clot retracts, pulling together the edges of the traumatized vessel to allow repair.

47. **Correct answer - D**

Calcium is essential for proper functioning of most of the intrinsic pathway. However, serum calcium levels can never fall low enough to interrupt proper clotting, because death will first ensue from muscle tetany. When blood is removed from the body during hemodialysis or extracorporeal circulation, clotting is prevented by binding the calcium with citrate or oxalate.

48. **Correct answer - D**

Cold agglutinins are part of an autoimmune process in which IgM autoantibodies react with the RBCs, specifically complement, causing agglutination and possibly hemolysis when exposed to cold. Agglutination ranges in severity, depending on how high the cold agglutinin titer is. Usually beginning in the hands and feet, agglutination may progress to massive hemolysis, or the agglutination RBCs may instead be cleared from the blood by splenic or hepatic macrophages. It can occur by transfusion of cold blood or exposure to cold temperatures, is most common in elderly patients, and is associated with primary atypical pneumonia. Hemolytic anemia and Raynaud's phenomenon may result from peripheral intravascular obstruction by the agglutinated RBCs.

49. **Correct answer - C**

Crossmatching is the test for agglutination - the clumping of blood from incompatibility - of two blood specimens. ABO-compatible specimens, confirmed by typing, are crossmatched, or combined, to see if other antibodies incompatible with the donor's blood have formed. If more than one unit is transfused, donor bloods are crossmatched among themselves to determine incompatibility among transfusions.

50. **Correct answer - D**

Albumin does not require typing and crossmatching before administration. Prepared from plasma, it is used to increase intravascular volume. Fresh frozen plasma contains albumin, globulins, and coagulation factors, but no platelets and is used to replenish coagulation factors and antibodies. Because of the antibodies, it must be typed to the recipient's blood type, but crossmatching and Rh compatibility need not be determined. Platelets should also be typed because they may lead to febrile reactions. Platelets, which have a 9 to 12 day life span, are transfused to increase clotting ability in platelet deficiency. Cryoprecipitate consists of fibrinogen and Factors VIII and XIII and must be typed. It is used for such bleeding disorders as disseminated intravascular coagulation and hemophilia .

51. **Correct answer - C**

Type O blood contains no RBC antigens but both anti-A and anti-B antibodies. Antigens are responsible for blood agglutination; hence absence of these in Type O makes it the universal donor. When anigens are absent on the red blood cell antibodies form against them. Type A blood has A antigens and anti-B antibodies. Type B blood has B antigens and anti-A antibodies. Type AB has both A and B antigens and no antibodies, making it the universal recipient. Care must be taken in transfusing Type O to A, B, or AB, because it contains antibodies and may cause tranfusion reactions if antibody titers are high enough.

52. **Correct answer - B**

RBC transfusion increases the hemoglobin and hematocrit levels faster than whole blood transfusions. Packed RBCs are erythrocytes with 80% of the plasma removed, decreasing the incidence of plasma protein reaction. RBC transfusion increases the hemoglobin and hematocrit twice as fast as whole blood because its hematocrit value is about 65%; it also decreases incidence of volume overload and congestive heart failure because it has less volume. However, because RBCs are so concentrated, they must be administered at a slower rate and are indicated for slow blood loss, whereas whole blood is indicated for faster, more severe blood loss.

53.   Correct answer - C

Stored blood becomes deficient in clotting Factors V, VII, and IX and platelets, so platelets and fresh frozen plasma may also need to be transfused. Adding sodium citrate - which binds serum calcium - to the stored blood to prevent clotting may cause hypocalcemia. Hyperkalemia may result from degradation of red blood cells, which releases intracellular potassium. Metabolic alkalosis may occur as the sodium citrate, which is used to prevent clotting in banked blood, converts into bicarbonate.

54.   Correct answer - B

Blood transfusion reactions due to ABO incompatibility are usually hemolytic. Antigens A or B may be present on a red blood cell, while antibodies against foreign antigens exist in the plasma. Transfusion of blood with foreign ABO antigens triggers the antibodies to agglutinate the antigens, causing hemolysis, or destruction of the RBCs . This may cause renal failure, shock, pulmonary edema, and disseminated intravascular coagulation. Anaphylactic reactions typically follow incompatible plasma protein transfusion, specifically IgA-containing plasma to IgA-deficient plasma, which has developed IgA antibodies. Urticarial reactions also typically occur from incompatible plasma protein transfusions but are less serious. Febrile reactions, also benign, are caused by an incompatible transfusion of leukocytes or platelets.

55.   Correct answer - A

Sodium bicarbonate may be administered in treating a hemolytic blood transfusion reaction, one that destroys the RBCs with large amounts of hemoglobin clogging the renal tubules, possibly leading to renal failure. Administering sodium bicarbonate alkalizes the blood and dissolves the hemoglobin. Treatment may also include fluid and diuretic therapy to flush the hemoglobin out of the tubules. Epinephrine and diphenhydramine are administered to treat an anaphylactic blood transfusion reaction; antipyretics, such as aspirin, are given to combat a febrile blood transfusion reaction.

56.   Correct answer - D

Hemoglobinemia - free hemoglobin in the plasma - is visible after an acute hemolytic blood transfusion reaction. The plasma appears pink or red. An acute hemolytic reaction occurs from ABO incompatibility when donor RBCs are attacked by the recipient's RBCs. Hemolysis may also occur if the transfusion is primed with intravenous fluid other than normal saline solution. In ABO incompatibility, antigen-antibody complexes activate complement, which causes the hemolysis. Other laboratory findings include hemoglobinuria and positive direct antiglobulin test.

57.   Correct answer - B

Obstetric incidents leading to disseminated intravascular coagulation (DIC) are caused by fetal and placental tissue activating the clotting mechanism. Pregnancy is a normally hypercoagulable state because amniotic fluid causes clot-promoting activities. However, dead fetal tissue and placental tissue also cause clot-promoting activities and may be released into the maternal circulation in such conditions as retained dead fetus and abruptio placentae, systemically activating the clotting mechanism. In those conditions, incidence of DIC approaches 50%. Treatment involves factor replacements and removal of fetal material.

58.   Correct answer - B

Tissue injury activates the extrinsic clotting mechanism. Extrinsic mechanisms occur outside the blood vessel; intrinsic mechanisms occur within it. Activation of the extrinsic mechanism occurs when blood contacts injured tissue, releasing tissue factor and phospholipids. These, along with Factor VII, activate Factor X. Factors X and V form prothrombin activator, which converts prothrombin to thrombin, triggering the final clotting mechanism of thrombin - the activation of fibrinogen to form fibrin threads. The intrinsic mechanism is involved in the above steps to form the common pathway of both mechanisms.

59.   Correct answer - C

Partial thromboplastin time studies the functioning of the intrinsic mechanism and the common pathway. This test initiates activation of Factor XII, the first step in the intrinsic mechanism; a normal partial thromboplastin ensures a normal intrinsic mechanism. The intrinsic mechanism is activated by injury to the blood vessel, releasing Factor XII and plasma phospholipids (or platelet factor 3). These activate Factor XI, which activates Factor IX. Along with Factor VIII, Factor IX activates the pathway common to both intrinsic and extrinsic mechanisms (Factors V and X) to convert prothrombin to thrombin, which converts fibrinogen to fibrin.

60.   Correct answer - A

The liver produces most blood-clotting factors, including fibrinogen, prothrombin, and Factors VII, IX, and X. Factor VIII is produced by many other organs. Liver diseases can prolong blood coagulation by decreasing production of factors or through malabsorption of vitamin K. Vitamin K is necessary for synthesis of prothrombin and Factors IX, and X. Liver disease results in decreased bile production, which allows fat and fat-soluble vitamins, such as K, to be absorbed from the GI tract.

61.   Correct answer - B

Fibrin split (fibrin degradation) products are increased in DIC and reflect an abnormal breakdown of fibrinogen by plasmin. This causes an increase in end products from fibrinogen and fibrindestruction and is associated with a decrease in coagulation factors. Accumulation of these products inhibits platelet aggregation and prolongs bleeding time. A normal fibrin split products value is less than 10 mcg/ 100 ml.

62.   Correct answer - D

Cryoprecipitate replenishes clotting factors, specifically Factors VIII and XIII and fibrinogen, and is used to treat coagulation deficiencies, such as in hemophilia, von Willebrand's disease, and DIC. Cryoprecipitate must be typed to the recipient's blood.

63.   **Correct answer - D**

Heparin neutralizes thrombin, preventing further clot formation. In DIC, the clotting mechanism is activated and bleeding results when a deficiency in clotting factors occurs. Replacement of clotting factors with the administration of blood and blood components does not stop clotting activation. Heparin, however, stops clotting by neutralizing thrombin, which activates fibrinogen to form a fibrin clot. Thrombin is also involved with prothrombin; Factors V, VIII, and XIII; and platelets. Amicar, an antithrombolytic agent, should be used only as a last resort in catastrophic bleeding and only with heparin. Used alone, it promotes clotting.

64.   **Correct answer - B**

Heparin interferes with coagulation by inactivating thrombin, thereby preventing conversion of fibrinogen to fibrin. Heparin also prevents a stable clot from forming by inhibiting fibrin-stabilizing factor; it does not interfere with platelet function or lyse existing clots. Proper anticoagulation therapy is evident when the partial thromboplastin time is twice normal. Heparin is reversed by protamine sulfate; 1 mg of protamine is administered to neutralize 100 units of heparin.

65.   **Correct answer - A**

Anemia associated with prosthetic heart valves is caused by the rupture of RBCs when they hit the valves. Turbulent flow against foreign material, such as Teflon, produces a mechanical anemia - not caused by an intrinsic defect of the RBCs. The degree of hemolysis depends on the valve and its size. Aortic prosthetic valves tend to increase incidence of hemolysis because of increased pressure and speed of blood flow on the heart's left side; smaller valves also tend to increase hemolysis. Lactic acid dehydrogenase levels may rise and iron may be lost in the urine (as hemosiderin) from RBC and hemoglobin destruction. This anemia cannot be reversed, but iron supplements may help. A new valve may be necessary in severe cases.

66.   **Correct answer - A**

Hypoxia stimulates release of erythropoietin, or erythropoietic-stimulating factor, into the blood; erythropoietin then acts on stem cells in the bone marrow to increase RBC production. Hypoxic states causing increased erythropoiesis include high altitudes, lung and cardiac diseases, and anemia through hemorrhage or destruction of bone marrow. Erythropoietin, produced by the kidneys, is decreased in renal disease, causing the typical anemia seen in chronic renal failure.

67.   Correct answer - B

Development of antibodies after a hepatitis vaccine is called active acquired immunity; in this strong, long-lasting immunity, a person develops antibodies after directly contracting the disease or receiving an injection of the attenuated virus. Passive acquired immunity lasts a short time and occurs when a person develops antibodies after exposure to someone else or from a vaccine. Passive immunity is involved when a mother passes immunity to a fetus or a breast-fed baby or when a person receives gamma globulin to fight the risk of hepatitis. Natural immunity, such as the inability to contract distemper, is genetic. Autoimmunity is a disturbance of the immune system, causing it to attack the self.

68.   Correct answer - D

In Hodgkin's disease, many blood cell types proliferate, including the Reed-Sternberg cell, lymphocytes, eosinophils, neutrophils, and plasma cells. The disease typically arises in one site, beginning in the lymph nodes; the immune system becomes disordered, and the patient may become infected with unusual organisms. Radiation is usually successful when the disease is confined, and chemotherapy can be effective with more extensive disease. The disease may spread to the lungs, liver, spleen, or bone marrow.

69.   Correct answer - B

Hypercalcemia may occur in lymphoma and in leukemia when the bone marrow is infiltrated. In lymphoma, hypercalcemia is typically associated with the T cell type. Demineralization of bone occurs when calcium is released into the blood. The patient is at risk of developing pathologic fractures, cardiac dysrhythmias, and renal failure from caliculi. Treatment usually consists of fluid administration and diuretic therapy, which flushes calcium through the kidneys, and phosphate administration, which binds the calcium.

70.   Correct answer - C

The body element responsible for clot lysis is plasmin, a fibrinolytic enzyme that attacks fibrin and clotting factors, producing fibrin split products. Plasminogen, a precursor to plasmin, is situated in the clot and is activated to plasmin by tissue a few days after the clot has formed. Over several days, the clot slowly dissolves. Streptokinase, which also lyses clots, may be produced by streptococcal bacteria during an infection to declot lymph and tissue.

71.   Correct answer - A

A direct or indirect Coombs' test may be performed when crossmatching blood to detect any immune antibodies in the recipient's blood and any hemolytic anemias caused by antibodies. A direct Coombs' test determines whether RBCs are coated with antibodies. An indirect Coombs' test assesses whether antibodies are present or spill over into the serum, indicating insufficient room for the antibodies on the RBCs.

72.   Correct answer - D

Preventing bone fractures is part of patient care in multiple myeloma, a malignancy of plasma cells causing anemia, leukopenia, and thrombocytopenia, with serum protein abnormalities. Plasma cells proliferate in the bone marrow, causing soft, spongy bones. Pathologic fractures may occur with possible compression of the spinal cord; one of the presenting symptoms of multiple myeloma is skeletal pain. Hypercalcemia may result from bone decalcification. Infection may occur with a decreased white blood cell (WBC) count and a disordered immune response. Renal failure is also a concern because of chronic hypercalcemia and plasma protein buildup in the renal tubules.

73.   Correct answer - D

Anemia is associated with cancer. Usually not severe, the anemia commonly results from iron or folic acid deficiency, blood loss in cancer, or bone marrow involvement. Anemia is also associated with chronic infections and inflammatory diseases. Chronic obstructive pulmonary disease and congestive heart failure may lead to increased RBC production from erythropoietin stimulation by hypoxia. Dehydration may lead to increased hematocrit values because of hemoconcentration, although levels are really normal; the amount of RBCs does not drop, but their relative percentage in the blood increases because dehydration lowers the percentage of fluid in the blood.

74. Correct answer - D

The spleen performs the hematologic function of producing antibodies. During fetal development, the spleen also forms RBCs; after birth, it produces lymphocytes and monocytes. The spleen also cleanses the blood, removing damaged and old RBCs from circulation. The kidney stimulates erythropoiesis in response to hypoxemia, and the liver produces most of the clotting factors. Vitamin K is synthesized by bacteria in the GI tract, or is found in the diet, such as in green, leafy vegetables.

75. Correct answer - B

Aplastic anemia, which can be congenital or acquired, is associated with agranulocytosis and thrombocytopenia. Hypoplasia of bone marrow occurs, usually from cytotoxic treatment for such diseases as leukemia or lymphoma. The WBC count may be below 500/mm3 and the platelet count below 20,000/mm3. The patient is at risk for infection and hemorrhage. Drugs implicated in the development of aplastic anemia include chloramphenicol, phenylbutazone, sulfonamides, and gold. The treatment of choice is bone marrow transplant.

CHAPTER 8

MULTISYSTEM PATIENT CARE PROBLEMS

Case Study

Questions 1-4 refer to the following case study:

Mr. S. is transferred to the intensive care unit (ICU) from a surgical floor. He had a transurethal prostatic resection (TURP) 3 days ago and is now hypotensive. A diagnosis of septic shock is made.

1. Which of the following actions receives the highest priority for Mr. S.?

    A. Obtaining an allergy history
    B. Drawing blood for cultures, then administering antibiotic therapy
    C. Initiating antibiotic therapy after obtaining urine culture results
    D. Inserting a Foley catheter to monitor urine output

2. A patient admitted to the ICU in the early stages of septic shock presents with:

    A. Weak, thready pulses and low blood pressure
    B. Decreased urine output and elevated serum creatinine level
    C. Warm, flushed, moist skin
    D. Hyperventilation and pulmonary congestion

3. In an assessment of Mr. S.'s respiratory system, which of the following findings indicates *early* septic shock?

    A. Increased mucous production
    B. Bilateral crackles
    C. Hyperpnea
    D. Respiratory acidosis

4. Increased cardiac output, dysrhythmias, normal urine output, increased need for fluids to maintain blood pressure, and confusion are:

A. Early signs of septic shock
B. Late signs of septic shock
C. Normal signs of any illness
D. Early signs of all shocks states

Case Study
Questions 5-10 refer to the following case study:

Mr. P., age 72, has been a patient in the ICU for 3 days after undergoing cancer surgery for a colon resection with formation of a loop colostomy. He has had a fever of 100.8° to 102.4° F. (38.2° to 39.1° C.) for the past 12 hours and on initial assessment is warm and flushed. His blood pressure is unchanged at 134/76, but he is tachycardic. Urine output from his indwelling urinary catheter is 40 ml/hr.

---

5. Based on the above data, Mr. P's condition can be described as:

A. Dehydration caused by intestinal fluid shifts from the surgery
B. The early phase of septic shock
C. The late phase of septic shock
D. Dehydration and normal postoperative fever

---

6. To collect more data, the physician converts Mr. P.'s central line to a pulmonary artery catheter. Which pressure readings would be expected?

A. Cardiac index of 2.1 liters/minute/m_2 and pulmonary capillary wedge pressure (PCWP) of 4 mm Hg
B. Cardiac index of 2.1 liters/minute/m_2 and PCWP of 20 mm Hg
C. Systemic vascular resistance of 600 dynes/second/cm_5 and cardiac index of 4.0 liters/minute/m_2
D. Systemic vascular resistance of 2,100 dynes/second/cm_5 and cardiac index of 2.1 liters/minute/m_2

7. Based on the physical findings and hemodynamic data, the physician would be expected to order:

A. Fluid boluses and dopamine (Intropin) drip
B. Fluid boluses and nitroprusside (Nipride) drip
C. Dopamine drip only
D. Nitroprusside drip only

8. Two hours later, Mr. P.'s skin is cool and clammy. His blood pressure is 92/56, his cardiac index is 1.8 liters/minute m_2, and his PCWP is 6 mm Hg. This change in Mr. P.'s condition has been initiated by:

A. Release of bradykinins
B. Effective drug and fluid administration
C. Increased capillary permeability
D. Massive vasodilation

9. The *most* effective treatment during this phase would be:

A. Fluid boluses and dopamine drip
B. Fluid boluses and nitroprusside drip
C. Dopamine drip only
D. Nitroprusside drip only

10. The physician orders naloxone (Narcan) 0.8 mg I.V. bolus. Narcan may be effective in this situation because it:

A. Reverses hypotension caused by opiates
B. Reverses hypotension caused by endorphins
C. Decreases capillary permeability caused by histamine
D. Decreases cellular damage and the likelihood of death

Questions 11-15 refer to the following case study:

Mr. J., age 72, is admitted to the ICU with a diagnosis of urosepsis and septic shock. He is confused and slightly restless. His white blood cell count is 32,000/ul, with an increase in metamyelocytes and band neutrophils and a decrease in segmented neutrophils. His erythrocyte sedimentation rate is 44 mm/hour.

11. Which of the following phrases *best* describes shock?

    A. The inability of the body to excrete metabolic waste products
    B. The collapse of the respiratory system
    C. The collapse of the sympathetic nervous system
    D. A state of impaired tissue perfusion

12. Mr. J. is in early septic shock. The nurse would most likely find which of the following acid-base values?

    A. pH 7.2; HCO_3 14 MEq/L
    B. pH 7.52; HCO_3 32 mEq/L
    C. pH 7.24; pCO_2 51 mm Hg
    D. pH 7.5; pCO_2 29 mm Hg

13. A patient in septic shock is depleted of intravascular volume. Which factor does *not* cause hypovolemia in septic shock?

    A. Fluid leakage into tissues from increased vessel permeability
    B. Fluid loss associated with infections, such as sweating during fever, and respiratory losses during hyperventilation
    C. Sequestering of plasma fluid in the extravascular spaces
    D. Increased vascular resistance compromising blood flow to vital organs

14. Which rationale is *not* responsible for the change in a patient's mental status during septic shock's early stages?

A. Decreased cerebral perfusion because of the low flow state
B. Elevation of metabolic waste products, such as blood urea nitrogen and creatinine, because of decreased kidney perfusion
C. Alkalosis that results from hyperventilation, causing cerebral vascular constriction
D. Endotoxins acting directly on the central nervous system

15. Mr. J.'s white blood cell count and differential indicate:

A. A normal response to infection
B. Acute leukemia as the cause of sepsis
C. Overwhelming infection
D. Inflammation

16. The erythrocyte sedimentation rate measures the:

A. Amount of foreign particles on the red blood cells
B. Velocity of red blood cells settling out of the plasma
C. Rate at which an antibody agglutinates the red blood cell
D. Fragility of the red blood cell

Case Study
Questions 17-19 refer to the following case study:

A woman is admitted to the ICU from the ER with a suspected drug overdose. The ER staff was unable to obtain any history as to the amount or type of drugs ingested because of patient obtundation. A toxicology screen was performed in ER.

17. The patient awakens in the ICU and admits to taking ½ liter of alcohol and about 25 tablets of acetaminophen (Tylenol). The physician orders the antidote acetylcysteine (Mucomyst). Prior to administration of the antidote, it is important for the nurse to know if which of the following medications was given in the ER?

A. Naloxone (Narcan)
B. Activated charcoal
C. Dextrose
D. Ipecac syrup

18. The nurse evaluates the patient's laboratory values, expecting which level to be abnormal in an acetaminophen overdose?

A. Serum bilirubin
B. Creatinine kinase
C. pH, bicarbonate level
D. Serum potassium

19. The day after admission, the patient develops nausea, vomiting, sweating, elevated vital signs, and agitation. The nurse should suspect:

A. Alcohol withdrawal
B. ICU (intensive care unit) psychosis
C. Acute myocardial infarction
D. Sensory deprivation

Case Study
Questions 20-22 refer to the following case study:

Mr. T., is admitted to the ICU with a suspected salicylate over-dose. Besides taking aspirin regularly for arthritis, the past two days he was also taking Alka Seltzer and Pepto Bismol (bismuth subsalicylate) for the flu. He presently is slightly lethargic and complaining of nausea and tinnitus.

20. The nurse would expect Mr. T to presently have which of the following blood gases?

   A. pH 7.49, HCO₃ 22 mEq/L, PCO₂ 29 mm Hg
   B. pH 7.24, HCO₃ 18 mEq/L, PCO₂ 55 mm Hg
   C. pH 7.30, HCO₃ 24 mEq/L, PCO₂ 52 mm Hg
   D. pH 7.31, HCO₃ 19 mEq/L, PCO₂ 30 mm Hg

21. The nurse, would in addition, monitor Mr. T.'s laboratory values for:

   A. Hyperglycemia
   B. Hyperkalemia
   C. Hypernatremia
   D. Prolonged Prothrombin time

22. As Mr. T.'s condition deteriorates, which nursing diagnosis would apply?

   A. Fluid volume deficit related to bleeding from impaired coagulation
   B. Potential for injury related to seizures
   C. Hypothermia related to drug effects
   D. Diarrhea related to administration of antidote

Case Study
Questions 23-26 refer to the following case study:

Mr. W., age 26, is admitted to the ICU from the ER after sustaining a near-drowning episode at the beach about 30 minutes ago. On his honeymoon at a local resort, he was swimming in the ocean in rough waters and was pulled out to sea by the current. He was rescued by local fishermen after 15-20 minutes submersion. Current core temperature is 34.2 degrees F.

23. The nurse would expect Mr. W. to have which of the following blood gases?

A. pH 7.19, HCO_3 18 mEq/L, PCO_2 60 mm Hg
B. pH 7.34, HCO_3 28 mEq/L, PCO_2 55 mm Hg
C. pH 7.30, HCO_3 24 mEq/L, PCO_2 52 mm Hg
D. pH 7.31, HCO_3 19 mEq/L, PCO_2 30 mm Hg

24. A high priority treatment for Mr. W. At this time is:

A. Sodium Bicarbonate IV
B. Hemodialysis
C. Electrolyte replacements
D. 100% O_2

25. A high priority nursing diagnosis for Mr. W. at this time would be:

A. Decreased renal perfusion related to shock state
B. Hyperthermia related to infectious process
C. Impaired gas exchange related to aspiration
D. Fluid volume excess related to aspiration

26. A diving reflex occurs in near-drowning victims in order to shunt blood to the heart and brain. Which heart rhythm is associated with this reflex?

A. Supraventricular tachycardia
B. Sinus bradycardia
C. Atrial fibrillation
D. Ventricular fibrillation

Case Study
Questions 27-30 refer to the following case study:

Ms. O., age 48, is admitted to the ICU after suffering burns from a house fire. She is presently awake, responsive, with stable pulse and blood pressure.

27. Which of the following findings is most often associated with the presence of inhalation injury in the burn patient?

A. Facial burns
B. Arterial pO_2 of 80 mm Hg
C. Inspiratory force of 22 cms H_2O
D. The presence of burns that are red, without blisters, and painful to touch

28. The nurse assesses Ms. O.'s burns to be pale, yellow-white, slightly moist and without blanching. Ms. O. feels pain upon deep pressure but not to pinprick. The nurse correctly documents these burns as:

A. Superficial partial thickness, first degree
B. Superficial partial thickness, second degree
C. Deep dermal partial thickness, second degree
D. Full thickness, third degree

29. The nurse anticipates that Ms. O. should receive which type of fluid therapy?

A. Crystalloids and colloids together the first 48 hours
B. Crystalloids the first 24 hours, with the addition of colloids the second 24 hours
C. Colloids the first 24 hours, with the addition of crystalloids the second 24 hours
D. The immediate institution of total parenteral nutrition

30. Which of the following assessments indicates adequate fluid resuscitation during the first 24 hours postburn?

A. Serum sodium 148 mEq/l
B. Hematocrit 65%
C. Cardiac index 2.1 1/min/mL
D. Urine output 30-50 ml/hr.

1. **Correct answer - A**

   Obtaining an allergy history from the patient has the highest priority because antibiotics can cause anaphylaxis more often than a n y other substance. Next, obtain all culture specimens before giving the first drug dose. Initiating antibiotics before collecting c u l - tures is a serious error. Accurately identifying the infecting organ- ism is important to provide optimal antibiotic treatment. A switch to a more appropriate therapy can help ensure patient survival.

2. **Correct answer - C**

   As septic shock develops, the patient's earliest signs and symptoms are those of the warm (early or hyperdynamic) stage. These include warm, flushed, moist skin; tachycardia with full bounding pulses; tachypnea; confusion; normal or slightly increased urine output; and normal or slightly decreased blood pressure.

3. **Correct answer - C**

   Hyperpnea is seen in early sepsis, sometimes to a point of respira- tory alkalosis, and is caused by the respiratory response to lactic aci- dosis and by the release of endotoxins, which stimulate the medul- lary respiratory control center. Advanced shock is characterized by pulmonary edema, which produces bilateral crackles. Additionally, adult respiratory distress syndrome (ARDS) has been associated with gram-negative sepsis.

4. **Correct answer - A**

   Increased cardiac output, dysrhythmias, normal urine output, in- creased need for fluids to maintain blood pressure, and confusion are early signs of septic shock. In the early phase of shock, powerful sympathetic stimulation produces catecholamines that increase con- tractility and heart rate to maintain cardiac output, normal urine out- put, and blood pressure. Cerebral ischemia from vasoconstriction and buildup of metabolic toxins may cause confusion.

5. **Correct answer - B**

   The patient is in early phase of septic shock (also known as warm, high-output, or hyperdynamic shock). Septic shock is caused by the effects of endotoxins released from bacteria infecting the blood. Endotoxins release bradykinin, a vasodilator. During this phase, blood pressure may be low or normal as compensatory mechanisms continue to work. The skin is warm, and tachycardia results from fever and vasodilation.

6. **Correct answer - C**

Normal systemic vascular resistance is 800 to 1,200 dynes/second/cm^5; this drops in early septic shock because of vasodilation. Cardiac index (normally 2.5 to 4.0 liters/minute/m^2) may be normal or high because of low impedence to left ventricular ejection. The pulmonary capillary wedge pressure (PCWP, normally 8 to 12 mm Hg) may be low or normal because of low preload from venous pooling.

7. **Correct answer - A**

Besides antibiotics, fluid boluses and dopamine are indicated in the early phase of septic shock. Fluid and dopamine help raise systemic vascular resistance and increase preload, thereby maintaining an adequate circulatory volume.

8. **Correct answer - C**

The late (also called cold or hypodynamic) phase of septic shock occurs when endotoxins release histamine, increasing capillary permeability. Fluid leaks out of the intravascular space, creating a relative hypovolemia. Preload is further impaired, resulting in a low PCWP and diminished cardiac output and tissue perfusion. Hypotension develops as endotoxins release endorphins.

9. **Correct answer - B**

Treatment for late septic shock includes antibiotic therapy, fluid administration, and vasodilator therapy. Fluid boluses are still indicated, and if the fluid deficit is corrected, the shock may revert to the hyperdynamic phase. Vasodilator therapy, such as a nitroprusside drip, may decrease the vasoconstriction associated with hypotension and impaired tissue perfusion.

10.   Correct answer - B

Naloxone (Narcan) is effective in septic shock because it can reverse the hypotension caused by the release of endorphins by endotoxins. Naloxone may displace the endorphins from the receptor site
on the cellular membrane. A bolus of 0.8 mg I.V. is given, followed
by a drip of 0.2 mg/hour.

11.   Correct answer - D

Shock is a state of impaired tissue perfusion caused by decreased
blood flow or impaired cellular metabolism. Septic shock is a combination of these states. Cellular damage occurs from the endotoxins, making cells unable to extract nutrients from the blood. As shock
progresses, vasoconstriction develops, leading to impaired blood flow.

12.   Correct answer - D

Respiratory alkalosis develops in the early phase of septic shock.
Tachypnea, a compensatory mechanism, is initiated as peripheral tissue perfusion decreases, causing hypoxia. In early shock, the patient
hyperventilates to increase oxygenation, thus blowing off CO_2. During progressive stages, excessive and prolonged vasoconstriction
causes lactic acid levels to increase within the body, producing metabolic acidosis.

13.   Correct answer - D

Several factors contribute to hypovolemia in septic shock. Fluid
and electrolytes can leave the body through events associated with
infection, such as sweating during fever, vomiting, diarrhea, and respiratory losses during tachypnea. Also, plasma fluid can be seques-
tered in the extravascular spaces because of a local or generalized
increase in vessel permeability secondary to the production of histamine, bradykinin, and other agents.

14.   Correct answer - B

In early septic shock, the sensorium may decrease because of decreased cerebral perfusion caused by endoxin-induced vasodilation,
which increases blood pooling within the venous system. Endotox-

ins act directly on the central nervous system to alter mental status and increase stimulation of the respiratory center. The resulting hyperventilation produces alkalosis. Cerebral vasoconstriction, occurring in response to alkalosis, decreases cerebral blood flow and produces a change in mental status. Whereas the blood urea nitrogen level may be elevated in the early stages of septic shock, the creatinine level rises in later stages as organ damage occurs from vasoconstriction.

15.   **Correct answer - C**

A white blood cell count of 32,000/ul with increased metamyelocytes and band neutrophils and decreased segmented neutrophils indicates overwhelming infection. Metamyelocytes and "bands" are immature neutrophils released in response to infection (sometimes referred to as a "shift to the left" because, historically, immature cells were recorded on the left side of the report sheet). Segmented and polymorphonuclear neutrophils (or "polys"), the mature forms, perform phagocytosis in infections and inflammations. A rise in all the levels indicates a normal response to infection (regenerative shift to the left), whereas a rise in immature cells and a decline in mature ones indicates that the polymorphonuclear neutrophils are being consumed at the active site of infection (degenerative shift to the left). (See *Normal White Blood Cell Values*, below).

Normal White Blood Cell Values

16.   **Correct answer - B**

The erythrocyte sedimentation rate measures the velocity of red blood cells (RBCs) settling out of the plasma and is normally 0 to 10 mm/hour. Because the rate can be elevated in infections (acute and chronic), inflammation, tissue damage, and autoimmune diseases, the test is nonspecific. The speed with which RBCs settle out of the plasma is probably controlled by serum proteins because the erythrocyte sedimentation rate changes whenever the serum protein level does.

407

17. **Correct answer - B**

Before giving acetylcysteine, the antidote for an acetaminophen overdose, it is necessary to ascertain if activated charcoal was given. Activated charcoal will bind the acetylcysteine, negating its desired effects.

18. **Correct answer - A**

Since acetaminophen toxicity can damage the liver, monitor for elevated bilirubin levels, as well as elevated serum aspartate aminotransferase and serum alanine aminotransferase levels. A prolonged prothrombin time may also result.

19. **Correct answer - A**

Alcohol withdrawal should be suspected if a patient develops nausea, vomiting, sweating, elevated vital signs, and agitation the day after admission. Withdrawal signs occur 12 to 48 hours after drinking stops and can last as long as 5 days. A patient at risk can develop cardiac and respiratory problems, liver failure, electrolyte imbalances, or seizures. Confusion, uncooperation, and hallucination can occur. Sedation, reorientation, and treatment of dehydration and electrolyte imbalances help the alcoholic patient over the acute phase; counseling and emotional support are key to long-term management.

20. **Correct answer - D**

Since salicylates are acid in nature, anticipate a primary metabolic acidosis with a compensatory respiratory alkalosis.

21. **Correct answer - A**

Hyperglycemia can result from a salicylate overdose because of activation of the stress response. Hypokalemia and hyponatremia are also seen. Impaired coagulopathy does not usually result from a salicylate overdose.

22. Correct answer - B

As Mr. T.'s condition deteriorates, seizures may ensue from irritation of the central nervous system. Hyperthermia and noncardiogenic pulmonary edema may also appear.

23. Correct answer - A

Victims of near-drowning will present with a mixed respiratory and metabolic acidosis. The respiratory acidosis is associated with hypoxemia and aspiration. The metabolic acidosis occurs from lactic acid production due to hypoxemia and an increased metabolic demand.

24. Correct answer - D

100% O_2 is necessary to combat the hypoxemia. Sodium bicarbonate is initially needed until if, after the respiratory acidosis has resolved, acidosis is still present. Hemodialysis may be required later in the course of therapy if renal insufficiency results. Electrolyte imbalances rarely occur from aspiration in near-drowning victims but may occur if a large amount of water has been swallowed.

25. Correct answer - C

Impaired gas exchange is a high priority nursing diagnosis due to aspiration. Adult respiratory distress syndrome is a common occurrence after a near-drowning episode either due to loss of surfactant or fluid-filled alveoli. Hypothermia is also a concern at this time. Impaired renal perfusion may occur days after the incident from shock or hypoxia. Fluid volume excess rarely results from aspiration but may result if a large volume of water has been swallowed.

26. Correct answer - B

Bradycardias may be seen in association with the diving reflex that is initiated when the face is submerged in water. Atrial fibrillation and, later, ventricular fibrillation are dysrhythmias associated with more profound degrees of hypothermia than Mr. W. presently has.

27. Correct answer - A

Inhalation injuries should be strongly suspected in the presence of facial burns. Pulmonary vasoconstriction is a normal physiologic response after a thermal injury, producing mild hypoxia and loss of compliance. Red burns that are without blisters and painful to touch are partial thickness, first degree burns that cause injury to the outer layer of epidermis and are most often associated with sunburn.

28. Correct answer - C

Deep dermal partial thickness, second degree burns are pale, yellow-white, slightly moist and do not blanch. Pain is felt upon deep pressure but not to pinprick. Damage occurs to the entire epidermis and to parts of the dermis. Superficial partial thickness, second degree burns appear bright red or pink with weeping blisters and are very painful to touch. Damage is limited to the epidermis. Full thickness, third degree burns cause damage through the entire layers of skin and into subcutaneous fat and, possibly, muscle and bone. Such burns appear charred, dry and are without feeling.

29. Correct answer - B

The first 24 hours post-burn is characterized by massive fluid loss and protein leak through damaged capillaries. Most burn formulas recommend crystalloid solutions to be infused the first 24 hours for fluid replacement. Colloid administration during this time would only result in more protein leak. When capillaries seal after the first 24 hours, colloids are then added to replace lost protein and promote movement of fluid into the intravascular space. The recommended route of feeding is enterally, if possible.

30. Correct answer - D

A urine output of 30-50 ml/hr indicates adequate fluid resuscitation. Other indicators are a normal to high cardiac index, low to normal serum sodium and a normal or slightly elevated hematocrit.

Selected References

AACN Staff, *Core Curriculum for Critical Care Nursing*, 4th ed. Philadelphia: W.B. Saunders Co., 1991.

AACN, *Clinical Reference for Critical Care Nursing*, 3th ed. St. Louis: Mosby - Yearbook, 1993.

Ahrens, T.S. "Effects of Mechanical Ventilation on Hemodynamic Waveforms, *Critical Care Nursing Clinics of North America*, 3 (4): 629-639, December 1991.

Alspach, G.J., *Core Curriculum for Critical Care*, 4th ed. Philadelphia: W.B. Saunders, 1991.

Blanford, N. "Renal Transplantation: A Case of the Ideal," *Critical Care Nurse*, 13 (1): 46-55, February 1993.

Burgess, M.C. "Initial Management of a Patient with Extensive Burn Injury," *Critical Care Nursing Clinics of North America*. 3 (2): 165-179, June 1991.

Cardma, V., Hurn, P. and Bastnagel, Moson, P. *Trauma Nursing: From Resuscitation Through Rehabilitation*. 2nd ed. Philadelphia: W.B. Saunders, 1994.

Cinetta, J., Taylor, R., and Kirby, R. *Critical Care*, 2nd ed. Philadelphia: J.B. Lippincott, 1992.

Cioffi, W.C. and Rue, L.W. "Diagnosis and Treatment of Inhalation Injuries," *Critical Care Nursing Clinics of North America*, 3 (2): 191-198, June 1991.

Conover, M.B. *Understanding Electrocardiography: Arrhythmias and the 12 Lead ECG*, 6th ed. St. Louis: The C.V. Mosby Co., 1992.

Cunningham, N, et al. "Renal Transplantation." *Critical Care Nursing Clinics of North America*, 4 (1): 79-88, March 1992.

Daily, E. *Hemodynamic Waveforms: Exercises in Identification and Analysis*, 2nd ed. St. Louis: Mosby Year Book, 1990.

Dantyker, D., *Cardiopulmonary Critical Care*, 2nd ed. Philadelphia: W.B. Saunders, 1991.

Eisenberg, P.G., "Pulmonary Complications from Enteral Nutrition," *Critical Care Nursing Clinics of North America*, 3 (4): 641-649, December, 1991.

Greenspan, F., and Forsham, P., eds. *Basic and Clinical Endocrinology*, 3rd ed. East Norwalk, Connecticut: Appleton and Lange, 1990.

Guyton, A., *Textbook of Medical Physiology*, 8th ed. Philadelphia: W.B. Saunders Co., 1990.

Guzzetta, C., *Cardiovascular Nursing Assessment and Intervention*. St. Louis: Mosby Year Book, 1991.

Halperin, M.E., Goldstein, M. *Fluid Electrolytes and Acid-Base Physiology: A Problem Approach*. 2nd ed. Philadelphia: W.B. Saunders, 1994.

411

Hartshorn, J., Lamborn, M., and Noll, Mary, *Introduction to Critical Care Nursing*. Philadelphia: W.B. Saunders, 1993.

Hazinski, M.F., et al. "Epidemiology, Pathophysiology and Clinical Presentation of Gram Negative Sepsis," *American Journal of Critical Care*, 2 (3): 224-235, May, 1993.

Henneman, E.A. "The Art and Science of Weaning from Mechanical Ventilation," *Focus on Critical Care*, 18 (6): 490-501, December, 1991.

Hickey, J.V. *The Clinical Practice of Neurological and Neurosurgical Nursing*, 3rd ed. Philadelphia, J. B. Lippincott, 1992.

Hudak, C., et al. *Critical Care Nursing: A Holistic Approach*, 5th ed. Philadelphia: J.B. Lippincott Co., 1990.

Klein, A., Lee, G and Manton, A. *Emergency Nursing Core Curriculium*, 4th ed. Philadelphia: W.B. Saunders, 1994.

Kokiko, J. "Septic Shock: A Review and Update for the Emergency Department Clinician," *Journal of Emergency Nursing*, 19 (2): 102-106, April 1993.

Kuhn, Merrily. *Pharmacotherapeutics: A Nursing Approach*. 3rd ed. Philadelphia: FA Davis, 1994.

Muirhead, J. "Heart and Heart-Lung Transplantation," *Critical Care Nursing Clinics of North America*. 4 (1): 97-110, March, 1992.

Richless, C.I. "Current Trends in Mechanical Ventilation," *Critical Care Nurse*, 11 (3): 41-50, March, 1991.

Rippe, J. et al. *Intensive Care Medicine*. 2nd ed. Boston: Little Brown.

Rue, L.W. and Cioffi, W.G. "Resuscitation of Thermal Injuries," *Critical Care Nursing Clinics of North America*, 3 (2): 181-89, June 1991.

Sparks, S.M. and Taylor, C.M. *Nursing Diagnosis Reference Manual*. Springhouse, Pennsylvania: Springhouse Corp., 1991.

Timby, B.K. "Pneumocystis in Patients with Acquired Immunodeficiency Syndrome," *Critical Care Nurse*, 12 (7): 64-71, October, 1992.

Weldy, N.J. *Body Fluids and Electrolytes*, 2nd ed. St. Louis: Mosby Year Book, 1991.

Wilson, R.F., *Critical Care Manual - Applied Physiology and Prinicples of Therapy*. 2nd ed. Philadelphia: FA Davis, 1992.

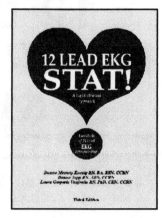

The Title Says It All...

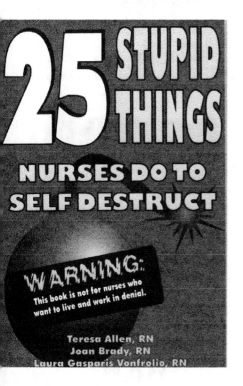

WARNING: This book is not for nurses who want to live and work in denial.

Teresa Allen, RN
Joan Brady, RN
Laura Gasparis Vonfrolio, RN

Our hope is that with this book, you will first, become aware of the 25 mistakes that have put nurses into the vulnerable position we are now in. Second, that it will provide guidelines to correct these 25 mistakes. It is only then that we can transform nursing into the rewarding profession it was meant to be.

Allen, Brady and Gasparis-Vonfrolio are armed with experience and should be considered extremely dangerous to the status quo.

They are the public's most ardent advocate, the staff nurse's staunchest ally, and hospital administration's worst nightmare!

Thank you, thank you for putting into words what I've been thinking for 20 years in nursing!

K. Karra Chicago, Il

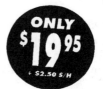

ONLY $19⁹⁵ + $2.50 S/H

Call 1-800-331-6534
& Charge To MC/VISA

Table of Contents

Make check payable to Power Publications & send to 56 McArthur Avenue, Staten Island, NY 10312.

Name_____

Address_____

City_____ State____ Zip_____

Please send me ____ copies of *25 Stupid Things Nurses Do To Self Destruct.* Enclosed is $_____. Date_____

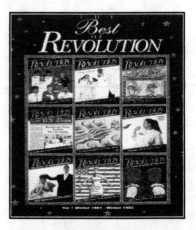

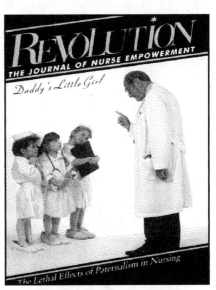
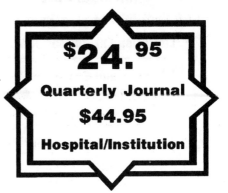

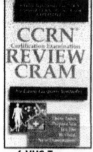